Medical Ethics in the Catholic Tradition

This book is a comprehensive survey and a sustained treatment of the major topics in contemporary medical ethics from within the Roman Catholic tradition. It brings together perspectives from philosophy, theology, medicine, and law to explore the traditions that undergird Catholic medical ethics.

The authors of this book are, respectively, a philosopher, theologian, physician, and attorney. Their commitment to the Roman Catholic tradition provides the foundational principles for addressing a wide range of issues in contemporary medical ethics. These topics include abortion, reproduction, cloning to produce children, cloning for biomedical research, embryonic stem cell use, genetics as screening, testing, therapy, enhancement, engineering, specific special relations such as maternal/fetal, physician/patient, mentally ill/caretakers, health care, and end of life issues. Furthermore, the book elaborates on the ways in which the authors' professions and disciplines act in service to medicine as an instrument for real human flourishing.

Medical Ethics in the Catholic Tradition is for the physician who would like to know more about the philosophical/theological/legal traditions that undergird the Catholic position. It is for the attorney who would like to know more about the philosophical/theological/medical traditions that undergird the Catholic position. Similarly, the philosopher or theologian can find here the appropriate information to understand how science and law contribute to the development of the Catholic position on major issues in medical ethics.

Margaret M. Hogan is the inaugural holder of the McNerney-Hanson Endowed Chair in Ethics at the University of Portland. She is also the Founding Director of the Garaventa Center for Catholic Intellectual Life and American Culture. She is a fellow of the Notre Dame Center for Ethics and Culture.

Edward M. Hogan is the Academic Dean and Associate Professor of Systematic Theology at Kenrick Glennon Seminary, USA. He was the Director of the Pontifical Paul VI Institute for Catechetical and Pastoral Studies for the Archdiocese of Saint Louis, served on the Vision Team for the Archdiocese, and managed Imprimaturs for the Archdiocese.

Annique K. Hogan is a practicing pediatrician in Philadelphia, Pennsylvania and an Associate Professor of Clinical Pediatrics at the Perelman School of Medicine at the University of Pennsylvania, USA. She serves as a member of the faculty for the Medical Humanities Program in the Collegium Institute at the University of Pennsylvania.

Matthew J.D. Hogan is an attorney and compliance professional in Philadelphia, Pennsylvania. He was a partner at Morgan Lewis & Bockius. He served as an Assistant U.S. Attorney in the Eastern District of Pennsylvania.

Routledge Annals of Bioethics

Series Editors Mark J. Cherry
St. Edward's University, USA
Ana Smith Iltis
Wake Forest University, USA

The Limits of Parental Authority
Childhood Wellbeing as a Social Good
Johan Bester

Bloody Bioethics
Why Prohibiting Plasma Compensation Harms Patients and Wrongs Donors
James Stacey Taylor

Agency, Pregnancy and Persons
Essays in Defense of Human Life
Edited by Nicholas Colgrove, Bruce P. Blackshaw, and Daniel Rodger

Voluntary Consent
Theory and Practice
Maximilian Kiener

An Ethics of Clinical Uncertainty
Lessons from the COVID-19 Pandemic
Mary Ann G. Cutter

Medical Ethics in the Catholic Tradition
Perspectives from Philosophy, Theology, Medicine, and the Law
Margaret M. Hogan, Edward M. Hogan, Annique K. Hogan, and Matthew J.D. Hogan

For more information about this series, please visit: https://www.routledge.com/Routledge-Annals-of-Bioethics/book-series/RAB

Medical Ethics in the Catholic Tradition

Perspectives from Philosophy, Theology, Medicine, and the Law

Margaret M. Hogan, Edward M. Hogan,
Annique K. Hogan, and
Matthew J.D. Hogan

Routledge
Taylor & Francis Group
NEW YORK AND LONDON

First published 2026
by Routledge
605 Third Avenue, New York, NY 10158

and by Routledge
4 Park Square, Milton Park, Abingdon, Oxon, OX14 4RN

Routledge is an imprint of the Taylor & Francis Group, an informa business

ISBN: 978-1-041-04175-7 (hbk)
ISBN: 978-1-041-04174-0 (pbk)
ISBN: 978-1-003-62719-7 (ebk)

DOI: 10.4324/9781003627197

Typeset in Sabon
by Apex CoVantage, LLC

Contents

Foreword

From antiquity to modernity, the Rod of Asclepius, a staff with a single serpent coiled around it, has been the symbol of medicine. The imagery, and the meaning borne by the ancient symbol, is strikingly similar to the staff carried by Moses as he tended sick Israelites in the wilderness. The fashioning of the bronze serpent and its placement on a pole is recounted in the book of *Numbers* as Moses followed the command of God: "Fashion a serpent of bronze, and set it up on a staff, bringing life to all who look toward it as they lay wounded" (*Numbers* 21:9). Allusion to this text and its amplification can be found in the Gospel of John which reads: "And this Son of Man must be lifted up, as the serpent was lifted up by Moses in the wilderness; so that those who believe in him may not perish, but have eternal life" (*John* 3:14–15). In these renderings, healing of human brokenness is held to be a divine gift serving the complex lives of human beings in sickness and in health, attending the living and the dying, and as well, healing of the body and the soul.

This rich understanding of medicine is the sheet anchor to the humane practice of medicine in modernity. It requires the understanding of all human life as embedded in relationships which define rights and obligations that are to be protected and fulfilled if human beings and human society are to flourish. The first and final relationship is that of human beings to God as creator, giver of gifts, and end of human life. Isomorphic to that relationship are the real and rational relationships of human beings to each other. These human relationships are to be actualized in the image of God, that is, to act as God would act. This understanding counters the contemporaneous claim that human beings are autonomous, rights-bearing individuals free to define and act on freely chosen values claimed as privacy rights or liberty rights or the right to be burden-free. An examination of human lives as embedded in relationships suggests the following: (a) autonomy is always a limited accomplishment achieved over time after a long period of dependency and often followed by another period of dependency; (b) living the rich human life often places human beings in asymmetrical relationships of varying degrees of dependency throughout life; (c) living the rich human life often places human beings in symmetrical relations, that is, relations as equals to each other; (d) autonomy is constrained by the relationships which define one's life; and (e) relationships to others sometimes require the acceptance of disadvantages – sometimes as providential obligation in generous and gracious giving and sometimes as grateful and humble receiving – for the sake of the other. It is our existence as related beings that is the source of our traditions of community and hospitality, of mutual respect, and of liberty as ordered. These relationships constitute the links in the web of sociality. These links need recognition and support, guided and directed by the principles of subsidiarity and solidarity.[1] This guidance is primarily the task of the principal anchors of the important asymmetrical relationships such as parents, teachers, physicians, lawyers, professors, lawmakers, and judges to make possible the good life. Insufficient attention to these links provides only a partial sense of reality.

The book is intended to provide a comprehensive survey of some of the major topics in contemporary medical ethics from within the Roman Catholic tradition as understood by the authors. This particular perspective of the tradition provides the foundational principles for addressing these topics. The book is cast toward the educated lay Catholic, lay in respect to professions other than one's own, and toward others interested in what the Catholic tradition holds on these contemporary issues. It is for the physician who would like to know more about the philosophical/theological/legal traditions that undergird the Catholic position. It is for the attorney who would like to know more about the philosophical/theological/medical traditions that undergird the Catholic position. Similarly, the philosopher or theologian can find here the appropriate information to understand how science and law contribute to the development of the Catholic position on major issues in medical ethics. The book is intended for a readership that is interested in the deep issues embedded in the contemporary practice of medicine. Examples of these issues include the notion of potentiality as it relates to the conceived unborn, the biology of conception and development, the effect of the law as instrument of social change, and the mutuality of sign and reality as indicators of meaning. While the explication of the notion of potentiality lies in the wheelhouse of the philosopher, its presentation for physicians, attorneys, and theologians supplies them with the concepts and language that allow them to grasp the distinction between a potential human being and a human being with potentiality. Similarly, the science of embryonic development provides the foundation for the appropriate ascription of the term human being as the foundation for legal protection and for an adequate metaphysics. The role of law as an instrument of social change, as evident in the effect of Court decisions such as *Roe v. Wade* and *O'Connor v. Donaldson* on the practices such as elective abortion and care of the mentally ill, reminds attorneys and discloses to physicians, philosophers, and theologians of the power of law and the necessity of its truth. The theological account of sacramental signs as disclosures of divine love and of human reality indicates both the privileged place of human beings as recipients of that love and their obligation to be instruments of that love in the world. It is the task of the theologian to facilitate that understanding so that the physician, philosopher, and attorney, as well as the theologian, may be in their practices a sign of the reality of God's love.

It is not the intention of this book to serve as a catalog of the extensive secondary literature in medical ethics. It is not the intention of this book to engage all contemporary Catholic commentators in the field of medical ethics. While it is appropriate for a tradition committed to faith and reason to continue study and dialogue and while the discussions of the philosophers and theologians contribute to the development of doctrine, these discussions are not settled doctrine. Nonetheless, references to significant secondary literature are indicated in footnotes for readers who might want to go deeper into the contemporary debates within the tradition regarding some issues.[2] It is not the intention of this book to take sides in the debate between the relatively conservative and relatively liberal positions within the tradition. While the former focuses on faith and the latter focuses on reason, the authors here are committed to faith and reason.[3] And, finally, it is not the intention of this book to address the vexing question of the role of the scholar within the tradition of contemporary Catholicism.

The authors – Margaret M. Hogan, Edward M. Hogan, Annique K. Hogan, and Matthew J.D. Hogan – are, respectively, philosopher, theologian, physician, and attorney. We are mindful of our need to speak out of our own competencies, out of our particular understanding of the tradition, and of our need to listen to and respect the competencies of the other professions.[4] The authors have had the experience of years of consultation with physicians in their practices as medical ethicist for a major hospital and a major hospital system, in conferences where they served as faculty for physicians, and in personal one-on-one encounters with physicians in the care of their patients. We have tried to include those voices in the book. The book arose from years of shared conversation over the dinner table and in the kitchen, from shared research, from teaching together, from requests for the expertise of each other, and from familial situations that required the wisdom found in consultation. In addition, the lives and practices of these authors are enriched by a particular tradition, Roman Catholicism, and the sets of principles, practices, and values that have their source in that tradition. As a consequence, this tradition, which penetrates the practice of their professions, amplifies and magnifies the intersection. The modern situation in medicine requires the gifts of all those professions and disciplines in service to medicine as an instrument for real human flourishing. The condition of humankind as fragile and finite requires the recognition of the dependence of each human being on others as each person traverses through the trajectory of life from absolute dependence to temporary autonomy to absolute dependence again to finally rest in God. The authors are also mindful that they speak out of their particular tradition and its values.

The completion of a book marks the occasion for the authors to look back with thanks to all who made the work possible. I am grateful to my husband, Tom, for his patience and encouragement. As a scholar, gratitude must be extended to all who nurtured that scholarship. I have been privileged to have been taught by scholars, both in the classroom and in their works, who have been or are giants in the field of medical ethics. Among these, now gone to God, are Richard A. McCormick, S.J., Edmund D. Pellegrino, M.D., H. Tristram Engelhardt, Jr. M.D., Ph.D., the Honorable John T. Noonan, Jr., Ph.D., J.D., and Patrick J. Coffey, Ph.D. Among those senior scholars who continue to share their wisdom with me are Gilbert T. Meilaender, Ph.D., Mark Siegler, M.D., and John Young, C.S.C., M.D. I have been privileged to have enjoyed the engagement of hundreds of physicians in the annual Medical Ethics Conferences at Notre Dame for more than 25 years. I am especially grateful to Wm. David Solomon, Ph.D. and O. Carter Snead, J.D. for that experience. For decades, David gathered together physicians, theologians, philosophers, and attorneys at Notre Dame and in Rome to enrich the practices of these domains and the lives of the practitioners. Carter continued this practice for many years. Other scholars who shared their knowledge and excitement in this amazing complex field include Ana S. Iltis, Ph.D., Farr Curlin, M.D., Brian Pilkington, Ph.D., Mark Cherry, Ph.D., Lauris Kaldjian, M.D., Ph.D., Jeffrey Bishop, M.D., Ph.D., and Jason Eberl, Ph.D. I am grateful to my faculty team in the Medical Humanities Seminar in The Collegium Institute at the University of Pennsylvania, to the students who populated the seminar for their wisdom-rich discussions, and to Daniel Cheely, Ph.D., Executive Director of The Collegium Institute, who convened the seminar. Members of the team include Ralph Rosen, Ph.D., Stacey Ake, Ph.D., Philip Gehrman, Ph.D., Thomas Kolon, M.D., Anthony Luberti, M.D., James Callahan, M.D., Lyndsay Mihoko Hoy, M.D., Adam Rizzo, Kristen Rock, M.D., and Horace M. DeLisser, M.D. Carolyn Chow (now Dr. Carolyn Fernandez del Castillo) and Lisa Eshleman, University of Pennsylvania students in the seminar, reviewed the text and offered many helpful suggestions. During the many years of my service as Medical Ethicist at Wilkes-Barre General Hospital, now and then called The Wyoming Valley Health Care System, and at Allied Health Care System in Northeastern Pennsylvania, I was privileged to work hand and heart with many physicians. I am grateful for the trust we shared in our attempts to serve the good of the patients who entrusted their lives and health to our care and judgment. (*MMH*)

I am grateful to my wife (Jen) and children (Brother Jean-Marie, O.S.B., Michael, Daniel, Peter, Margaret, and Mary) for reminding me, in concrete terms, why both principles and distinctions matter. I am grateful to my mother and father (Peg and Tom), for teaching me how a life of scholarship and diligence can be joyful and fruitful. I am grateful to my teachers – especially E. Springs Steele, Susan Mathews, Fred Lawrence, Fr. Michael Buckley, Charles Hefling, and Pat Byrne – for inviting me and challenging me to move to ever-deeper levels of theological analysis, synthesis, and application. I am grateful to my friends and colleagues at the Institute for Priestly Formation and Kenrick-Glennon Seminary for showing me that spiritual, intellectual, and pastoral integration is not only necessary but possible. And I am grateful to friends and colleagues who have been involved in the Science for Seminaries initiatives for helping me remember the joy of staying engaged at the intersection of disciplines. (*EMH*)

I have been formed as a physician by the many experiences, teachers, mentors, patients, and families that I have encountered on my journey. I cannot name them all, but I would like to acknowledge and thank Dr. Patrick Pasquariello, Jr. for modeling the kind of pediatrician I would like to be, Dr. Allison Ballantine for introducing me to the field of pediatric Complex Care medicine and her contagious passion for the work that has forever captivated me, Dr. Louis Bell for giving me my first opportunities as a new faculty member, Dr. Chris Feudtner for teaching me how to sit quietly to listen to a family's story and the many faculty of the Notre Dame Medical Ethics conference who taught me how to step back and think about complex ethical issues. I would like to thank Dr. Margaret Hogan for her sage wisdom and guidance throughout my career from its very beginning. I would like to thank my Compass Care and Complex Care teams for inspiring me daily in the work of caring for children with medical complexity. I would like to thank my family for believing in my dream to be the first physician in our family, and my husband for supporting my journey. Finally, I would like the thank the patients and families that have allowed me the privilege to care for them, whom I will not name to protect their privacy, but who hold a permanent place in my heart. (*AKH*)

Thank you to my wife Annique and our children, Matt, Annika, and Aidan as we continue to develop and support each other. Thanks to my parents who have always been our advocates and encouraged our education and discourse at the dinner table and beyond. Thanks to my siblings as we strive to "do better next time;" and as we have challenged each other. Thank you also as you have opened doors for me to walk through and windows for me to see better. (*MJDH*)

Notes

1 The terms solidarity and subsidiarity, along with the principles of the dignity of human persons, the common good, the universal destination of goods, and the preferential option for the poor, appear in the modern social teaching of the Roman Catholic Magisterium. In the late nineteenth century, the Magisterium began to address these principles as a matter of the proper ordering society. The principles received specific definition in *The Compendium of the Social Doctrine of the Catholic Church* (2004) prepared by the Pontifical Council on Justice and Peace for Pope John Paul II. Subsidiarity directs decision-making and administration toward smaller and more local units of society. Responsibility falls first to the individual, then, in order, to the family, the neighborhood, and the village. The larger and higher level units such as the government, the state, and the nation provide appropriate help and support when necessary (186). Subsidiarity encourages proper and essential participation by individuals and intermediate groups, which fosters freedom and initiative, and it protects against abuses by higher level authorities (187). The encyclical *Quadragesimo anno* of Pius XI is cited as developing the limiting function of subsidiarity in the following:

> Just as it is gravely wrong to take from individuals what they can accomplish by their own initiative and industry and give it to the community, so also it is an injustice and at the same time a grave evil and disturbance of right order to assign to a greater and higher association what lesser and subordinate organizations can do. For every social activity ought of its very nature to furnish help to the members of the body social, and never destroy and absorb them.
>
> (§79)

Solidarity is a "firm and persevering determination to commit oneself to the common good" (193) [in a manner that provides for] "the equality of all in dignity and rights" (192) [in a manner that reflects] "the living image of God the Father" (196). *Compendium of the Social Doctrine of the Catholic Church.*

2 *Contemporary Controversies in Catholic Bioethics* (Springer, 2017) edited by Jason T. Eberl, Ph.D. provides a fine summary of the contemporary discourse within the Catholic tradition. Topics included in the book are the moral status of the embryo and the fetus, appropriate life-saving interventions, contraception in special circumstances, ethical genetics, issues at the end of life including determination of death and the provision of nutrition and hydration, organ donation, and, finally, health care ethics and public policy. Professor Eberl provides an introduction to each section.

3 Religious traditions which have a scriptural component are usually marked by degrees of commitment to the letter of the scripture and the use of reason in the presence of the scripture. Within the religions which reverence the Scriptures, there is a range of interpretations of the texts found within those traditions. The interpretations range from the orthodox to the progressive and various expressions in between. The orthodox, for the most part, hold that the words of the text are binding, that is, commanding or forbidding, even though there is usually a scholarly tradition to aid in the interpretation. The progressive allows for the wider application of reason in interpreting the scriptures in a particular situation. Examples of the range are between Haredi Judaism and Reform Judaism and between Traditional and Progressive Catholics. While the theological and

philosophical foundations in Islam are different from Judaism and Christianity, there is some revelation/reason tension as exemplified in the premodern Ash'arites and Mu'tazalites echoed in the contemporary fundamentalist and rationalist traditions in Islam (Emon, A. M. (2004–2005). Natural law and natural rights in Islamic law. *Journal of Law and Religion*, *20*(2), 351–395).

4 None of the authors hold positions within the ecclesial structure of the Roman Catholic Church. Our contributions are those of lay people who have taken to heart the contributions of Saint John Henry Newman and Fr. Bernard J. Lonergan, S.J. to the enterprise of the commitment to and development of doctrine. Newman wrote,

> The development then of an idea is not like an investigation worked out on paper, in which each succeeding advance is a pure evolution from a foregoing, but is carried on through and by means of communities of man and their leaders and guides; and it employs the mind as its instruments, and depends upon them while it uses them.
>
> (*An Essay on the Development of Christian Doctrine*, p. 38)

Lonergan wrote of the development of theology as an ongoing recurrent process that requires the continuous, reciprocal, contributions of research ↔ interpretation ↔ history ↔ dialectic ↔ foundation ↔ doctrines ↔ systematics ↔ communication/implementation (*Method in Theology*).

1 The Point of Departure

The *Book of Genesis* presents an account of creation which reveals several essential features about human life. The author of the text wrote: "God made man in his own image, made him in the image of God. Man and woman both he created them. And God pronounced his blessing on them, Increase and multiply and fill the earth, and make it yours" (*Genesis* 1, 27–28).[1] The first essential feature is that all human beings are created; hence, they are dependent upon God for their very existence. This dependency establishes as a fact of human existence that human beings begin life in a relationship as related to God. Second, as created by God in His image, all human beings possess intrinsic dignity. Third, inasmuch as God is creative, humanity, as manifesting the image of God, is called to be creative. Fourth, God created human beings embodied in a particular way as man and woman. God blessed them as man and woman, and then God doubly charged them to be fruitful and to be responsible. Fifth, God gave humanity dominion over the created world, that is, to make the whole earth yours. This dominion given by God to human beings is to be understood as responsibility – stewardship and providence – for God's creation (Catechism of the Catholic Church, 373). As in a house, so in a book, the foundations matter. These five points serve as the fundamental building blocks of all that follows.

This introductory chapter will continue in the following order:

(A) The Anthropological Foundation
(B) The Roman Catholic Context
(C) The End of Modern Medicine Within This Context
(D) Going Forward – The Chapters in Outline
(E) Afterword

DOI: 10.4324/9781003627197-1

(A) The Anthropological Foundation

Understanding human life as embedded in relationships is essential to any appropriate anthropology. Attendance to the content of these relationships gives definition to human responsibilities and duties. Fulfillment of these responsibilities and duties serves human flourishing; failure to attend these results in decline for the individual, the family, and ultimately the community. The relation of human beings to God is the ultimate marker of human existence. It marks the beginning of human life and the end as goal to which humans are called, that is, from God to God. It is a temporal journey from absolute dependence through limited autonomy to absolute dependence. It is an eternal journey from human autonomy to participated theonomy, that is, "free obedience to God's law [which] effectively implies that human reason and human will participate in God's wisdom and providence" (John Paul II, *Veritatis splendor,* 1993, §41). It is only in the participation in the wisdom and providence of God that human beings are truly and effectively free. The God–human being relationship is, however, not the only relationship that defines human life. It is evident that human beings come into and exist in the world as related. In the normal course of events, the embodied existence of every human being originates in the relationship between parents and the ensuing mother–child relationship in pregnancy. From these specific relationships, concrete duties arise and are defined. Human relations vary. Some relationships are derived from the very nature (φύσης)[2] of human beings and the specific manner in which they are related. Some relationships derived from human agreement or consensus are conventional (νόμος).[3] Some are quite close – even intimate. Some are distant – so distant that it takes a concerted effort to experience and acknowledge them. Some are problematic; some are so effortless as to appear natural. Some of the relations are physical; some are moral. Some are freely chosen; others occur without choice. Some are symmetrical; others are asymmetrical. Some of the more obvious relationships are those of husband and wife, mother and fetus, parent(s) and family, the self as embodied, family and community, physician and patient, attorney and client, experimenter and subject, teacher and student, the community of scholars, political leaders and their constituents, judges and those seeking justice, and the members of the global community. These relations give definition and content to responsibilities and duties. These relationships limit and structure the activity of choosing. It is our existence as related beings that is the source of our traditions of community and hospitality, of mutual respect, and of liberty as ordered. These relationships constitute the links in the web of sociality. Failure to attend to these relationships risks undermining not only the continuation of the ordered social structure but the very freedom as effective freedom that permits the emergence of appropriately limited autonomy.[4]

At the same time, human beings who anchor these relationships possess individual identity, that is, their lives do not receive definition only in terms of their relations. They have significance in themselves quite apart from the relationships. An adequate ethics attends both the beings who constitute the relationship and the link which defines the relationship. While this text is anchored in a religious tradition, knowledge of these human relations and the beings who are the terms of the relationship does not depend on the belief in a creator God as the source of nature as normative. Furthermore, knowledge of these relationships does not depend on a privileged intuitive power to recognize a nature as morally normative. Knowledge of these relationships and their terms arises from the cumulative and ongoing work of experience, observation, inquiry, understanding, and judgment of human living. It is the end of an empirical inquiry. Knowledge of these relations and their terms provides a foundation to derive prescriptions from descriptions in the same way that knowledge of the role of a quarterback offers direction to the aspiring athlete or knowledge of the role of the Snow Queen offers guidance to the fledgling ballerina or knowledge of the structure of the human heart offers direction to the rising surgeon.

This text locates the practice of medicine in a complex set of relationships. While the most obvious relationship is that of the physician to the patient, the grounding relationship is that of the individual to God. Catholic physicians and all members of the healing professions, who are adherents to the biblical religious tradition, have a special vocation to serve creation in the image of God. They are called upon to practice medicine in a manner that is worthy of their image as created in the likeness of God, that is, to be creative, to be responsible, and to be providential. All patients, having also been created in the image and likeness of God, are to be seen as possessing intrinsic dignity. Physicians and health care providers have the responsibility of offering appropriate care – care that represents the best of the profession – in the treatment of patients. Physicians and patients recognize the reality of death for every human being, but acknowledge death as a passage to God.

For much of human history, the practice of medicine, as well as its efficacy, was limited. The codes surrounding its practice were appropriately limited: do good; do not harm; do not kill; practice within your competence; keep confidences; be mindful of your obligations; do not abuse anyone. The practice of medicine in the contemporary era, marked by incredible advances in science and technology, is complex. This complexity requires not only internal direction and regulation of the profession by its practitioners but also augmentation by complementary disciplines of ethics, law, and theology inasmuch as they turn their attention to the task of medicine as it serves the ultimate good of patients and practitioners. If this is the correct understanding of the end of the healing art, then this understanding requires attendance to medicine as practice and as science; to ethics as the study of the human good; to the law, as it guides and regulates human life in the public square; and to theology, as it directs medicine both in the practitioners and the patients to their ultimate end. Inasmuch as the end of human life is union with God, then the proper context for medicine is a theological one. All of these are required disciplines in service to the overarching goal of human flourishing. The working together of these professions recalls the words of Paul Ramsey at the birth of medical ethics: "Just as man is a sacredness in the social and political order, so he is a sacredness in the natural, biological order" (*The Patient as Person, xiii*). It is for these reasons that this text is cast within the collaborative creativity made possible by the dialectical exchange of medicine, theology, law, and philosophy. Moreover, inasmuch as medicine requires social structures to support its advance, it requires that its practitioners recognize their debt to that society by serving the social good – individual and common – as well as their individual private good.

(B) The Roman Catholic Context

The theological context operative for this work is Roman Catholicism. This sets the work apart from secular bioethics and from bioethics ordered by different theological traditions. An example of the former can be found in such works as the many editions of *Contemporary Issues in Bioethics* by Beauchamp et al. whose guiding principles are free informed consent, scientific progress, and legal approbation and whose measure is adherence to consensual procedure. An example of the latter can be found in *The Foundation of Christian Bioethics* by H. Tristram Engelhardt, Jr. This latter is contextualized by Engelhardt's confidence in Eastern Christian Orthodoxy – Orthodox Catholicism – of the first millennium which Engelhardt describes as continuous and unbroken through the faith as carried by the patriarchs, the bishops, and the faithful.

The theological context of Roman Catholicism frames advancement within the matrix structured by faith and reason. Adherents to the Catholic tradition acknowledge that both faith and reason are gifts of God. Faith provides a particular framework that enriches as well as guides moral judgment. This understanding is as old as the Scriptures of the New Testament and as new as the encyclicals of the contemporary Roman Pontiffs. In the first century, Saint Peter admonished his followers, "If anyone asks you to give an account of the hope which you cherish, be ready at all times to answer for it, but with courtesy and due reverence" (I *Peter*, 3:15). In the fifth century, Saint Augustine explicates this understanding in his commentaries on the Gospel of Saint John in the following: "*Non quia cognoscerunt ut crediderunt, sed ut cognoscerunt crediderunt. Credimus enim ut cognoscamus, non cognoscamus ut credamus*" ("It is not that they believed because they knew but that they knew because they believed. We believe in order that we may know, we do not know in order that we believe.") (Augustin, p. 291). Saint Anselm repeats this in the eleventh century in the original title of his *Proslogion* – *Fides Quaerens Intellectus*. The Scholastics of the medieval period recast the work of the earlier Councils into a philosophical framework to elucidate Christian beliefs to serve as a guide for the lives, both intellectual and practical, in a world expanded by the presence of the great universities and the proliferation of literacy by word and book.

In the twentieth century, the dialectic of faith and reason was the central theme of the encyclical – *Fides et Ratio* – of Saint Pope John Paul II. It continues today as the finite human capacity to understand faith and to encounter the infinite grows in the presence of a developing culture. Acknowledgment of the finite possibilities of human beings requires recognition that participation in the life of the Church requires prayer and participation in the liturgy and, as well, the study of the Scriptures and the study of the development of the teachings of the Magisterium. In these practices, the faithful acknowledge the gifts of faith and reason. Through liturgy and prayer, humans acknowledge and are drawn to the transcendent and are transformed in heart and mind. Through rigorous and continuous study, the development of doctrine and the application of doctrine move forward to address the exigencies of the contemporary world.

Roman Catholics accept the rich deposit of faith and the teachings of the Magisterium, and yet at the same time accord great respect to the ongoing work of the Holy Spirit as the truth of religious tradition is understood and developed in the dialectic of the truth of the tradition with the advance of knowledge in the sciences and in the contemporaneous culture. While there is great stability in Catholic teaching, particular teachings of the Church have developed over time. This claim should present a problem for no one who has studied the history of the church. Development in teaching has, as a matter of historical fact, occurred in both the speculative and practical domains of theology. On the speculative side, attempts to find appropriate language to express the mystery of the Trinity and to express the dignity of Mary serve as two examples. Attempts to give an account of the Trinity using material symbols failed. The account of the Trinity proffered by Saint Augustine, based on the understanding of the operations of the mind and the procession of the interior words, was more satisfying. The Augustinian account, while not dispelling the mystery, afforded the mind some repose. Contemporary theologians continue this task of making mystery more accessible. The understanding of the role of Mary has advanced as her role as Mother of God, her perpetual virginity, her Immaculate Conception, and her Assumption have been proclaimed. Catholic feminists, such as Gertrud von Le Fort and Edith Stein, of this postmodern period offer reflections on Mary as model and on her dignity in her real consent to take on her role in salvation history.

On the practical side of theological development, there is an extensive list of changes including the transitions: (a) from the acceptance of slavery to its condemnation; (b) from the prohibition of usury to the acceptance of the capitalist, but not materialist, principle of the right of the individual to use money to make money; (c) from the indissolubility of marriage to the dissolution of certain marriages for the sake of the faith; and (d) from the requirement of the persecution of heretics and from the teaching that "outside the Church there is no salvation," to the declaration of religious freedom (Noonan, 1993, p. 669). More recent evidence of change can be found in the transition from the acceptance of capital punishment as an appropriate societal means of self-defense to the reluctant acceptability of capital punishment in only the rarest of circumstances, that is, circumstances which are "very rare, if in fact they [the circumstances] occur at all" (John Paul II, *Evangelium vitae,* 1995, §56). And more recently a potential development can be found in the claim of Pope Francis that capital punishment is a matter of vengeance rather than justice. This would render capital punishment an intrinsically evil act and hence never permitted.[5]

How are these changes to be understood? That is, how can it be maintained that, at one and the same time, the Church is the repository of truth and that there is development of doctrine? That these changes represent development in doctrine cannot be denied. However, the advance in teaching is not a change in truth but a change in the understanding of the truth, that is, "Insight grows both into the words and the realities that have been handed on" (Paul VI, *Dei verbum* 8, 430). And in that new insight, sometimes the change is development and sometimes the change is correction. Changes in the understanding of usury, slavery, marriage, and religious freedom have come about as the core principles regarding their understanding have been contextualized and deepened.

In the nineteenth century, Saint John Henry Newman in his *An Essay on Development of Doctrine* described the developmental change not as a matter of deduction but as the result of the hard work of men and women utilizing the powers of the mind to approach a better understanding of truth. He offered the following:

> The development then of an idea is not like an investigation worked out on paper, in which each successive advance is pure evolution from

> a foregoing, but it is carried on through and by means of communities of men and their leaders and guides; it employs their minds as its instruments and depends upon them while it uses them . . . . It is the warfare of ideas under their varying aspects striving for mastery.
>
> (Newman, p. 38)

In the twentieth century, John Noonan described the change in this way:

> These principles were replaced by principles already part of Christian teaching: in the case of usury, that the person of the lender, not the loan, should be the focus of evaluation; in the case of marriage, that the preservation of the faith is more important than the preservation of a human relationship; in the case of slavery, that in Christ there is "neither free nor slave" (Gal.3:28); and in the case of religious liberty, that faith must be free. In the course of this displacement of one set of principles, what was forbidden became lawful (the case of usury and marriage); what was permissible became unlawful (the case of slavery); and what was required became forbidden (the persecution of heretics).
>
> (Noonan, 1993, p. 669)

What Noonan is describing here is a dialectical method in which the capacity to understand and apply the doctrines developed from the Scriptures by the Church Fathers, the Councils, and the Magisterium of a particular historical period replaces the partial and limited understanding of the past. This dialectical method refines and develops doctrine in the presence of the advances and challenges of the new context. Note that each instance of development is the occasion of the recovery of an essential notion of the tradition. These notions include the dignity of every human being, the importance of the preservation of the faith, the essential role of freedom in the life of everyone, and freedom of religion.

Vatican II in an effort to respond to renewal, which eschews both a theological positivism which simply repeats culturally and historically specific admonitions and a rationality anchored only in free choice, called for a moral theology that is not only nourished by Scripture and linked to dogma but also is scientifically and philosophically grounded (Pinckaers, pp. 4–5). The call for progress is tethered to reality and faith. It is wise to realize that in human affairs there is no guarantee of uninterrupted progress. Recall the warning of philosopher Bernard Lonergan, "while there is progress and its principle is liberty, there is also decline and its principle is bias . . . to ignore the fact of decline was the error of the old liberal views of automatic progress" (Bernard Lonergan, *Insight*, p. 260).

(C) The End of Modern Medicine Within This Context

Medicine, if it is to be able to serve the flourishing of human beings, must recognize human complexity and in this recognition realize that an organized and ordered set of sciences and practices is required to tend to that flourishing. Human beings have functions that are physical, physiological, psychological, and spiritual. Human needs are individual as well as social. Human beings are finite and material. Human beings are spiritual and yearn for the infinite. Human beings have their origin in God through their parents and, as well, have an ultimate end in union with God. Once, the practice of medicine tended all these multifaceted ends. Now, these tasks are parceled out among distinct professions – although sometimes united institutionally. By and large, contemporary medicine tends to focus on the physical, physiological, and psychological needs of the person, while remaining mindful of the social and spiritual needs, and, as well, the legal protections of the person. Medicine as a science uses its skills in and with and through the body to care for patients. Sometimes this care is the restoration of health so that that person may be or may become the optimally functioning human person. Sometimes this care is amelioration of a condition that, while it cannot be cured, its symptoms or disabilities can be abated. Sometimes this care can be only solicitous attention in the face of dying. This obligation to care is a proscription as well as a prescription. Certain actions such as ordinary care are required; certain actions such as killing are forbidden.

The ethics that serves and guides the practice of medicine as it strives to contribute to human flourishing is a complex science and a complex practice as well. There is an ethics that is intrinsic to the practice of medicine even as it draws wisdom and strength from other professions and disciplines including philosophy, theology, and law. As a science, medical ethics is a set of rational judgments that directs and guides the professions within medicine and informs the practical judgments that its practitioners must make. As a practice, it has as its focus – as an end – the care of patients who seek the aid of physicians. Moreover, as a practice, it forms and shapes the character of those who aspire to and participate in the profession of medicine, even as the science of the practice of medicine enriches and amplifies the set of necessary judgments. Medical ethics is rooted in the practice of medicine, which in turn is dependent upon scientific progress. Advances in science facilitate progress in medicine and progress in the refinement of the set of judgments that constitute medical ethics while at the same time fixing the gaze of the science and medical practice on human beings and the conditions of their flourishing. Inasmuch as human life has its origin from God and its end in union with God, medical ethics, if it is to tend authentic human flourishing, is a theological study. As theological, it has a particular place in the functional specialties of theology where it is dependent on the lower specialties and directive of the higher. Because the practice of medicine has a social end as well as an individual end, it benefits from public and private programs that wisely administer the distribution of its goods. Because in its history medicine has been an instrument of good as well as a tool of tyranny, it benefits from the pedagogical guidance of laws and codes and the corrective force of law as well as the aspirations of medicine, law, philosophy, and theology.

(D) Going Forward – The Chapters in Outline

There is an internal movement to the book which moves from the background of foundations and historical development to the foreground of the examination of particular issues. Each chapter is designed to move the discussion in an ongoing, cumulative way. The movement of the chapters begins with the foundations to provide a framework for particular topics. The more theoretical discussion examines, for the most part, essential points in the contemporary debates. The practical application is guided by the theoretical to proper means and ends. Each chapter closes with an *Afterword* that offers a reflection on future directions, complex issues, and lingering questions.

Chapters 2 and 3 lay out the foundations – the principles and rules – that are essential to guide the pursuit of medicine and medical research. Consideration of the foundations is necessary, if the discussion is not to be reduced to bare casuistry – a case-by-case consideration – and if the tradition developed from the foundations is to serve as a guide for the present day and for issues not yet within the contemporary horizon. In Chapter 2, the delineation of the foundations will be presented in the following order: (A) the historical background in the ancient world out of which medical ethics grew; (B) the intersection of the practices and texts of the ancient world with the Judeo/Christian religious tradition; (C) the ends and limits of the fields of medicine, philosophy, theology, and law as they intersect to serve human flourishing; (D) the position of Catholic Medical Ethics – its general and specific principles – in its encounter with the contemporary world; (E) the contemporary challenges to Medical Ethics in the matrix formed by the intersection of medicine, philosophy, theology, and law; and (F) a reflection on the continuing task of the tradition.

Chapter 3 addresses the issue of research ethics involving human subjects and patients. The chapter includes: (A) a presentation of the sources of danger inherent in research projects; (B) the exploration of historical instances of abuse by citing two concrete instances of abuse – one in the United States and the other in Germany; (C) the presentation, beginning with the Nuremberg Code, of some of the efforts to provide guidelines for researchers; (D) the examination of the ongoing efforts in the United States to guide and regulate research; and (E) reflection on the underlying principles operative in ongoing medical research in order to present some conclusions.

Chapter 4 examines the issues at the beginning of life and treats those issues within the context of the contemporary abortion debate. The treatment of the beginning of human life appears relatively early in this text so that the conclusions developed here can guide the responses to subsequent questions. The question of the beginning of life within the abortion context continues, in the contemporary culture, to be an emotion-filled and value-laden issue. While a great deal of the public debate has centered on the justification for abortion, this chapter focuses on the object of abortion, with particular focus on what is destroyed when an abortion is procured. This appropriate re-centering, while still recognizing the fact of problem pregnancy, serves to correct the main bias in the contemporary debate. The examination of the issue of abortion will be presented in the following order: (A) some observations will be offered; (B) some historically interesting information will be presented; (C) the object of the act will be considered; (D) the specific claims of the contemporary debate will be outlined and responses will be presented; and (E) the Afterword will bring this chapter to a closure with the consideration of some suggestions on how to move forward in the transformation of the culture.

Chapter 5 addresses the issue of reproduction – both its accomplishment and its avoidance. It proceeds in the following order: (A) framing the issue; (B) description of advances in reproductive technology to ameliorate infertility and to accomplish conception; (C) description of advances in understanding of the reproductive process and cycle to prevent conception; (D) the presentation of the teaching of the Catholic tradition as it guides the reproductive finality; (E) an examination of practices and problems that have arisen in the contemporary culture which accepts scientific progress and human desires as the only significant criteria in determining the goodness of an act; and (F) the Afterword – challenges facing forward.

Chapter 6 will address the issue of human cloning in the following manner: (A) a brief history of cloning; (B) an introduction to two significant reports on cloning; (C) a clarification of terms and a description of the process; (D) an examination of the ethical issues and the opposing views surrounding human cloning-to-produce-children; (E) an examination of the issues and the opposing views surrounding human cloning-for-biomedical-research, that is the use of human embryonic stem cells; and finally (F) some conclusions will be drawn and some lingering questions will be raised.

The focus of Chapter 7 is genetics. It begins with (A) a bit of history about eugenics as a reminder of the perennial hope of improving the quality of the human race, and as well, the past history tainted by eugenics programs which were egregious violations of human dignity; it then presents (B) an account of the development and progress in genetic testing and screening; which is followed by (C) a description of modern efforts at eugenics under the topics of gene therapy and genetic enhancement in somatic cells and germ cells; then (D) a sketch of the remarkable recent advancements in genetic engineering; and finally (E) a reflection on the promise, power, and peril of the new genetic technologies.

The focus of Chapter 8 is relationships. It begins in (A) by framing the issue in the following facts: (1) human lives are lived in a variety of relationships; (2) the unequal distribution of gifts results in sets of asymmetrical relations; and (3) specific obligations fall upon the recipients of special gifts to serve others if individual human life and human society are to flourish. This chapter will be limited to the examination of four relationships: in part (B), the maternal–fetus relationship; in (C) physician–patient relationship; in (D) that of the mentally ill to their families and society; and in (E) that of the human person in relation to the gift of the body. The first three relations can be described, isomorphically, as the relation between the powerful and the vulnerable and each relationship can guide – serve as an exemplar for – the direction of other relationships encountered in society. The asymmetry of these essential relationships is obvious. One member has power; the other is vulnerable. Power has its source in position, competency, and knowledge; vulnerability derives from a variety of limitations such as inadequate knowledge, immaturity, and the deficit caused by illness. The fourth, as a relationship of whole to part, simultaneously empowers and limits the individual in the use of his or her body understood as a gift from God.

Chapter 9 examines the issue of the provision of health care. This chapter will proceed in the following fashion: (A) an examination of the current challenges in the provision and distribution of medical care; (B) a consideration of the role and limits of Catholic Health Care Institutions; (C) a consideration of scarce resources in ordinary and extraordinary times; and (D) the Afterword.

Chapter 10 addresses issues at the end of life. It will progress in the following order: (A) observations on the progression of the human encounter with dying and death; (B) examination of the very modern issue of the medical determination of death; (C) discussion of the contemporary medical, ethical, and legal issues dealing with the end of life; and (D) reflection on the Catholic understanding of death as it responds to the challenge of dying in the face of medical, ethical, and legal pressures in the contemporary culture.

(E) Afterword

When a Catholic woman philosopher enters into the discussion of medical ethics, she enters with a variety of tools and experiences that provide the perspective and the requirements for her examination. She enters with the tools of her disciplines – here philosophy and science. In the pursuit of both, it is truth and the Truth that draws and frames her endeavors. She, because she is Catholic, has been formed by the stories of the scriptures – the Annunciation, the Visitation of two women each with a problem pregnancy, the Nativity, the Crucifixion, and the Resurrection – and she is formed by the scriptural theme of "love for the least of these" as well as the formative practices of Christian life. When, in addition, she is a mother, she enters the discussion of life issues with the memory of her experience and awareness of nascent human life developing within her body. As a wife, she is aware that these experiences are those of her marriage and she shares them with her husband. As a daughter, she has been privileged to accompany her parents as they journeyed from this life into eternal life. These are important experiences which enrich her perspective and which she ought not to cast aside.

When a Catholic man who is a theologian and father enters the discussion, he does so with the tools of the theologian and out of the particularity of his religious tradition. As a theologian, he understands his tasks are to *reason* about God, to *point* to the presence of God, and to *manifest* the presence of God. He understands theology as a kind of science with a disciplined method analogous to all the sciences. Theology has a dynamic method that moves systematically and cumulatively through research to interpretation to understating to judgment to verification or revision under the relentless pressure of the operations of the mind to be attentive, to understand, to judge, and to be responsible as it attempts to fashion higher and more complete accounts. As a discipline, theology has a place in both the theology-science dialogue and the interreligious dialogue. In regard to the former, inasmuch as physicists can, within the confines of their domain, present an account of light as a wave or a particle based on observations of activities in a particular field, the theologian claims that the supernatural is factual and, with the method proper to his science and focused on its domain, he will face the difficulties of that claim. In regard to the latter, he will acknowledge that the divine shows forth as in individual and historical experiences that confront and beckon all of humankind not just Christians. This last presents an invitation to religious dialogue not as an exercise in toleration of difference and agreement in minimal claims but as an opportunity to examine deeply, listen carefully, and bear witness fully to the claims of each tradition. Finally, as a father, he understands that his children have been entrusted to him and his wife by a loving God who desires them to be a gift to the world, and also desires their return. As a teacher, he acknowledges an analogous vocation in his relationship with his students.

When a Catholic woman who is a physician, a pediatrician, and a mother enters the discussion of medical ethics, she enters with the tools of her discipline – here medicine and science. She understands medicine as practical and theoretical, and she acknowledges the necessity that she be competent in both. As practical her work occurs in the clinical encounter with a vulnerable human being – a child, and as well those who love this child. As theoretical, her work calls upon her to apply the science of her practice to the particularities of this child. As a mother, she is well aware that this child is as loved by the child's parents as her children are loved by her and their father. As a Catholic, she is aware of the stories of the Scriptures that depict the special care that Jesus manifested for sick and dying children as He healed the daughter of Jairus (Mark 5:21–43) and the son of the royal official (John 4: 51–54). These remind her of the importance of healing as God's gift and of her human limits as a practitioner.

When a Catholic man who is an attorney and father enters the discussion, he does so with the tools of his profession and its practices as well as an understanding of the role of law, because it is rooted in human nature as apprehended by human reason, in fashioning a flourishing society. He understands that law has a function as an agent of social control positively through legislation and negatively through punishment. The latter provides for the security of the commonwealth and the former provides fixed basis and opportunities for ordered growth in the commonwealth. He recognizes, moreover, that the law has higher functions also. Among the higher functions is the teaching function of the law which instructs the uncertain as to what is required, what is permitted, and what is forbidden. In its aspirational function, the law inspires toward the accomplishment of justice. The law shares its tools with medicine in the codes and regulations that guide medical practice. He is mindful of the fact that his respect for the law requires his adherence to its careful, exacting application and its prudential discretionary power as they apply to him, to his clients, and to the community. As a father, he is aware of the fragility, the strength, and the wonder of human life. He is mindful that he and his wife must teach by word and example the children who have been entrusted to their care so that their lives may be ordered to the good, the common good, and finally to God.

This dialogue across the professions provides a safeguard for those whom medicine serves, a structure for facing the as-of-yet-unknown issues in medicine, and, at the same time, a safeguard against the powerful human tendencies to allow compassion to overwhelm reason or to allow power to overwhelm compassion and reason.

Questions for Reflection

1. Where one begins an inquiry matters. What examples have you encountered by taking different starting points – physically or intellectually – and what are the implications of those different starting points?
2. What are some examples from the multiple roles in your own life of how relationships define responsibilities?
3. Think of some examples of how (a) the science and (b) the practice of medicine advance. How do those changes enter into medical ethics? How do these changes enter into moral theology?
4. How do you understand development in knowledge in science, law, medicine, and theology? What are some of the effects of this new understanding?
5. What examples have you experienced, or can you think of, that show how medical *practice* stands at the intersection of science, philosophy, theology, and law?

Notes

1 All Scriptural quotations found in this book are taken from THE HOLY BIBLE, A Translation from the Latin Vulgate in the Light of the Hebrew and Greek Originals by Ronald Knox. New York: Sheed & Ward, Inc. 1944, 1948, 1950.

2 The Greek term here is φύσης – physis. The English terms "nature" and "natural" generally translate this concept as nature or norm as something given.

3 The Greek term here is νόμος – nomos. The English terms "natural" and "norm" generally translate this concept of nature as something consented to as in a social construct.

4 The term "freedom" has different meanings in the philosophical and theological tradition. See, for example, Catechism of the Catholic Church in 1732 and 1733. *Liberum arbitrium* – free will – means the capacity to choose one thing or another. *Libertas* – freedom – means the capacity to choose the good. It is freedom in the "libertas" sense that is of concern here.

5 This would still leave open the question of lethal defense against a lethal aggressor.

2 The Foundations

The miracles of healing – both those witnessed and those reported – were a key element of what drew crowds to Jesus. This text from the Gospel of Saint Matthew focuses attention on this healing role of Christ. Matthew wrote the following:

> As evening drew on, they brought him many who were possessed. He expelled the spirits by a simple command and cured all who were afflicted, thereby fulfilling what had been said through Isaiah the prophet, "it was our infirmities he bore and our sufferings he endured."
>
> (*Matthew*, 8: 16–17)

The promise of Christ to be with humanity is fulfilled, in part by his healing of us, in part by bearing our sufferings in imitation of Christ, in part, by letting go of our lives to Christ to bear us to God, and in part by relieving the suffering of those who journey to God with us. This last is to be accomplished in the work of our professions and our lives guided by the Holy Spirit who is the promise of Jesus.

The first task required for developing medical ethics for the Catholic tradition is that of establishing the foundations. Consideration of the foundations is necessary, if the discussion is not to be reduced to bare casuistry – a case-by-case consideration – and if the tradition developed out of the foundations of the practice of medicine itself is to serve as a guide for now and for issues not yet within the contemporary horizon. The exploration and delineation of the foundations will be presented in the following order:

(A) The historical background of the practice of medicine in the ancient world out of which medical ethics grew;
(B) The intersection of the practices and texts of the ancient world with the monotheistic religious traditions of Judaism and Christianity;

DOI: 10.4324/9781003627197-2

(C) The ends and limits of the fields of medicine, philosophy, theology, and law as they intersect to serve human flourishing;
(D) The foundational sources including the Scriptures, Natural Law, the requirements of the integrally good act, the principle of the sanctity of human life, the principle of double effect, the ordinary/extraordinary distinction, and the principle of totality that supply the general and practical principles of Catholic Medical Ethics in its encounter with the contemporary world;
(E) The contemporary challenges to medical ethics in the matrix formed by the intersection of medicine, philosophy, theology, and law; and an
(F) Afterword: a reflection on the continuing tasks of the tradition.

(A) The Historical Background – The Ancient World

From the beginning of the practice of medicine in antiquity, its practitioners pondered the appropriateness or the inappropriateness – the morality – of their practice. For centuries, these discussions of medical intervention, even when conceived as lying in the domain of philosophy as natural philosophy, were carried on as embedded within a religious tradition and, hence, the human good – as health and virtue – was the end. In the world of classical antiquity – in Greece, Egypt, and Rome – medicine was practiced under the guidance of the gods and goddesses who were invoked to heal and to assist in healing. Judaism and later Christianity, the religions that revere the Scriptures, found in those books the wisdom to guide human life and the practices which serve human life. While there are significant differences within these traditions, there are important truths they hold in common. The beliefs they share include that of life as the gift of God, of human living as life lived in covenant with God, and of a people called to exercise stewardship in the image of God – creative stewardship – in the created and finite world. If these traditions that reverence the Scriptures are not to operate as forms of fundamentalism, then the work of reason – and the consequent advance of knowledge – is to be numbered among the gifts of a loving God alongside the gift of Revelation.[1] If these traditions are to be directive of human flourishing, then they are required to bring the truth to bear in a culture always in need of repair.

In ancient Greece and ancient Rome, the practice of medicine was a priestly art connected with Asclepius. The symbol of Asclepius became and continues to be the symbol of the practice of medicine. The Code and Canons of Hippocrates, which date from the fifth century B.C. and which guided a set of practices of a particular guild, have long associated healing with priestly office. In the Code, the physician prays for divine guidance, acknowledges debt to those who transmitted the art of medicine, and swears to use treatment in the following manner:

> I swear by Apollo the Healer, by Asclepius, by Hygieia, by Panacea, and by all the gods and goddesses, making them my witnesses, that I will carry out, according to my ability and judgment, this oath and this indenture.
>
> To hold my teacher in this art equal to my own parents; to make him partner in my livelihood; when he is in need of money to share mine with him; to consider his family as my own brothers, and to teach them this art, if they want to learn it, without fee or indenture; to impart precept, oral instruction, and all other instruction to my own sons, the sons of my teacher, and to indentured pupils who have taken the physician's oath, but to nobody else.
>
> I will use treatment to help the sick according to my ability and judgment, but never with a view to injury and wrong-doing. Neither will I administer a poison to anybody when asked to do so, nor will I suggest such a course. Similarly I will not give to a woman a pessary to cause abortion. But I will keep pure and holy both my life and my art. I will not use the knife, not even, verily, on sufferers from stone, but I will give place to such as are craftsmen therein.
>
> Into whatsoever houses I enter, I will enter to help the sick, and I will abstain from all intentional wrong-doing and harm, especially from abusing the bodies of man or woman, bond or free. And whatsoever I shall see or hear in the course of my profession, as well as outside my profession in my intercourse with men, if it be what should not be published abroad, I will never divulge, holding such things to be holy secrets.
>
> Now if I carry out this oath, and break it not, may I gain for ever reputation among all men for my life and for my art; but if I break it and forswear myself, may the opposite befall me.
>
> (*Hippocrates*, pp. 299–301)

While the Oath itself contains much more and the Hippocratic Corpus contains more than the Oath, there may be noted, at least in inchoate form, the ends[2] and limits of medicine. Among them are the following 12 commitments. The first is a covenant with the deities, who are the gods of healing. The second is the covenant with teachers, and this is done with the pledge of collegiality and financial support. Next is the commitment to students by the promise to teach those who swear the Oath. After the commitment to students comes the covenant with patients, and this is the physician's pledge to use their best ability and judgment. The fifth area is appropriate means with the use of standard dietary care; this is using the established and accepted practices to treat their patients. Appropriate ends are next. A doctor is to do what is best for the patient, rather than what is best for the physician. The seventh area is the limit on ends. The limit on ends prohibits killing, that is, a physician would not help a woman have an abortion and the physician would not administer a lethal drug if asked. The next area is limits on means. This refers to the leaving of surgeries and specialty care to those who have been trained in that particular specialty. Action is limited by competence. Next is justice; upon taking the Oath, the physician is swearing that they will avoid any voluntary act of impropriety or corruption. After justice comes chastity, which states that a physician will not have any sexual contact with their patients. The eleventh area covered is confidentiality; this simply says that a doctor will not repeat anything that is seen or heard. The final area of the Oath is accountability, which is a prayer that the physician be favored by the gods if the Oath is kept and punished if it is broken.[3]

(B) The Religious Historical Background

In the Jewish tradition, medicine was practiced, and still is practiced by many Jews, out of the steadfast fidelity to the covenant with God and to the covenant of life – *L'Chaim*. In both Moses of Mount Sinai and in Moses Maimonides, who are often referred to as the temporal poles of the golden age of Judaism, there is to be found the combination of healing power and priestly office. The staff of Moses – the staff with the single snake coiled around the shaft of the staff – is recorded to have had healing power. Moses Maimonides, the Jewish philosopher-physician who practiced medicine in the twelfth century in the regnant Muslim society that reached from Spain to Morocco and finally in the Sultan's Court at Cairo in Egypt, is credited with writing a prayer that is often considered to contain a moral code for the practice of medicine.[4] The following is an excerpt from the prayer of Maimonides:

> Inspire me with love for my art and with love for Thy creatures. Do not allow thirst for profit, ambition for renown and admiration, to interfere with my profession, for those are the enemies of truth and of love for mankind and they can lead astray in the great task of attending to the welfare of Thy creatures. Preserve the strength of my body and of my soul that they may be ever ready cheerfully to help and support rich and poor, good and bad, enemy as well as friend. In the sufferer let me see only the human being. Illumine my mind that it recognize what presents itself and that it may comprehend what is absent or hidden. Let it not

> fail to see what is visible, but do not permit it [the mind] to arrogate to itself the power to see what cannot be seen, for delicate and indefinite are the bounds of the great art of caring for the lives and health of Thy creatures. Let me never be absentminded. May no strange thoughts divert my attention at the bedside of the sick, or disturb my mind in its silent labors, for great and sacred are the thoughtful deliberations required to preserve the lives and health of Thy creatures.
>
> (attributed to Maimonides, translated by Harry Friedenwald, Bulletin of the Johns Hopkins Hospital 28: 260–261, 1917)

Note carefully in the prayer of Maimonides the following: the acknowledgment by the physician of dependence on God; the practice of medicine as informed by love of God; the practice directed to the good of the patient and, moreover, practices described as care for life and health and the preservation of life and health; the universal application of the art of medicine to rich and poor, and as well to friend and foe; the recognition of the distinction between the physical and the spiritual; the tie of the practice to truth and love; the warning against those things such as desire for profit and ambition for renown which detract from the practice of medicine; a warning against arrogance and a plea for attentiveness (which can never be taken for granted).

Of the material elements that inform the Christian tradition, the most important are those rooted in the Scriptures, especially in the New Testament accounts of the ministry of Jesus, and in the teaching Magisterium which is entrusted with presenting the meaning of the Scriptures in each age. Among the most frequently recurring stories in the New Testament are those of the healing miracles of Jesus. That healing ministry of Christ is part of the identity of the Catholic physician, the Catholic health care provider, and Catholic health care institutions. They cite rightly, as an apothegm "to heal as Jesus healed" and they ought to appropriate that apothegm into practice. Examples of the healing by Jesus abound in the scriptures. The healing acts include the healing of the leper, the servant of the centurion, and the mother-in-law of Peter, the restoration of sight, the restoration of bodily integrity, the restoration of life, and of speech and of mobility. It is said in the gospel of Matthew that in this healing mission Jesus fulfilled the prophecy of Isaiah, "He took away our infirmities and bore our diseases" (Is 53:4). Yet, Jesus as healer of physical illness is just one dimension of His healing ministry. His radical healing ministry extended beyond the healing of bodily infirmity. He healed those who suffer from sin as well as those who suffer from physical infirmity. He drove out demons and forgave sinners and condemned hypocrisy. Medical practice worthy of the name Catholic would, through appropriate partnering with clergy, keep alive the multidimensional healing that our human nature with its contending powers requires.

In terms of theological and philosophical foundations, the case of Islamic ethics is different from Judaic and Christian ethics. The Muslim tradition of medicine, which flourished in the Middle Ages, was renowned for its technical skills and its intellectual advances. Medicine was practiced within an ethical code derived from Islamic teaching and philosophy. God was acknowledged as the author of life and death. Physicians were admonished that they did not control life or death. Those who were physicians had grave obligations – to be expert in their art, to be humanitarian in the distribution of their practices, to respect human life, to keep confidences, and to do no harm. The physician/philosopher Avicenna (980–1037) is among the most famous of the Eastern Islamic Scholars of the medieval period. He integrated religion and science and philosophy, especially the philosophy of Aristotle, in his works. His *Canon of Medicine* was considered a standard medical text in Europe and Asia until the seventeenth century. In the *Canon,* he described medicine as the art whereby health is conserved and the art whereby health is restored after being lost.

In contemporary times, the Islamic Code of Medical Professional Ethics continues this tradition and calls for Muslim physicians to practice medicine within the framework of belief in God and belief in Islamic teaching. They look to the *Qur'an* to inspire the Muslim physician in practice and to keep before the physician the obligations and limits of the practice of the medical art. In an oath which bears some similarity to the Oath Of Hippocrates, the Muslim physician makes these commitments: to acknowledge his faith and his dependence upon God; to be grateful to his teachers and parents; to be competent in his field; to remember that human life is a gift from God; to refrain from administering anything harmful to a patient; to respect his patients by appropriate communication with the patient and by keeping in confidence information about the patient; to be modest in his practice; and to seek wisdom in decisions.

(C) The Ends of Medicine, Philosophy, Theology, and Law

The tradition of medical ethics is a rich one whose material elements are drawn from sound medical practice and scientific research, whose formal elements are derived from ethical principles, from the Natural Law tradition, and whose limiting elements are derived from legal theory, as all of these, enriched by the religious tradition, interact to serve the human good and the human pilgrimage through life and by death into eternal life. Each of these specialties is defined by a particular end but all claim a method of inquiry directed by the imperatives of the mind, namely, research (be attentive), understanding (be intelligent), judgment (be reasonable), and action (be responsible).[5]

(1) Medicine: as a practice is directed to the care of the sick in curing disease and infirmity, in restoring optimal functioning, and in attending the dying. In its practice, medicine begins in a temporary one-to-one relationship between the physician and the patient. Appropriate care is the immediate goal of medicine and it is competence in the practice that shapes medical training. The one-to-one relationship is still the case even in the presence of multiple specialists and physician extenders as the primary physician guides and coordinates practices and care. The relationship is complex because it is a temporary relationship and because it is simultaneously a symmetrical relationship and an asymmetrical one. It is symmetrical because it is a relationship between two human beings, so the appropriate attitude is respect between equals. It is asymmetrical because the physician has knowledge and power while the patient is vulnerable because of illness and, very often, lack of appropriate knowledge. Even in those instances in which the patient is a physician, the vulnerability, because of illness, often presents an obstacle to knowledge and judgment.[6] Hence, the relationship remains asymmetrical. The relationship is temporary because it lasts only as long as the patient requires the care of the physician and only as long as the patient accedes to this care. If the patient no longer accedes to the care, the patient has broken the relationship and the physician ought not to continue. If the patient no longer needs care, then this particular relationship ceases to exist at that time.

(2) Philosophy has as its end, its goal, wisdom – *Sophia* in Greek and *Sapientia* in Latin. Its end is not merely skill in argument, even as philosophers use the necessary tools of rhetoric and dialectic as methods in assisting philosophy in the accomplishment of its goal. The journey of reason toward wisdom is long and arduous. The journey takes decades of study and traverses the disciplines of the liberal arts, the natural sciences, and mathematics long before the work of the philosophic dialectic can be initiated. It is to be understood that there is both (a) content to be mastered and (b) a skill set to be developed. Time and the discipline of learning not only provide a body of material to be understood but also transform the subject as knower to be appropriately situated to encounter the real in awe and wonder. Saint John Paul II recalls this in *Fides et Ratio*, wherein he described the proper role of philosophy and its particular integrative and corrective role in the Catholic intellectual life in the following:

> To be consonant with the word of God, philosophy needs first of all to recover its *sapiential* dimension as a search for the ultimate

> and overarching meaning of life. This first requirement is in fact most helpful in stimulating philosophy to conform to its proper nature. In doing so, it will be not only the decisive critical factor which determines the foundations and limits of the different fields of scientific learning but will also take its place as the ultimate framework of the unity of human knowledge and action, leading them to converge towards a final goal and meaning. This *sapiential* dimension is all the more necessary today, because the immense expansion of humanity's technical capability demands a renewed and sharpened sense of ultimate values. If this technology is not ordered to something greater than a merely utilitarian end, then it could soon prove inhuman and even become potential destroyer of the human race.
>
> (John Paul II, 1998, *Fides et Ratio, §81*)

In the encyclical *Spe salvi*, Pope Benedict XVI also directed attention to the danger of technological progress without wisdom in the following:

> First we must ask ourselves: what does "progress" really mean; what does it promise and what does it not promise? In the nineteenth century, faith in progress was already subject to critique. In the twentieth century, Theodor W. Adorno formulated the problem of faith in progress quite drastically: he said that progress, seen accurately, is progress from the sling to the atom bomb. Now this is certainly an aspect of progress that must not be concealed. To put it another way: the ambiguity of progress becomes evident. Without doubt, it offers new possibilities for good, but it also opens up appalling possibilities for evil – possibilities that formerly did not exist. We have all witnessed the way in which progress, in the wrong hands, can become and has indeed become a terrifying progress in evil. If technical progress is not matched by corresponding progress in man's ethical formation, in man's inner growth (cf. Eph 3:16; 2 Cor 4:16), then it is not progress at all, but a threat for man and for the world.
>
> (Benedict XVI, 2007, *Spe salvi*, §22)

The wisdom-seeking role of philosophy serves to temper the research imperative and the therapeutic imperative by focusing the attention of medicine and science on the good of the particular patient at hand and the flourishing of human society. It carries a constant reminder of the dignity of the person and the elements that are required to affirm that dignity. Those trained in philosophy are able to assist the medical team as the team focuses on the good – both as care and as end – of the patient in the presence of conflicting pressures and interests. Those trained in philosophy are able to assist the research team in determining the appropriate use of persons, in understanding the limitations of consent in vulnerable populations, and in attenuating the particular power of money. In addition, those trained in philosophy are able to assist physicians and patients in determining the appropriateness of treatment and limits of care for a particular patient.

(3) Theology has an end in knowing God, in knowing all things in relation to God, and reaching God. Theology operates in this text within a matrix framed by the Roman Catholic tradition as it attempts to apply the meaning of that tradition to the culture and its practices. The cultural context includes contemporaneous scholarship and requires the collaboration of theology with that scholarship. It is anchored in its observations of the human relationship to God and the natural relationships observed in the created order. Theology is empirical in that sense and, as empirical, it is subject to progression as well as regression – as is the case with all the sciences – as it pursues its goal. The religious tradition includes revealed truths as found in the Scriptures and the infallible teachings of the Church. Its method is "a normative pattern of recurrent and related operations yielding cumulative and progressive results" (Lonergan, 1972, *Method in Theology*, p. 4). Theology's interrelated and reciprocally influencing tasks include: research, interpretation, history, dialectic, foundations, doctrines, systematics, and communications (Lonergan, 1972, p. 127). In accomplishing its ends, it witnesses truth in teaching and practice in a manner capable of assimilation in the culture and transformation of the culture. In the dialogue of Roman Catholicism with culture, it communicates its tradition – the doctrines – and it listens to the scholarly advances of the culture. The method of communication is as varied as the research is limited. Research contributes to the development of doctrine and doctrine directs and limits research. The advance of both requires the renewal of communication.

Historically, the initial contact with culture was found in the preaching of the word and the life of the community. Over time, the work of the councils in the scholarly study of the meaning of the word augmented the understanding of the Scriptures. As scholarship grew, the medieval universities began to contribute to this interpretive work. This task continues as the universities of the contemporary era offer their contributions. The tradition speaks both from the heart and the head. To neglect the heart is to fail to bear witness to the human condition and to fail to attempt the repair of its brokenness. To neglect the head is to risk the possibility of overwhelming reason by undisciplined feelings of compassion. The *Ethical and Religious Directives for Catholic Health Care Services*, in various iterations, display this ongoing theological work.

(4) Law has an end in justice – the right ordering of the civil community – and laws have multiple ends: (a) in their contribution to discovering and articulating the needs and delivering the goods required for sustaining the civil community; (b) in maintaining the order without which justice cannot be achieved; (c) in teaching citizens what the law requires and forbids; and (d) in protecting citizens from those who would disrupt and threaten the order of community and the lives of the citizens. While as a profession medicine maintains that it regulates itself, the influence of law is evident not just in the sanctions of malpractice but in the legal direction of medicine through the proliferation of regulatory agencies of administrative law and in the power of the legislatures to accomplish the health and healing goals of the state. Medicine is thereby subjected to the force of politically organized agencies. In the modern era, the most striking entry of law into medicine occurred at the conclusion of the Nuremberg Trial of Physicians with the presentation of a ten-point code, the *Nuremberg Code*, to regulate the relationship between physician researchers and subjects. Subsequent to the Trial and the *Code*, regulation has, of necessity, become more complex as medicine has advanced. The Code of Federal Regulations of the Health and Human Services Agency provides one instance of the reach of administrative law as regulatory into medicine. In addition, the legislative role of law provides another instance of the operation of law in medicine. What began as an ideal to provide basic medical care to all has been extended into a complex system of sickness insurance that requires new professions such as health care navigators and facilitators to maneuver patients successfully to care while avoiding their financial ruin. Finally, the judiciary has entered medicine through Court decisions, for example, *Roe v. Wade* (1973) and *Washington v. Glucksberg* (1997). The same goal of legal reasoning to provide for growth and stability has the capacity to expand or contract these experiments in the social engineering role of the law as it contributes to the practice of medicine.

Because medical ethics is developed at the intersection of medicine, ethics, and law, a few notes on the move from morality to law, the limits of each, and the functions of law are appropriate. It is often claimed that the assertions of a moral tradition are binding only on those in the moral tradition and ought not to crossover into law. Now that claim is partly right and partly wrong. There are some claims of the tradition that are binding only on those who accept the tradition, but there are some claims that are universal in their application. An example of the former is the form of liturgical celebration within the tradition. An example of the latter is the prohibition of the taking of life. The protection of human life is one of the most important functions of the law. Here, the moral standards of the tradition and civil law overlap. Only those elements of the tradition which are necessary for the survival and functioning of the individual and the good community are to be embodied in the law.

It is important to note in any treatment of law that law has more than one function. Law functions to coerce, to forbid, to permit, and to instruct. One of the most important functions of law is its teaching function. Law instructs those in the civil community of the standards of right and wrong and of the rights and responsibilities of citizens. Furthermore, if it is the case, that the moral development level of most people rarely rises above the level of concordance to the law, then the essential role of law in maintaining order and well as in facilitating human flourishing must be acknowledged.

(D) Contemporary Catholic Medical Ethics

Catholic physicians often embrace, with appropriate modifications, the commitments articulated in the Code of Hippocrates. For many, the experience of reciting the Oath of Hippocrates at the completion of their Medical School training created a singular memory. And the Catholic tradition continues to keep its tradition alive through the careful examination, in the light of the tradition, of the practices of medicine and the gains of science, and through the timely publication of the results of that study.

Evidence of this commitment to ongoing study and reflection can be found in activities that range from Pontifical institutions to local conferences and committees. The Pontifical Institute of Science which was established in 1936 and which traces its ancestry to the *Academia Lincei* established in 1603, and whose international membership includes renowned scientists, Catholic and non-Catholic, among them many Nobel laureates, is committed to the study of the advances of science so that science and religion may advance together to serve human good. In recent years, the academy has addressed such issues as the environment, neurological research, human fertility, the origins and the evolution of life, the formation of galaxies in the young universe, the beginning of life, the implications of genetics, and the food needs of the developing world. In addition to the Pontifical Academy, the bishops of various national conferences study, through commissions created for precisely that purpose, issues in the practice of medicine and issue guidelines to assist in the formation of the individual conscience and of institutional conscience.

The Ethical and Religious Directives for Catholic Health Care Institutions (ERDs), prepared by the United States Conference of Catholic Bishops in the United States (USCCB), provide one example of the ongoing efforts of the tradition to interact with and transform contemporary medicine and the contemporary world. The sixth edition of the document presents 77 directives to guide the Catholic community in respect to appropriate health care. The directives are ordered around the six themes of social responsibility, pastoral and spiritual responsibility, the health care professional and patient relationship, care at the beginning of life, care at the end of life, and the formation of health care alliances. These directives that inform and give shape to Catholic medical ethics and to medical practice are rooted in the Scriptures. The meaning of the Scriptures has been developed by the philosophical, theological, historical, and anthropological study that attempts to understand the wisdom of the scriptures in a manner that allows that wisdom to be brought forward to apply to the advances within the horizon of the contemporary world. The communication of the results is the task of the Magisterium. A summary of the essential elements of the tradition will be presented, then the Natural Law foundation of the tradition will be made explicit, and finally, the more specific principles, some material and some formal, will be presented.

(1) The Scriptures

The Catholic tradition holds that the Scriptures record the words and the deeds by which God reveals himself to humankind and communicates the divine life to us (Catechism of the Catholic Church, #53 and 236). Words and deeds, not either alone: words give us something to believe in, and deeds give us a reason to believe it. This revelation in words and deeds does not happen all at once, but unfolds gradually over time – God being the master teacher. Among the things that the Scriptures reveal that are foundational for Catholic medical ethics are the following. The Scriptures reveal that human beings are created in the image and likeness of God. Human beings are called upon to exercise power in the world in a manner that manifests human dignity as the image of God. Human creative power is limited. Human creative power is to be providential as God is providential. It is to be stewardship, not control. God as a loving Father continues His guidance over human affairs. God entered into history with Divine Law, for example, through the giving of the Ten Commandments, the Eight Beatitudes, and the great commandments of love, to assist humans so that they might reach the end for which they were created. While God created human beings in such a way that they have a share in God's eternal reason through Natural Law, revelation is the gift of God to guide His fragile creatures to their end.[7] The covenant of God with humanity is the model for human beings to relate to each other. The covenant is faithful – *hesed*; it is patient; it is merciful; it is compassionate. Each human life, inasmuch as every human being is created by God in God's image, is equal in dignity. Human life is finite, vulnerable, and dependent. It comes from God and is drawn back to God. Every human being receives life from God and from their parents – to share in the joy of life; to experience suffering; and, finally, to die. Life and sickness are sometimes to be healed and sometimes to be patiently endured in faith and hope. The source of that faith and hope is centered in a firm grasp that our incarnate God took upon Himself our human nature, lived, suffered, and died in expiation for our sins. Death marks the end of the earthly pilgrimage for each and every human being. But, just as Jesus departed from this life to go to His Father, so we hope to journey to be united to a loving Father who now awaits us.

(2) The Natural Law Tradition

The historical antecedents of the Natural Law tradition lie in the Stoic philosophy of ancient Greece and Rome. The Natural Law tradition, as foundational for the Catholic tradition, was systematically developed in the thirteenth century in the *Summa theologiae* of Thomas Aquinas.[8] Aquinas displays here the synthesis of the religious tradition with the philosophical tradition that developed out of Stoicism. The theory of Natural Law, as described by Thomas Aquinas, delineates the subjection of human beings to God's providence in a most excellent way – "in so far as it partakes of a share of providence by being provident for itself and for others" (ST, I-11 Q.91. a.2). In the treatment by Aquinas, he presents the self-evident principle of practical reason and he provides a mechanism for the generation of more specific precepts to guide prudential decision-making for ethics generally. This mechanism assists in the formulation and in the application of the principles in medical ethics. Natural Law theory makes these fundamental claims: (1) there is a natural order or rule in the universe; (2) this natural order or rule is accessible to human reason as (a) known by reason and (b) as directed by reason; and (3) human flourishing is accomplished in following the directives of practical reason.

It is essential to the understanding of the Natural Law tradition to locate and to understand its remote source and its proximate source. The remote source of Natural Law is Eternal Law – the plan of God for the created world. The proximate source of Natural Law for human beings (here and now) is human reason as human reason comes to understand human nature. Human reason experiences the inclinations which manifest human nature; human reason apprehends the inclinations of human nature as good; and commands that these goods be accomplished under the command of human reason. Because the remote source of Natural Law is the mind of God, the tradition remains confident in its claim that there is truth to be achieved. Because all things in the universe, inasmuch as they have being, have their ultimate source in the mind of God, they have specific natures which are open to be understood by human reason over time. Nonetheless, because the proximate source of understanding the Natural Law lies in the activity of fallible human reason and its grasp of nature, including human nature, the tradition recognizes this grasp as limited and open to revision of the more specific precepts in the advance of knowledge. The general principles and the general precepts are, of course, not open to revision.

A closer examination of this theory as explicated by Aquinas in the *Summa theologiae* illustrates the principles and the generation of the precepts of Natural Law. Aquinas maintains that good is apprehended by human reason and that the first precept of Natural Law, based on the principle that all things seek good, is "good is to be done and pursued and evil is to be avoided" (ST I-II, q. 94, a. 2). In the derivation of the several more specific precepts, Aquinas, working from within an empirical context, holds that practical reason apprehends the natural inclinations or tendencies of human nature as good. These inclinations or tendencies are dynamic principles which press for actualization and which are ordered to the flourishing and conservation of human life. Aquinas lists a methodical ordering of the inclinations identified as moving from more extensive instantiation to more specific. The first more specific and most extensive precept is the precept to preserve human life. It is derived from the inclination in human beings to continue in existence – to live. This inclination is one that is common to all living organisms, for example, trees put down roots which seek water and turn their leaves to the sun to receive energy necessary for photosynthesis. Practical reason apprehends the inclination to continue in existence as good and orders the preservation of existence and the pursuit of the means of preserving human life. The application of this precept is central to medical ethics in the Catholic tradition. It is controlling in issues at the beginning and the end of life such as abortion, euthanasia, appropriate care for the dying, and medically assisted suicide. The second set of inclinations identified by Aquinas is the set of those that are common to human beings and to animals. They include the inclination of male and female to unite in sexual intercourse and to nurture offspring. Reason grasps the inclinations; apprehends them as good; and commands that they be fulfilled under the rule of reason. The Natural Law precepts, which have their foundation in these inclinations, are controlling in the theology of marriage as the institution within which it is reasonable to actualize these inclinations. In addition, these Natural Law precepts are controlling in such medical ethical issues as the governance of the reproductive finality.

The third set of inclinations includes those that are proper to human beings alone. Among them, Aquinas lists the pursuit of truth and the pursuit of life in community. In summary, the principles of Natural Law and the precepts of Natural Law identify objects (ends) of human flourishing. The ordering of the Natural Law precepts moves from the more essential, that is from sustaining life, to the more excellent, that is to knowledge of God.

Human living is, of course, complicated and its goods are multiple. Some other distinctions are helpful to order the pursuit of goods. The first is the realization that the move made from the general principles to the command of a specific act is fraught with difficulty because of the complexity of human action, the fallibility of human reason, and the ordering of the passions. Aquinas reminds us that practical reason is concerned with contingent matters and as we descend from universal truth to the rightness of action in contingent matters, it may be the case that because of some peculiarity of detail the more general principle does not apply in this situation. For example, the Natural Law precept to have sexual intercourse does not apply to those who have been called to a vocation which embraces celibacy and it applies to those who are married within certain limits and it applies to those who are unmarried by informing them to refrain from intercourse. In addition, the Natural Law precept to preserve human life applies in a manner different for the soldier from the way it applies to the ordinary citizen. Furthermore, it is to be noted that the general principles of Natural Law may fail to be operative in a particular human being because of the lack of rectitude or because of the lack of knowledge. In regard to rectitude, the passions may have been trained, either by persistent choices of the individual or by the effects of the environment, that is, having been raised in a household where such abuse was common, in such a way as to pervert rectitude. While this does not make the abuse right, it makes it understandable why the actions of the person are not governed by Natural Law. It is very difficult for these human beings not to be blinded by the press of disordered passions. In regard to knowledge, it is clearly understood that the achievement of knowledge is a long process and when achieved at all is achieved only late in life. Examples of lack of knowledge abound. An example from the history of the development in knowledge is found in the transition in understanding of human reproduction from the preformationist[9] perspective to the understanding found in the germ cell theory. Within the preformationist account, destruction of the germ cell would be considered the destruction of a human being. An example from the development of culture can be found in the difficulty for a child who was raised in the era of slavery or in the era of segregation to come to an understanding that slavery or segregation is wrong and a violation of Natural Law. Likewise, a child who is taught by his father that pornography is natural may have a hard time coming to an understanding that pornography is wrong. The lack of knowledge does not make the behavior right. It does, though, make it understandable that the person's actions are not in accord with Natural Law.

(3) *Integral Goodness of a Human Act*

Another helpful distinction that assists in the ordering of the human pursuit of goods is the recognition that the specification of an act alone or of an intention alone or of a circumstance alone is not sufficient for the moral determination of an act. The moral goodness of an act requires that the object, the intention, and the circumstances all be good for an act to be good and hence morally permissible (*Catechism of the Catholic Church*, 1755). If either the object or the intention behind the act or the circumstances of the act is not good, then the integral goodness of the act is lost.

Some examples are provided in the following. An example with respect to the object is telling a lie. It is a lie to tell a flat-out, bald-faced lie about someone. That action is wrong at the level of object.[10] An example with respect to intention is a) telling the truth about someone, but b) telling them in order to humiliate them rather than to help them grow in virtue. A person might say "But I told the truth!" That may be the case, but that by itself does not make the act moral. The act became immoral at the level of intention, rather than at the level of object. Finally, an example with respect to circumstances is telling the truth about someone with respect to a bad habit of theirs but telling them in front of a large audience of people who will simply make fun of them for their bad habit. Here, the action is immoral not on the level of object or intention but on the level of circumstance.

Other examples from within the contemporary culture abound. It is good for married couples to have children, however, if the circumstances of their marriage are not conducive to the nurturing of children, then they ought to refrain from having children. An example in regard to the object as ordered to procreation is the following. If one of the partners of the marriage is infertile, they cannot, even for the good of procreation, use material from outside the marriage to accomplish the intrinsic contingent procreative end. Procreation is limited to the marital union. An example in regard to intention is the following. It is good for married couples to engage in marital intercourse. However, if one of the partners engages in intercourse as an act of power over the other, then the act loses its integral goodness.

Another example in regard to intention, one that is very powerful in the contemporary culture, is the intention of compassion. It has been suggested, out of compassion, that the stem cells, gathered by way of the destruction of the human embryo, of one human being be used to serve the well-being of another human being or that, out of compassion, the life of the dying be terminated. The goodness of the intention – compassion – does not obviate the evil of the object that is the direct destruction of human life as a means.

In addition to the contributions of the Scriptures, the Natural Law tradition, and the understanding of the essential requirements of good action, there are several principles that function in the discernment of the good. Among the more specific principles operative in medical ethics in the Catholic tradition, the most important are the principle of sanctity of human life, the principle of double effect, the ordinary/extraordinary distinction, and the principle of totality.

(4) Principle of Sanctity of Human Life

The principle of sanctity of human life is the fundamental principle in medical ethics. It recognizes that other goods may be secured only in virtue of having life. Life is not, however, an absolute value. There are circumstances under which the sacrifice of life is justified. The principle of the sanctity of human life has its source in the acknowledgment of God as the author of life and in recognition of the reality that human life is finite, vulnerable, and dependent. In addition, it has a foundation in common sense, in positive law, and in Natural Law. In regard to common sense, it is only within the continuation of life that autonomy or choice or any good can be exercised. In regard to the positive law, the protection of life is required for order in the civil community. Life within the community permits the pursuit of the good life. If life is not protected, the community cannot flourish. In regard to Natural Law, the precept "preserve human life" is the first of the more specific and the most extensive of the Natural Law precepts. It is the fundamental building block of ethics just as the nucleus is the fundamental building block of the atom and the cell the fundamental building block of life.

In contemporary medical ethical literature, there are several different and even conflicting renderings of the principle of the sanctity of human life. Among them are the following: (1) human life has absolute value and may never be taken; (2) innocent human life may never be directly taken; (3) human life has relative value and may be taken for other significant values; and (4) conflict of life situations are inevitable; whenever conflict occurs, minimize the taking of human life. The Catholic tradition aspires to the first of these understandings. Such affirmation is found in the seamless garment rendering of Cardinal Bernardin and in the great Gospel of Life of Saint John Paul II. However, for most of its history, the Catholic tradition, acknowledging human frailty and the right of self-defense, has affirmed the second of these principles. In this affirmation, there is special emphasis on the qualifying terms "innocent" and "direct" and in the acknowledgment that in a fallen and broken world – in a world in which there is evil – human aspirations fall short of the ideal. Instances of killing in self-defense and in just war, when no other remedy is available, are instances of the application of the second understanding. This principle is operative in medical decision-making in instances of the use of particular medications at the end of life and in certain types of abortion decisions.

The third interpretation of the principle is operative in those philosophical positions that do not recognize human life as having fundamental value or do not distinguish human life and its particular dignity from other forms of life, or tend to ignore the human life issue in the pursuit of other goods. This understanding of the principle is operative in the claims of some feminists who rank the choice of a woman to have a career or education or financial well-being over the continued existence of nascent human life. The fourth interpretation has been put forward to account for the claim that some action which directly takes innocent human life may be permissible in some extraordinary circumstance beyond those permitted in the second rendering. The bombing of Hiroshima is sometimes offered as an example and is defended in this interpretation. This defense is not without controversy.[11]

(5) *The Principle of Double Effect*

The Principle of Double Effect is a purely methodological principle. It rests on the common sense perception that the human agent is responsible for acts and omissions and also, to some degree, for the consequences of action. It recognizes that in this imperfect and complicated world, the same action may have more than one effect. The foreseen effects of an action may be both good effects and bad effects. The principle attempts to clarify the conditions under which it is permissible to engage in an act which has two foreseen effects – one good and one bad.[12] The application of the principle of double effect operation requires knowledge of the probable effects. The principle of double effect does not apply in those instances in which the consequences are unknown. For example, if an action has unknown consequences and the consequences could not have been known, the result is understood as accidental. And, if the consequences are unknown but should have been known, then the result is understood as caused by negligence. The conditions are (a) the act itself must be good or indifferent; (b) the good effect is not produced by means of the bad effect; (c) only the good effect and not the bad effect is directly intended; and (d) there is a proportionate reason for taking the action and permitting the bad effect. A recent application of this principle is the use of particular medications at the end of life. In order to relieve pain in the dying patient, medications are morally permitted which have as the intended effect the mitigation of the pain of the patient and the bad, although not intended, effect of depressing the respiratory system resulting in the death of the patient. The physician and family know that morphine will have these two effects. But the medication can be used under the principle of double-effect: (a) the act of relieving pain is good or indifferent; (b) the suppression of breathing is not the means to the end of relieving of pain; (c) the relief of pain is intended, the suppression of breathing is not; and (d) there is a proportionate reason for administering morphine to relieve the pain. The good of the mitigation of the pain is permissible, even though death may be the foreseen result.[13]

(6) *Extraordinary/Ordinary Distinction*

The distinction between extraordinary and ordinary means is critical for the determination of obligation. Human beings in the exercise of stewardship of their lives are morally obliged to take ordinary means in the care of life. Ordinary means are all medicines, treatments, and operations which offer a reasonable hope of benefit for the patient and which can be obtained and used without excessive expense, pain, or other inconvenience. Extraordinary means are all medicines, treatments, and operations which cannot be obtained without excessive expense, pain, or other inconvenience or if used would not offer a reasonable hope of benefit. The distinction between ordinary and extraordinary means shifts generally as technology advances as well as specifically and individually depending on the prognosis of a patient and the invasiveness of the treatment. What, in the past, might have been extraordinary means such as almost any surgery, has, because of medical advances such as antibiotics, anesthesia, heart and lung machines, and immunosuppressant drugs, become ordinary means. What might be ordinary means for one patient might be extraordinary means for another. The hinge element here is a benefit to the person. It might be appropriate, hence ordinary care, to use a ventilator to support, temporarily, the respiration of a patient recovering from an injury or illness, and it might be inappropriate, hence extraordinary care, to use the same ventilator modality for a patient actively in the dying process.

(7) *The Principle of Totality*

The most general statement of the principle of totality is the part can be used for the good of the whole; the part is subordinate to the good of the whole. The principle of totality recognizes that the individual person is the steward of body and soul. In exercising stewardship, the person is permitted the use of the faculties and powers of the body and soul in accord with the immanent finality of the faculties or the powers in the service of the whole.

The person may not destroy the faculties or powers or limbs or organs unless their destruction is required for the good of continued existence or that of mending or avoiding serious injury. This principle, aided by the distinction between ordinary and extraordinary means and the principle of double effect, governs treatment decisions which require that function or powers be rendered useless or that body parts be destroyed. In applying this principle, however, there is an important distinction to be made. The distinction depends upon a determination of the nature of the organism to which the principle is to be applied. The distinction is between a physical organism and a moral organism, and there is a corresponding limitation of the application of the principle. An organism, for example, a human body, is a physical whole if it has a unity subsisting in itself. It has a unity on the level of essence. The relationship of part to whole exists if the part is an integral part of the physical unity, that is, the part by its very nature has no finality outside the whole. As Pope Pius XII noted, "It is wholly absorbed by the totality of the organism to which it is attached" (Pius XII, 44,786). For example, it is morally justifiable to amputate a diseased arm in order to save the life of a person. The person is a physical unity where the part – the arm – serves the whole and can be disposed of as necessary for the sake of the survival of the person.

The case is different for a moral organism. A moral organism, for example, a community is a whole which is not a physical unity subsisting in itself but a union of individuals bound together for the realization of some common good or action. Individuals who are members of a moral community such as citizens of a polity have meaning in themselves and meaning outside that determined by their role as collaborators in the common enterprise that unites the group. A moral organism has a unity on the level of action. From the distinction of organisms as either a physical or a moral totality, there follows the corresponding limitation of action in the application of the principle of totality. In the case of a physical whole, such as an individual human being, the person seeking the good of that particular person may dispose directly of the parts and organs within the scope of their natural finality. Common examples include the amputation of a diseased limb or a cancerous uterus when the life of the person is at risk. The person may "intervene, as often as and to the extent that the good of the whole demands to paralyze, destroy, mutilate and separate the members" of the body (Pius XII, 1952). On the other hand, if the organism is a moral whole, the application of the principle is limited to the activities of the members in the service of the whole. This understanding of the principle of totality, as it applies to moral organisms, clarifies the limits of the application of the principle of sociality in the political sphere. The application of the principle of totality exercises a limiting function in medical ethical issues such as limits on human subject use in medical research and medical therapies such as the use of human embryonic stem cells.

(E) The Challenge in the Contemporary Culture

Consideration of the foundation of medical ethics, however, is not unproblematic. The religious tradition, despite these challenges, continues its role of informing the practices of individuals and institutions who claim the tradition and developing its responses in the presence of new knowledge and advancing technologies. In the last quarter of the twentieth century, a deliberate effort was made to separate medicine from its moorings in religious commitment and even from the traditional ethics that guided its practice through centuries. The lean to the latter is found in a set of claims, namely, (1) medicine ought to be limited only by what technology and medical skill enable medical practitioners to do and (2) medicine's primary purpose is to enhance human life by whatever means are legal and can be devised to relieve suffering. Evidence of the former may be found in the effort to develop a more general and, hence, more universal set of ethical principles to guide bioethics to serve a pluralistic community. The more general universal principles included such sets of principles as beneficence, non-maleficence, autonomy, informed consent, and justice. Autonomy is sometimes rendered as respect for autonomy or respect for persons. The requirement of informed consent is necessary for autonomy to be operational. Non-maleficence while originally understood as subsumed under beneficence is now sometimes claimed as the first principle of medicine in *Primum non nocere*. These principles were articulated in the Belmont Report and were made famous as the Georgetown Mantra in the work of Professors Thomas Beauchamp and James Childress in *Principles of Biomedical Ethics*. These principles were thought sufficient to direct a value-free science and a value-free medicine for a religiously and culturally pluralistic polity. Furthermore, these principles were wedded to a particular enlightenment and Western liberal account of human life that has, at its core, an inadequate philosophy of person – a philosophy which values an excessive individualism fueled by the will, unfettered by truth, of the autonomous rights-bearing individual and which respects only those individuals who are capable of exercising autonomous rights. Moreover, the principles are so general as to be empty, that is, what is the good to be achieved; what is the harm to be avoided; what are the limits of autonomy; what are the necessary and sufficient conditions of informed consent; and, finally, what is justice.[14]

The myth of a value-free science and medicine collapses in the wake of the revelation and subsequent scrutiny of the findings of the Nuremberg Trials, the revelations of the Japanese Biological Warfare Unit 731 experiments, and, in the United States in the disclosure of experiments such as the Tuskegee Syphilis Studies, the Willowbrook hepatitis studies on disabled children, the injection of cancers cells into elderly patients at New York's Jewish Chronic Disease Hospital, and the Radiation experiments in the United States. The underlying philosophy of the person found in these practices reveals a form of elitism which denies protection to those who are not like those in power. A more adequate philosophy of person reveals that we live most of our lives as related dependent human beings. Autonomy is always a limited accomplishment achieved over time, if at all, and achieved only after a long period of dependency and often followed by another period of dependency. Autonomy is always limited – constrained by the relationships which define one's life and these relationships oftentimes require that the powerful accept disadvantage for the sake of the dependent other. Human beings are dependent in the most absolute and radical way, first upon God and then upon each other. Living a rich human life places us in different relationships to each other throughout life. Some of these relationships are symmetrical and some are asymmetrical. The symmetrical relationships have their source in our being related to each other in fundamental equality as human beings. The asymmetrical relationships have their source in the fundamental inequality that we have on account of the obligations and duties that arise in our different vocations whereby we serve one another. In those relationships which are asymmetrical, such as physician/patient, professor/student, attorney/client, and parent/child, the model is God's relation to God's creatures. They are asymmetrical because one party of the relationship has knowledge, which is the source of its power and authority, and the other party of the relationship is in need of the skills of those with authority and power. These relations have definition and give content to duties and rights. The physician, professor, attorney, or parent exercises authority over the patient, student, client, and child; and the patient, student, client, and child have the right to the appropriate competence of the authority. Out of that competence and within the limits of the role, the physician serves the good of the patient; the professor serves the good of the student; the attorney serves the good of the client, and the parent serves the good of the child. The patient, student, client, and child submit to that authority until that authority is no longer needed. The exercise of power and authority is to be merciful, compassionate, and just as God is merciful, compassionate, and just. It is worth considering that perhaps the measure whereby we measure those in asymmetrical relations to us will be the measure of God toward us.

So in the face of the historical and systemic failure of the attempt to construct a value-free bioethics in the twentieth century, the religious traditions are called upon in the twenty-first century to recover their role as informing practices and institutions they claim as their own.[15] Dr. Edmund

Pellegrino – for many years, a leader among Catholic physicians and in Catholic medical care – speaking to and of the tradition of Catholic medicine and health care often cited Kierkegaard to remind medical practitioners of their calling to imitate Christ. These words of Kierkegaard are "Without imitation of Christ, the fruit of Catholic faith, Christianity becomes mere mythology or poetry or an abstract idea" (Pellegrino, 2008, p. 2). The Catholic physician then is called to imitate Christ – to heal as Christ healed.

The Catholic tradition, moreover, is reminded of its limits. Healing of physical illness is not always possible. The bodies of this temporal life are mortal and corruptible. Hence, an exclusive focus on healing is too narrow and too exclusive a center. It is to buy into what Professor Stanley Hauerwas calls the Promethean myth of modern medicine that offers the promise of human salvation in more and better medicine (Hauerwas, 2008, p. 270). Jesus healed but he also suffered and died. Here, Catholic medical practices, health care institutions, and patients have special obligations because of the Christ revealed in Scripture. Catholic practices and institutions must embrace methods and be places of caring for the dying that is inevitable. They must offer visible witness to both the truth of the finitude and the truth of the promise of human existence. In His suffering and dying, Jesus, from the depths of His humanity, called out for consolation. In Gethsemane, He asked to be rescued, "My Father . . . take this cup of suffering from me." He revealed to His friends His grief and anguish. Even while trusting, He said, "The sorrow in my heart is so great that it almost crushes me." He asked them to stay with Him and He was sorely disappointed by their failure to remain with Him. He experienced a sense of abandonment and, close to the end, He cried out to His heavenly Father, "*Eli, Eli, lema sabachthani* (My God, My God, why have you forsaken me?)." And, at last, He placed Himself into His Father's care. Catholic health care institutions have to be places and have to provide services and spaces within which human beings who are experiencing crushing sorrow, anguish, and abandonment will find in attendance caring people to touch, to wash, and to anoint their bodies, attentive people who do not turn away from them, loving people whose simple presence sustains them, and faithful people who do not abandon them in their dying. And Catholic people who are dying must come to terms, finally, with human nature as created, accept their dying in the hope of eternal life, and in the end, entrust themselves to God's infinite power.

(F) Afterword

The Catholic tradition values the contributions of medicine, science, and law, but it does not turn over its moral authority in medical ethics to the success of medical practice, to the advances in science, and to current renderings in the law. Technologies honed by medicine and science and public policies crafted within the law must serve the dignity and vocation of the human person. Science by itself cannot define that dignity and vocation. There is an extensive history of scientific and medical research, propelled by the research imperative, which treated human beings as means to the ends of progress and therapy. Religious authorities must respond appropriately and respectfully to the scientific and medical advances when they present opportunities for genuine human flourishing. Church leaders have on occasion stepped inappropriately into the domain of science, and scientists have more than once sought refuge in the claim that its pursuits are value-free. History has witnessed, on both sides of the science-theology debate, both hubris and authoritarianism. Both sides, in careful application of the canons appropriate to their respective fields, must accept the limitation of their expertise. Authority exercised rightly recognizes the power of the dialectical tension between fields and disciplines and between theory and practice in the pursuit of truth. Moreover, authority is not exercised for its own sake or for the sake of power but for the sake of truth. Recent history has also witnessed from both sides the incredible results of appropriate collaboration and cooperation. One particular example of such cooperation is to be found in Directive 58 in the Ethical and Religious Directives for Catholic Health Care Services. Directive 58 asserts a presumption in favor of providing food and water to patients as long as the food and water provide a benefit to the patient, that is, as ordinary care. The advance in the directive was accomplished in the presence of ongoing conversations by physicians, theologians, lawyers, and philosophers.[16] The physicians offered their medical judgment that there are some conditions of illness and decline in which food and water no longer benefit the patient. Philosophers and theologians offered their expertise in the careful application of the distinction between ordinary and extraordinary means of preserving human life, in their affirmation of life as a fundamental value, and in the distinguishing of continuation of biological existence from the continuation of human existence. Those tasked with the work of law held fast to the distinction between dying by way of lethal interventions and dying because of an underlying pathology and to the understanding that the exercise of liberty requires living. This discussion continues in current cases in the presence of advancements in diagnostic technology, of improvement in treatment and rehabilitative modalities, and as the focus shifts between the values of biological continuity and personal continuity. That this collaborative work continues is evidence of the reality, the necessity, and the goodness of the ongoing dialectic of medicine, philosophy, theology, and law in service to human flourishing. This discussion does not continue without debate about such topics as the object of the act and moral absolutes, the debate on the nature of nutrition and hydration as either ordinary or extraordinary means in the presence of a variety of conditions, persistent vegetative state, permanent vegetative state, and minimally conscious state, presented by patients, and the debate about the end of life.[17] To these debates must be added the reminder that inasmuch as Catholics believe that death marks the passage to eternal life, Catholics ought to behave as if they really believe that.[18]

Questions for Reflection

1. The *Oath of Hippocrates* enumerates duties and limitations on the practice of medicine. What are some of the consequences for physicians who would be guided in medical practice by the Oath? Do the same for the *Prayer of Maimonides*.
2. What do you think should be the *goals* and the *limits* of medicine? What would be an example of a practice that would violate the proper goals or limits?
3. The care of Jesus for the vulnerable is the model for the Catholic physician. How do the Gospel passages in *Matthew 8* and *9* guide physicians who would model their medical practices on the ministry of Jesus?
4. Reflect on the dignity of the human person as a free creation by God in the image of God. What are the consequences of this for the practice of medicine? What are the consequences of this for the patient?
5. Consider the medical principle "treatment and experiment require informed consent." Describe the intersection of Scriptural, natural law, historical, and legal principles in the establishment of that principle.
6. If treatment and experiment require informed consent, how can a patient – a sick person – truly give informed consent? How can a research subject be sufficiently knowledgeable and free to give informed consent?
7. The natural law tradition as presented by Saint Thomas Aquinas and Saint John Paul II requires the recognition of nature (*natura*) and the operation of reason (*ratio*). How can this tradition respond to the complexities of contemporary medicine?
8. The principle of sanctity of human life has been subjected to a variety of interpretations in the contemporary culture. Which interpretation would you defend?

9. Come up with your own example of how an act can be morally wrong because of its object, intention, or circumstances. Give an example where:

   (a) the object is wrong;
   (b) the object is right, but the intention is wrong;
   (c) the object and intention are right, but the circumstances are wrong.

10. What is the function of principles such as the principle of double effect or the principle of totality in medical ethics?

Notes

1 See the opening words of *Fides et Ratio* of Saint John Paul II:

> Faith and reason are like two wings on which the human spirit rises to the contemplation of truth; and God has placed in the human heart a desire to know the truth – in a word, to know himself – so that, by knowing and loving God, men and women may also come to the fullness of truth about themselves.
>
> (cf. *Ex* 33:18; *Ps* 27:8–9; 63:2–3; *Jn* 14:8; *1 Jn* 3:2)

2 The word "end" here takes its meaning from τέλος (telos) in Greek which is used to indicate a goal or objective.

3 The *Hippocratic Oath* in its classical form is sworn by very few medical schools in the United States. Sixty-seven of 141 contacted medical schools (48%) had medical students recite an oath. Fifty-nine (88% of responding institutions) had students swear an oath more than once during medical training and 30 (45%) used more than one oath. Responses show that 29 (43%) schools used the classic Hippocratic Oath or a modified version of it, 29 (43%) used oaths authored by students and/or faculty, and 28 (42%) used some other oath. All reporting institutions (67, 100%) incorporated an oath into a White Coat Ceremony (62, 92%), a ceremonial event where medical students are given short white coats to be worn during clinical rotations, or Commencement (62, 93%) (Dossabhoy, 139). The omission of the *Oath* is based on considerations of it as outdated (abortion and euthanasia are forbidden) and/or insufficient (no reference to medical research) and/or inapplicable (no tuition). Some medical schools use a modified form of the Oath such as that developed by Dr. Louis Lasagna; some use an oath constructed by the graduating class; some use a prayer such as the Prayer of Maimonides; and some have no oath at all. *Hippocrates' oath and Asclepius' snake* (OUP, 2018) by T.A. Cavanaugh and *Hippocratic, religious, and secular medical ethics* (Georgetown UP, 2012) by Robert Veatch provide, respectively, a history and a critique of the development of the medical profession.

4 It has been suggested that the prayer was written by the German physician Marcus Herz, the physician to Moses Mendelssohn.

5 This particular account of the dynamic structure of human knowing expressed as transcendental imperatives is the work of Bernard Lonergan. It can be found in summary form in Lonergan's "Cognitional Structure," found in *Collection*, edited by F. E. Crowe, S.J.; in full explication in *Insight*, and applied in *Method in Theology*.

6 A special case arises when a physician becomes a patient. The physician's knowledge can be an asset or a deficit in treatment. Moreover, illness can be transformative of the practice of physicians. David Fajgenbaum wrote about his research as an asset to his treatment in *Chasing My Cure* (New York: Ballantine Books, 2019). Robert Klitzman in *When Doctors Become Patients* (London: The Oxford University Press, 2008) wrote out of his own personal experience as a psychiatrist suffering from depression and out of the experiences of 36 patients he interviewed as they practiced medicine in the presence of serious illness. Klitzman suggested that through suffering these physicians acquired a double lens to serve their patients.

7 It was necessary for man's salvation that there should be knowledge revealed by God besides philosophical science built up by human reason. Firstly, indeed, because man is directed to God, as to an end that surpasses the grasp of his reason: 'The eye hath not seen, O God, besides Thee, what things Thou hast prepared for them that wait for Thee' (Isaiah 64:4). But the end must first be known by men who are to direct their thoughts and actions to the end. Hence it was necessary for the salvation of man that certain truths which exceed human reason should be made known to him by divine revelation. Even as regards those truths about God which human reason could have discovered, it was necessary that man should be taught by a divine revelation; because the truth about God such as reason could discover, would only be known by a few, and that after a long time, and with the admixture of many errors. Whereas man's whole salvation, which is in God, depends upon the knowledge of this truth. Therefore, in order that the salvation of men might be brought about more fitly and more surely, it was necessary that they should be taught divine truths by divine revelation. It was therefore necessary that besides philosophical science built up by reason, there should be a sacred science learned through revelation.

(*Summa Theologiae*, I, q.1. a.1)

8 While this understanding of the natural law tradition is taken from the text of the *Summa theologiae* I-II, QQ. 90–97 of Thomas Aquinas, there are different understandings of the natural law tradition and even of Aquinas within the Catholic tradition. See, for example, the exchanges between Ralph McInerny (McInerny, R. (1980). The principles of natural law. *American Journal of Jurisprudence*, *25*(1), Article 1) and John Finnis (Finnis, J. M. and Grisez, G. (1981). The basic principles of natural: A reply to Ralph McInerny. *American Journal of Jurisprudence*, *26*(1).) where each accused the other of misunderstanding each other and misunderstanding of Aquinas.

9 The theory of preformation in embryology holds that the completely organized body of every human being, the homunculus, is present in either the sperm or the egg. Development of this miniature human being is simply a case of enlargement over time. The germ theory in embryology holds that the union of germ cells, one from the sperm of the male and one from the ovum of the female accomplishes reproduction in human beings. The sperm penetrates the ovum and with the union of the gametes, the zygote is formed.

10 This is the case, even though there are several levels of nuance with regard to truth-telling in the Catholic tradition. For a short and interesting treatment, see Janet Smith's article "Fig Leaves and Falsehoods" (*First Things*, June 2011). For a more detailed treatment, see Note F (The Economy) and Note G (Lying and Equivocation) in John Henry Newman's *Apologia Pro Vita Sua*.

11 Anscombe, G. E. M. (1981). Mr. Truman's degree. In *The collected philosophical papers of G.E.M. Anscombe* (Vol. III, pp. 62–71). Blackwell.

12 The application of the principle of double effect assists in the discernment of permissible action where an action has both a good effect and a bad effect. It assists in the sorting of the intentions, consequences, and circumstances of an action. It is a methodological tool. It has no doctrinal content and should not be referred to as the Doctrine of Double Effect. There is widespread debate even within the Roman Catholic tradition as to its validity and applicability. Examples can be found in T.A. Cavanaugh's (2006). *Double effect reasoning: Doing good and avoiding evil.* Oxford University Press, and in Lawrence Masek's (2018). *Intention, character, and double effect.* University of Notre Dame Press. Cavanaugh develops the history and application of the principle as well as the controversies surrounding it. He locates its foundation in the Aristotelian/Thomistic tradition in the treatment of the distinction between intention and foresight in voluntary acts. Masek situates the principle within virtue theory and the way in which the application of the principle contributes to the character formation of the actor.

13 Chapter 10 deals with the difference between his action and physician-assisted suicide. In physician-assisted suicide, the negative effect – death – is the means to achieve the relief of suffering, and death is directly intended.

14 An alternative approach, rather than bracketing religious commitment in an attempt to reach agreement on value-free grounds alone, is to delve deeply *into* the religious commitments, and let practitioners of different religions discover points of agreement from within those commitments. Christian, Jewish, Muslim, and Hindu physicians often find themselves able to do so.

15 This can actually lead to more robust conversations among medical professionals of different religious traditions. It is not rare that Jewish, Muslim, and Hindu physicians work at Catholic hospitals precisely because of the commitment of the hospitals to Catholic principles such as the dignity of human life.

16 We have had the privilege of being part of some of those conversations.

17 For contemporary discussion among Catholic Bioethicists, see Tollefsen, C. (Ed.). (2007). *Artificial nutrition and hydration: The new catholic debate.* Springer, and Hamel, R., & Walter, J. (Eds.). (2007). *Artificial nutrition and hydration and the permanently unconscious patient: The catholic debate.* Georgetown University Press.

18 McCormick, S. J., Richard A. (1992, March 14). Moral considerations ill considered. *America*, pp. 210–214.

3 The Modern Codes

The Ethics of Research Involving Human Patients/Subjects

The *Psalms* in the ancient scriptures praise the glory of God as revealed in the created world. The Psalmist wrote: "Chant we the Lord's wondrous doings, delight and study of all who love him. Ever his deeds are high and glorious, faithful he abides to all eternity" (*Psalms*, 110, 2–3). This text recognizes the goodness of the created world as majestic, exquisite, and ordered. Enjoyment of the beauty of the world calls for contemplation of its grandeur and worship of God. It also implicates an ordering of the world as fashioned by God and as the object of human study. This last serves as a task. A faithful ordering of the world requires knowledge of the world as created and action in a world where disorder, such as sickness and injustice, is ever close at hand. Included in the wonders of God's creation is human reason, as speculative and practical, as it operates through its internal drives to experience, to know, to understand, to judge, to take action, to revise, to love, to do good, and to care out of that knowledge and love. Included in the wonders of God's creation is human nature, which, while created in the image and likeness of God, remains as created finite, vulnerable, and dependent. This condition as embodied is empirically verifiable and requires care. If there is to be a just ordering of the world, then vulnerable human beings, a category which includes every human being at particular times in their life trajectory, require the protection of the temporarily powerful, less dependent but still finite human beings whose lives are linked to theirs in particular real relations.[1]

Medicine as a human activity is pursued out of those imperatives, especially to know and to care. Medical research is one tool in the arsenal of medical practice. These imperatives, both the research imperative and the therapeutic imperative, operate within limits that are defined by the relation of physician to patient and the relation of researcher to subject and both sets of relations as ordered to God. The demands and limits of the imperatives are more complicated when the operative matrix is defined by a physician/researcher to a patient/subject.

DOI: 10.4324/9781003627197-3

Medicine requires knowledge that is to be gained through the ongoing dialectic and praxis of experience, research, knowledge, and practice. Research is an important component for the advancement of science and for the advancement of medicine. The imperative to do research arises out of the drive to know and the imperative to advance medicine arises out of the desire to heal. The drive to know and the desire to heal are to be acknowledged as gifts of God so that human beings, who are created in God's image and likeness, may exercise, through a better understanding of the created world, creative stewardship in that world. Both the desire to know and the drive to heal are to be appropriately directed toward human flourishing as the proper end of each. The means to accomplish the intended ends must also be instances of human flourishing. Hence, research, whether directed to the advance of knowledge or therapy, which requires the participation of human subjects, must respect the dignity of the human subject – a dignity which has its source in the fact that human beings have been created in the image and likeness of God and in the acknowledgment that human beings are ends in themselves. This chapter will address the issue of research ethics involving human subjects and patients in the following order:

(A) The examination of sources of danger in research projects;
(B) The exploration of concrete historical instances of abuse;
(C) The presentation of early efforts to provide guidelines for researchers;
(D) An inquiry into the ongoing efforts in the United States to guide and regulate research and care of the vulnerable;
(E) Afterword: reflection on the underlying principles operative in ongoing medical research in order to present some conclusions.

(A) Sources of Danger Inherent in Research Projects

The acknowledgment of the good of the advancement of science and the good of the advancement of medicine does not mean that the pursuit of these goods is unproblematic. There are several significant problems latent in the domain of research which includes the issue of human subjects in trials. The first lies in the tendency of scientists and physician-scientists to press and to defend their research as a value-free pursuit – a pure pursuit of knowledge without the confounding presence of bias. The study of the history of research involving human subjects, however, reveals that (a) the value-free claim cannot stand and (b) the vacuum resulting from the absence of directing principles resulted in instances of egregious abuses of human subjects. It has often been the case that the research imperative and the healing imperative are so strong that they drive the scientist researcher and the physician researcher past the appropriate limits of research. The second problem lies in the fact that the operative cultural climate within which the researcher operates is sometimes distorted such that the good intended is tainted by bias. A third problem is presented in the complication of the physician researcher for whom the person under care is simultaneously subject and patient.

(B) Historical Instances of Abuse

This section will present some examples of the abuse of human subjects in research in modern history. The examples will be drawn from the United States and from Nazi Germany. While there are numerous examples of human subject abuse in research in the United States, including the Willowbrook Study which infected institutionalized children of limited cognitive ability with hepatitis, the injection of cancer cells into elderly patients at the Jewish Chronic Disease Hospital in New York, and the radiation exposure of members of the American military, the Tuskegee study can serve as one egregious example. So too the studies of Nazi Germany can function as an international example while acknowledging at the same time the existence of other examples such as the Japanese Detachment 731 experiments in World War II and the Communist psychiatric experiments aimed at disabling dissidents during the Cold War.

(1) The Tuskegee Study

The first example of research abuse to be examined is the Tuskegee Syphilis Study. This study was carefully documented in 1977 by Allan M. Brandt in *Racism and Research: The Case of the Tuskegee Syphilis Study*. It is appropriate to begin here because the Tuskegee study appears chronologically earlier than the Nazi research projects and because it is proper to be aware of the mote in one's own eye before examining the beam in another's eyes. The syphilis study began in 1932 as a project of the United States Public Health Service. It is important to note that at the time the study started, the various regulating bodies in the United States, and the rest of the world as well, had articulated no formal position on human experimentation. The scientific purpose of the project was to study the natural course of syphilis in its progression from onset of symptoms through latency to death. On the first level, it was a study in nature. The research cohort, as described in the study, was made up entirely of black males. On the second level, then the social purpose of the study was to observe how the disease affected the lives of the men. The site of the study was Macon County, Alabama. There were 600 men involved initially in the study. Four hundred of them had been diagnosed with syphilis; the other 200 men were uninfected and they were to serve as controls. The men who were involved in the research were not informed that they were participants in a research project. They were told that they were ill and that the public health services would provide them care and that the public health services would even provide for their funeral expenses. It is important to note that at the inception of the study there was no effective medication to treat syphilis. In 1936, the first results of the study were published. Publication of the results of the study continued regularly every four to six years through the sixties. In 1969, the Center for Disease Control, through one of its committees, made the decision to continue the Tuskegee Study. The experimental study then continued until 1972 when the study was revealed by Dr. Henry Beecher and the national press published accounts of the study. Only then, in the midst of a public outcry, did the Department of Health Education and Welfare order the experiment halted.

There were two significant occurrences in the 40 years from the commencement of the Tuskegee Study until it was halted. One was the discovery of the effectiveness of penicillin in the treatment of syphilis and its ready availability after World War II. The other was the framing and publication of *The Nuremberg Code* in 1946 at the conclusion of the trial of Nazi physicians as war criminals. The American Justice, Robert H. Jackson, who presided over the military tribunal of physicians, presented *The Nuremberg Code*. Two American physicians, Dr. Andrew Ivy and Dr. Leo Alexander, assisted in the preparation of the Code. Although there is some disagreement between the two physicians regarding the role of each in the drafting of the code, there is enough independent corroborating evidence to show that each made a significant contribution. In the immediate wake of the Nuremberg Trial, the House of Delegates of the American Medical Association formally approved and adopted the principles of *The Nuremberg Code*. And in 1953, when the National Institutes of Health opened the Institute's clinic, a policy was put into place requiring the voluntary agreement, based on informed understanding, for all human research subjects.

Neither the discovery of penicillin nor the articulation of principles of *The Nuremberg Code* nor the adoption of the principles of the Code by various U.S.A. regulating bodies in medicine and science was sufficient to stop the experiment and to treat the infected men. The men in the Tuskegee Study were denied, in an explicit decision, penicillin. The application of the principles of the Code never became an issue. The cultural bias, which was fed by social Darwinism and supported by anthropologists, ethnologists, and biologists, viewed the American Negro as a primitive race doomed to disease, vice, crime, and inevitable early extinction. This assessment combined with the research imperative pressed for the completion of the study which required as an end point postmortem examination.

(2) *Medical Research in the Nazi Era*

The research efforts in Nazi Germany have been chronicled since the end of World War II. Accounts of the violations of human dignity in anthropological research and medical research appeared as early as 1949 with the publication by Dr. Leo Alexander of his observations of the Nuremberg Trial of Physicians. His paper, *Medical Science under Dictatorship*, appeared in the prestigious *New England Journal of Medicine*. A more recent and more expansive account by Robert Jay Lifton appears in his book, *The Nazi Doctors: Medical Killing and the Psychology of Genocide*, which was published in 1986. While the mass extermination projects that were executed by the Nazis between 1939 and 1945 are comparatively well known, less well known are the research projects undertaken for the advancement of science and the advancement of medicine. The following are two examples of the research imperative. Dr. Julius Hallervorden, renowned German neuropathologist, who was engaged in the study of diseases of the brain, was the eager recipient of materials – the brains of those who had been killed in the camps – for the advancement of his studies. He reported to Dr. Alexander that "There was wonderful material among those brains, beautiful mental defectives, malformations and early infantile diseases. I accepted those brains of course. Where they came from and how they came to me was really none of my business" (Alexander, p. 40). Dr. August Hirt, professor of anatomy at the University of Strassburg, enlisted the help of the camp officials in the procurement of specimens for the development of a collection of skeletons. He preserved them and used them in his anthropological work.

The medical therapeutic imperative in the Nazi era was tied to national security – the risks encountered by the military and efforts to ameliorate those harms. Two examples – one for treating wounded soldiers and the other for treated fliers downed in the ocean – will suffice. (1) In attempts to develop coagulants to stem hemorrhage on the battlefield, experimental coagulants were tested on live and conscious prisoners whose limbs were amputated in order to measure differences in coagulation time. (2) The concern for the risk of shock from exposure to the cold by pilots who suffered immersion in the North Sea, prompted a team of physicians headed by Dr. Sigmund Rascher to subject prisoners to exposure to brutally frigid temperatures, sometimes in ice vats, in order to measure the effects of the cold and devise care that would effectively treat the pilots.

(C) *The Nuremberg Code* and Its Progeny

In reaction to the atrocities revealed at the Nuremberg Trial, *The Nuremberg Code* was developed. The *Code* is appended at the end of this chapter.

The *Code* lists ten principles to guide research involving human subjects. The most important elements in the *Code* are the following. The *Code* requires the voluntary consent of the research subject. The *Code* explicitly defines what it means by voluntary consent. It says,

> the person involved should have legal capacity to give consent; should be so situated as to be able to exercise free power of choice, without the intervention of any element of force, fraud, deceit, duress, overreaching, or other ulterior form of constraint or coercion; and should have sufficient knowledge and comprehension of the elements of the subject matter involved as to enable him to make an understanding and enlightened decision.
>
> (*Code*, Article 1)

The three elements of informed consent – freedom, voluntariness, and knowledge – are made specific here. Among the other significant components of the *Code* is that it is the duty of the researcher to make certain that the appropriate consent is in place. Moreover, this is not a duty that the researcher may delegate to anyone else (*Code*, Article 1). The research is required to have as its goal "fruitful results for the good of society, unprocurable by other methods or means of study" (*Code*, Article 2). The research must be necessary and it cannot be random in its design. The design of the research, in order to increase the probability of useful results and in order to protect human subjects, requires that it be "based on the results of animal studies and a knowledge of the natural history of the disease or other problem under study" (*Code*, Article 3). A most important ratio of degree of harm to the research subject to degree of knowledge acquired in the research is found in the requirement that "No experiment should be conducted where there is an a priori reason to believe that death or disabling injury will occur; except, perhaps, in those experiments where the experimental physicians also serve as subjects" (*Code*, Article 5). If the continuation of the experiment is likely to bring harm to the research subject, the experiment must be terminated (*Code*, Article 10). Note well in keeping with an earlier medical tradition, the appropriate first subject of dangerous experiments is to be the experimenter.

The Nuremberg Code is not law and does not have the power of law. Nonetheless, it exercises powerful influence as an ideal. The limitations of *The Nuremberg Code* quickly became evident to the scientific and medical research community. In its narrow focus on the atrocities immediately before the Court, the *Code* made no distinction between research for the sake of the advancement of knowledge and medical research combined with medical care, that is, research to advance therapy for a particular patient. *The Nuremberg Code* attends the researcher–subject relationship, but not the physician/researcher//patient/subject relationship where research is coupled with therapy.

In 1964, the World Medical Association published *The Declaration of Helsinki*[2] to provide the needed expansion. Of particular interest in the *Declaration* is its affirmation of the good of the individual over the interests of society in research. The *Declaration* says, "In medical research on human subjects, considerations related to the well-being of the human subject should take precedence over the interests of science and society" (Article 5). The *Declaration* is particularly sensitive to vulnerable populations and lists some of those for whom special care should be taken in any research situation. Among the vulnerable populations are "the economically and medically disadvantaged". . ."those who cannot give or refuse consent for themselves, for those who may be subject to giving consent under duress". . ."those who will not benefit personally from the research, and . . . those for whom research is combined with care" (Article 8). Despite this declared sensitivity to vulnerable populations, the *Declaration* moves away from the strict informed consent requirements of *The Nuremberg Code* and from research focused primarily on the benefit of the particular patient at hand to research to benefit the population of patients of which this particular patient is a representative. It allows the participation or use of research subjects who are incapable of informed consent, such as those who are legally incompetent, whether physically or mentally, and legally incompetent minors. The *Declaration* permits the substitution of the informed consent of the participants with the informed consent of the legal representative of the incompetent, with the added limitation that the "research . . . [must be] . . . necessary to promote the health of the population represented and this research cannot be performed on legally competent persons" (Article 24). Another significant development is the addition of an assent requirement – displacing informed consent – on the part of children and other incompetent persons that permits their participation in any research project. The assent requirement avers that these populations are capable of a sufficiently appropriate understanding of the research project and their role in the project that enables them to express a willingness to participate that does not reach the high standard of informed consent (Article 25). Assent is understood to be an active agreement which takes into account the experience and level of understanding of the legally incompetent person. In articulating the principles for medical research combined with medical care, the *Declaration* begins with the requirement that the protocol has potential value – therapeutic or diagnostic or prophylactic – for the patient (Article 28) and then progresses to the permissibility, within the scope of the other relevant guidelines, for the use of new and unproven procedures for patients for whom proven procedures are ineffective (Article 32).

(D) Ongoing Efforts to Guide Research in the U.S.A.

After the public outcry in response to the revelation of the Tuskegee Study, the United States Department of Health, Education, and Welfare (now the United States Department of Health and Human Services) proposed its first set of regulations to protect human subjects in behavioral and biomedical research for those projects that are conducted by and supported by federal funds. These guidelines were published in May of 1974 as the Code of Federal Regulations, Title 45 Public Welfare and Part 46 Protection of Human Subjects (45 CFR 46). In 1979, the Belmont Report,[3] which sets out an ethical framework as the basis for regulation, was published. The framework lists as important principles: respect for persons, beneficence, non-maleficence, and distributive justice. It provides guidelines for the establishments of institutional review boards, guidelines for informed consent, assessment of risks and benefits, and the selection of subjects. In 1983, the Code of Federal Regulations specifically addressed the issue of research with children and added a section to protect the interests of children. The Federal Code of Regulations continues to be amended and revised in the face of multiple pressures.

The progression of science and medicine combined with the need for testing the products of its research, and as well, the occasional revelation of yet more abuses and missteps, require regular oversight of research by regulatory agencies and further refinement of the principles and regulations. The Council for International Organizations of Medical Science (CIOMS) has taken up the task of speaking for and to the international community. The progression of the field can be seen in the development of guidelines for research involving subjects in underdeveloped communities and countries. In the United States, the Department of Health and Human Services under the direction of its Secretary has the responsibility for the maintenance and development of its regulations. The power of the HHS derives mainly from the funding it provides or refuses.

A consideration of the current set of regulations in the Code of Federal Regulations for research projects that involve children who are patients as well as potential research subjects is illustrative of some changes since *The Nuremberg Code*. There are four guidelines in 45 CFR at §46.404, §46.405, §46.406, and §46.407, which require, as the research progresses from decreasing benefit to the child, an increasing degree of regulation. Regulation 46.404 addresses research not involving greater than minimal risk to the child and a direct benefit to the child. Regulation 46.405

addresses research involving greater than minimal risk and a direct benefit to the child. Regulation 46.406 addresses research that is likely to yield generalizable knowledge about the patient's condition or disorder, but does not directly benefit the child. Regulation 46.407 addresses research "not otherwise approvable which presents an opportunity to understand, prevent or alleviate a serious problem affecting the health or welfare of children." Regulations 46.404 and 46.405 are considered therapeutic research because there is direct benefit to the child with, respectively, either minimal risk or a favorable benefit/risk ratio; regulations 46.406 and 46.407 are considered nontherapeutic because, while they offer the possibility of an increase in knowledge or an increase in the understanding of disease, they offer no direct benefit to the child/research subject. To be in compliance with the federal code, all four types of research require review and approval by the institutional review board and all four require the assent of the child and the consent of a parent. Regulations 46.406 and 46.407 require consent by both parents if two parents are available. Regulation 46.407 requires additional approval by the Secretary of the Department of Health and Human Services who is required to consult with a panel of representative experts and who is required, furthermore, to provide the opportunity for public review. In addition, regulation 46.407 requires that the research be in accord with sound ethical principles.

(E) Afterword

Of course, no set of regulations is needed for the reputable responsible scientist and no set of regulations is sufficient for the unscrupulous scientist. Virtue is always more subtle than a list. So too is sin. There is always a need for a sensitive conscience. There is also always a need for a community of conversation if the navigation between the subtleties of virtue and the subtleties of sin is to be safely accomplished.[4] Good research is not achieved alone. Neither is ethical research. Nonetheless, regulations have a pedagogical function to serve as ideal and guide to the uncertain as well as to prescribe and proscribe courses of action. The regulations must function as a covenant between the researcher and the subject such that the protection of the subject remains paramount. The participation of human beings in research that benefits either themselves or others or that advances knowledge or understanding of human development or human illness is a morally permissible good, provided that respect for human dignity and respect for the gift of human life are maintained. Participation in research that benefits oneself is in accord with the natural law precept to preserve human life. Participation in research which benefits others is a sign of membership in the human community and a sign of solidarity with that community. Participation in research which advances knowledge is in itself a contribution to the progression of science. Participation in research is justified but limited by the application of the principle of totality, which allows the use of the part for the good of the whole. The principle requires the distinction between a physical organism and a moral organism with a consequent limitation on activities. The individual person may consent to participate in research which serves to benefit the life of the person even to the degree that the research may require the use of a part – or if the part is diseased the destruction of the part – that is not required for the good of the whole person. The individual person may participate in research which benefits the community, but only to a limited degree, that is, the relationship of the person to the community as part to whole is limited to the use of the activities, not the use of the life, of the person. Respect for human dignity requires careful attendance to the provisions for informed consent. The greater the risks attendant on the research and the more diminished the benefits for the patient subject, the more stringent are the essential requirements for informed consent – knowledge, voluntariness, and freedom. This development of the principle of totality with its distinctions and its applications was articulated by Pope Pius XII in the presence of the atrocities presented by the research programs of Nazi Germany.[5]

Just as there were horrific abuses in the past, there is always the danger that the drive for knowledge and the drive for effective therapies may overstep the ethical boundaries that are in place to guide the advances that are sought. This is how every effective temptation works: it does not propose a simple evil, but proposes one good such as the advance of knowledge at the expense of another good such as the dignity of the research patient. There are several populations that are especially vulnerable, therefore, susceptible to use and hence abuse. Among them are (1) those in underdeveloped countries; (2) those in developed countries who are marginalized by poverty, education, disability, race, gender, or legal status and, who are therefore, powerless[6]; (3) those who have been diagnosed with fatal illnesses; and (4) the dying – both children and adults. Each of those populations – or those who speak for them – are situated so as to call into question the possible application of the necessary elements of informed consent. When parents or a parent speaks on behalf of a child, the focus must be on the best interest of the child. Because a child is incapable of forming a set of guiding ethical principles, there can be no substituted judgment. The introduction of an assent requirement can be used as a kind of ethical sleight of hand offering the appearance of assent while unmindful of the dynamics of the developmental stage of the child who wishes to please or the child patient who wishes to comply. It is to be forgetful of children as children. In some instances, when assent is used without appropriate developmental awareness or without honesty, this becomes an example of effective temptation.

That is, for the good of moving the research or therapy forward, the dignity of the child is sacrificed.

Those in underdeveloped countries can be targets for drug testing that violates the protocols – including understanding the distinctions between different trial phases and being situated so as to be free to exercise consent – operative in developed nations. The situation of those in this group requires careful examination of the operational level of knowledge and the operative degree of freedom. The proposed use of research subjects who reside in or operate within total institutions such as residential homes for the cognitively challenged, prisons, or the military requires as a starting point the assessment of their freedom to consent. The changed existential situation of these potential research subjects requires special concern that coercion, whether that of third parties including family, the health care team, insurers, or even the subtle coercion of a final sacrifice, might present occasions for the sick or dying person to be considered a means only and hence abused.

There is, of course, a limit which cannot be traversed. The following minimal conclusions are (1) under no circumstance may the life of a human being be sacrificed for the good of research; (2) under no circumstance may research be carried out on any human subject without the assent and consent provisions in place; and (3) the greater the risk entailed by the research, the greater the necessity of fulfillment of the requirements of informed consent. The twentieth-century scholar, Hans Jonas, in his reflection on experimentation using human subjects, proposed a rule of the descending order and its counter-utility sense. Jonas's proposed rule requires that the research subject possess the maximization of identity, of understanding, and of freedom in regard to the research project at hand. Application of this rule would require physicians and scientists to be the first recruited and the first to volunteer as subjects. Jonas maintained that the greater the risk the more compelling is the requirement of maximization of identity, understanding, and freedom. He wrote:

> With the fact of self-solicitation the issue of consent in all its insoluble equivocality is bypassed per se. Not even the condition that the particular purpose be truly important and the project reasonably promising, which must hold in any solicitation of others, need be satisfied here. By himself the scientist is free to obey his obsession, to play his hunch, to wager on chance, to follow the lure of ambition.
>
> (Jonas, 1980b, p. 121)

The example of this dedication by scientists and physicians will, according to Jonas, generate a community which will trust the research community when it calls for participation by the wider community to take risks in the advance of medicine to protect the community.

The study of past abuses in the use of human subjects in research is no guarantee that abuses will not be repeated. The research imperative remains very powerful. Within the contemporary horizon, there are several movements that raise some concerns. The first is the movement in the U.S.A. from informed consent to presumed consent for organ removal and use as needed in transplantation therapies. Along with the controversies surrounding declaration of death, presumed consent seems to open the door to more aggressive harvesting of organs. The second is the twofold transition that has taken place in the use of sick children as research subjects. The transition is marked by the lack of informed consent on the part of the child; the other is the expanding target of the research. Children are incapable of giving informed consent so parental *consent* and child *assent* have been put into place. The research need no longer serve the good of the particular child or children similarly situated, but may now simply advance knowledge. The third is the rapid expansion of newborn screening in number of diseases and anomalies detected by screening, in the extension of screening beyond the category of treatable conditions, and in the storage, as well as use, of specimens and data. The fourth is the opportunity for genetic engineering, whether for therapy or enhancement, made possible by newly developing technologies of gene editing whose development ultimately requires research on human life at its earliest stages – the human embryo. The fifth is the ongoing emergency medicine research. This research, in its search for better treatment of trauma victims, employs experimental therapies including blood substitutes administered by emergency medical technicians on trauma victims whose consent cannot be obtained and for whom an explicit exemption from consent has been put in place. This ongoing research is supported by a variety of Canadian and American agencies.

Questions for Reflection

1. Research as a function of the desire and medicine as an aspect of the desire to heal are opportunities for human beings to exercise creative stewardship. Assess the opportunities and limitations of each. How do violations of ethical principles occur in the medical or research setting?
2. The Tuskegee Syphilis Study had both a scientific purpose and a social purpose. Identify these. Assess the study and the longevity of the study. In your assessment, pay careful attention to (a) cultural bias, (b) the availability of penicillin, (c) the provisions of the Nuremberg Code, and (d) the research imperative.
3. If you were responsible for setting up an ethical code for your institution, what would your core principle(s) be? How will you balance informed consent with the vulnerability of patients and the limitations of research subjects?

4 As you go forward with your practice or with a research project, what is your experience as you consider the rules now in place and your ethical commitments?
5. How can benefit to the patient and benefit to society be balanced?
6. What did the Nuremberg Code get right? What are its limitations? Can it be effective?
7. Hans Jonas demands a strict standard, that of maximization of (a) identity, (b) understanding, and (c) freedom, for medical experimentation. Is it reasonable to demand this in the contemporary period?
8. Is the distinction between informed *consent* and *assent* an appropriate distinction or is in impermissible as a violation of informed consent?
9. What are the dangers to the patient/research subject when the researcher is both the doctor caring for a particular patient and the principal investigator in the research project?
10. What are the major current threats to ethical research?

The Nuremberg Code

1. The voluntary consent of the human subject is absolutely essential. This means that the person involved should have legal capacity to give consent; should be so situated as to be able to exercise free power of choice, without the intervention of any element of force, fraud, deceit, duress, overreaching, or other ulterior form of constraint or coercion; and should have sufficient knowledge and comprehension of the elements of the subject matter involved as to enable him to make an understanding and enlightened decision. This latter element requires that before the acceptance of an affirmative decision by the experimental subject there should be made known to him the nature, duration, and purpose of the experiment; the method and means by which it is to be conducted; all inconveniences and hazards reasonably to be expected; and the effects upon his health or person which may possibly come from his participation in the experiments.

   The duty and responsibility for ascertaining the quality of the consent rests upon each individual who initiates, directs, or engages in the experiment. It is a personal duty and responsibility which may not be delegated to another with impunity.
2. The experiment should be such as to yield fruitful results for the good of society, unprocurable by other methods or means of study, and not random and unnecessary in nature.
3. The experiment should be so designed and based on the results of animal experimentation and a knowledge of the natural history of the disease or other problem under study that the anticipated results [will] justify the performance of the experiment.

4. The experiment should be so conducted as to avoid all unnecessary physical and mental suffering and injury.
5. No experiment should be conducted where there is an a priori reason to believe that death or disabling injury will occur; except, perhaps, in those experiments where the experimental physicians also serve as subjects.
6. The degree of risk to be taken should never exceed that determined by the humanitarian importance of the problem to be solved by the experiment.
7. Proper preparations should be made and adequate facilities provided to protect the experimental subject against even remote possibilities of injury, disability, or death.
8. The experiment should be conducted only by scientifically qualified persons. The highest degree of skill and care should be required through all stages of the experiment of those who conduct or engage in the experiment.
9. During the course of the experiment the human subject should be at liberty to bring the experiment to an end if he has reached the physical or mental state where continuation of the experiment seems to him to be impossible.
10. During the course of the experiment the scientist in charge must be prepared to terminate the experiment at any stage, if he has probable cause to believe, in the exercise of good faith, superior skill, and careful judgment required of him that a continuation of the experiment is likely to result in injury, disability, or death to the experimental subject.

Of the ten principles which have been enumerated our judicial concern, of course, is with those requirements which are purely legal in nature – or which at least are so clearly related to matters legal that they assist us in determining criminal culpability and punishment. To go beyond that point would lead us into a field that would be beyond our sphere of competence. However, the point need not be labored. We find from the evidence that in the medical experiments which have been proved, these ten principles were much more frequently honored in their breach than in their observance. Many of the concentration camp inmates who were the victims of these atrocities were citizens of countries other than the German Reich. They were non-German nationals, including Jews and "asocial persons," both prisoners of war and civilians, who had been imprisoned and forced to submit to these tortures and barbarities without so much as a semblance of trial. In every single instance appearing in the record, subjects were used who did not consent to the experiments; indeed, as to some of

> the experiments, it is not even contended by the defendants that the subjects occupied the status of volunteers. In no case was the experimental subject at liberty of his own free choice to withdraw from any experiment. In many cases experiments were performed by unqualified persons; were conducted at random for no adequate scientific reason, and under revolting physical conditions. All of the experiments were conducted with unnecessary suffering and injury, and but very little, if any, precautions, were taken to protect or safeguard the human subjects from the possibilities of injury, disability, or death. In every one of the experiments the subjects experienced extreme pain or torture, and in most of them they suffered permanent injury, mutilation, or death, either as a direct result of the experiments or because of lack of adequate follow-up care.

Obviously all of these experiments involving brutalities, tortures, disabling injury, and death were performed in complete disregard of international conventions, the laws and customs of war, the general principles of criminal law as derived from the criminal laws of all civilized nations, and Control Council Law No. 10. Manifestly human experiments under such conditions are contrary to "the principles of the law of nations as they result from the usages established among civilized peoples, from the laws of humanity, and from the dictates of public conscience."

United States v. Karl Brandt, et al., Trials of War Criminals Before Nuremberg Military Tribunals Under Control Council Law No. 10 (October, 1946–April, 1949).

Notes

1 *Exodus* provides a warning of the ever-shifting dependency/autonomy human condition in: "Do not oppress the alien; you know what it is to be an alien, since you yourselves were exiles in the land of Egypt" (Exodus 23:9). The relative autonomy of the competent adult was preceded by dependency which dependency will most likely be repeated in old age. All of us, physicians included, will be patients.

2 *The Declaration of Helsinki: Ethical Principles for Medical Research involving Human Subjects* was published by the World Medical Association at their 18th congress. The *Declaration* has been amended seven times since its origin. Its most recent revision in 2013 required that all participants in medical trials in every country be afforded the best standard of care.

3 The *Belmont Report* was the work of the National Commission for the Protection of Human Subjects of Biomedical and Behavioral Research.

4 The community of conversation must be marked by freedom of expression. There is a tendency in the contemporary culture to limit conversation to an accepted circle of opinion. This is a kind of tyranny of the majority that Tocqueville warned about in *Democracy in America*.

5 The essential distinctions for the Principle of Totality as developed by Pope Pius XII can be found in Chapter 2, Section D-7. The distinction between a moral union and a physical union controls action.

6 There is rich literature to serve (1) as an appropriate paradigm for the care of the vulnerable and (2) as an inspiration for the relatively autonomous. The work of Stanley Hauerwas in his writing, his lectures, and his life provides a rich and profound source of reflection. *Living gently in a violent world: The prophetic witness of weakness*. Madison: InterVarsity Press, 2008 written with Jean Vanier allows readers to enter that world and be changed. *Critical reflection on Stanley Hauerwas' theology of disability*. Routledge, 2004 by John Swinton examines the 30-year work of Hauerwas on the theological significance of those with developmental disabilities.

4 Abortion

In the Beginning

The writer of the *Psalms* avers that God creates us and knows us from the beginning. Moreover, that beginning is in our mother's womb. The scriptural text of *Psalm* 138 proclaims:

> Author, thou of my inmost being, didst thou not form me in my mother's womb? I praise thee for my wondrous fashioning, for all the wonders of thy creation. Of my soul thou hast full knowledge, and this mortal frame has no mysteries for thee, who didst contrive it in secret, devise its pattern, there in the dark recesses of the earth.
>
> (*Psalm* 138: 13–15)

Herein is to be found the repetition of the foundational claim of this book that human life is lived in a series of relationships. The two relations recalled here are the relationship of every human being to God and the relationship of each human being to the woman who sustained its existence from the beginning. While our beginning may be hidden from the created world, it is not hidden from the Creator who fashions each of us as a unique creation, and who knows each of us as a unique self from the beginning and calls each of us to Him. Furthermore, the beginning cannot be hidden from a pregnant woman.

Throughout much of history, the beginning of human life has been a mystery. This is no longer the case. The growth of technology and science has revealed much of what had long been speculation. The beginning of human life as individual, not as evolutionary, occurs with the union of the egg and sperm. To be more precise, every human life begins its unique existence with the penetration of the egg by the sperm to begin a specific process of cascading molecular events which culminates in the union of the chromosomal material carried in the male and female gametes to become the zygote. If this were not the case, then millions of hours of research energy and millions of dollars spent to replicate this process toward reproduction have been wrongly directed.

DOI: 10.4324/9781003627197-4

Nonetheless, some powerful voices in the contemporary culture cast doubt on the reality of the beginning of individual human life. As a consequence, the practice of the destruction of nascent human life in elective abortion has been given legal protection. The result has been almost 50 years of acrimonious debate. Some of the public debate sets the values of life and liberty as opposed to each other and each side tends to absolutize the centrality of its claim. Some of the public debate centers on the subjective pole of the act, the reasons why and the justification for abortion, and it is this that fuels the emotional debate. This focus has been so powerful that the objective pole of the act, that is, the reality of what is done when an abortion is procured or performed has been largely obscured. As a consequence, the public debate has been seriously skewed. On the other hand, much of the philosophical debate centers, as it should, on the ontological status of the conceived but not yet born human being – the *conceptus* – as a starting point.[1] This appropriate balancing, while still recognizing the fact of problem pregnancy and appropriate care for women in these situations, serves to correct the bias in the contemporary debate. While the focus of this chapter is on what it is that is being destroyed in the abortion procedure, the important subjective component of the issue, the woman and her reasons for seeking an abortion, will be examined in Chapter 8 which deals with special relations, including that of the pregnant woman and the *conceptus*. The examination of the issue of abortion here will be presented in the following order:

(A) Three observations will be offered;
(B) Some historical information will be presented;
(C) The object of the act will be considered;
(D) The specific claims of the contemporary debate will be outlined and responses will be presented; and
(E) An Afterword: a brief reflection on some elements that are critical to the transformation of the culture will bring the chapter to a close.

(A) Three Observations

The first observation is that there is a certain simplicity about the issue of abortion. If abortion takes the life of a human being, then abortion falls under the species of moral problems dealing with killing human beings, a kind of homicide, and the ethical injunctions that apply to other kinds of killing of human beings apply similarly to abortion. If, on the other hand, abortion is an act that destroys a life that is not a human life, then abortion is not the same as other acts of killing human beings and the ethical injunctions regarding abortion are to be attenuated as informed by principles appropriate to that circumstance. So a central issue here concerns the object of abortion, that is, what it is that is destroyed when an abortion is procured. The second observation is that the conclusions that are reached in regard to abortion have implications for other significant issues in medical ethics among them are cloning, the generation and use of stem cells, genetic testing and screening, genetic engineering, and assisted reproduction technologies. The third observation is that choices following these conclusions and the application of their principles in the practical order are determinants of the character of the agent and, hence, affect subsequent judgments and practices that are articulated and acted upon in regard to other life issues.

(B) A Bit of History

Abortion as a means of birth control is as old as the human race. There are other practices, such as stealing, murder, and rape, that are also as old as the human race and society rightly condemns these actions. The longevity of the practice of abortion is no more testimony to its moral acceptability than the fact that the continuous presence of the practices of stealing, murder, and rape would require their acceptance by society.

Despite the fact that throughout much of history there has been little regard for the hidden nascent human life, there are nonetheless some early instances of the condemnation of abortion. The Oath of Hippocrates (c. fifth century B.C.) which called a guild of ancient physicians to practice their art within a set of specific ethical constraints contains the pledge, "I will not give a woman a pessary to cause abortion" (Hippocrates, p. 299). While the meaning and the extent of application of that swearing have been subjected to varying interpretations in the contemporary world, its appearance in antiquity suggests that at least those most closely associated with the practice of Hippocratic medicine, perhaps the Pythagoreans as preformationists, expressed reservations regarding their participation in abortion practices.

On the other side of the issue, some philosophers of the same era including Plato, in pursuit of his ideal *Politeia*, encouraged or permitted abortion for pregnancy out of season and infanticide for unwanted and imperfect children. Plato admonished the citizens of the Republic that it was, "preferable not even to bring to light anything whatever thus conceived, but if they were unable to prevent birth to dispose of it on the understanding that we cannot rear such an offspring" (Plato, 5.461c).[2] Recall that for Plato the more important good is the good of the *polis*. The individual is subsumed under and expected to serve that larger good. In a more limited sense, Aristotle, in the *Politics*, permitted abortion provided that it be done before life begins. Aristotle wrote, "When couples have children in excess, let abortion be procured before life and sense have begun; what may or may not be lawfully done in these cases depends on the question of life and sensation" (Aristotle, 1335b, pp. 20–25). Note Aristotle's careful caveat "*before life and sensation.*"

While the Scriptures of the Old Testament record nothing about abortion in the modern medical sense as an elective medical intervention, they do testify to a profound regard for the human being developing in the womb of the woman. The prophet Jeremiah records God's love for the unborn in these words, "Before I formed you in the womb, I knew you, and before you were born, I consecrated you" (*Jeremiah* 1:15). The Psalmist acknowledges the careful creation and intimate love of God for God's creature in these words, "You formed my inmost being; you knit me in my mother's womb. My very self you knew; my bones were not hidden from you, when I was being made in secret, fashioned as in the depths of the earth" (*Psalm* 139:13–15). In addition, there is in *Exodus* 21:22 a passage that refers to the accidental injury to a pregnant woman and the possible occurrence of miscarriage as a consequence of the injury. In the Hebrew translation, it is said that if the woman is injured, the person who caused the injury suffers a punishment commensurate to the injury, that is, life for life, eye for eye, etc. If the woman is uninjured but the child is lost, a penalty is to be set by the husband of the woman. However, the Greek translation of the same passage prescribes the penalty of life for life for the death of the child if the child is formed (Noonan, 1970, p. 6). In the early Christian tradition, abortion is condemned as early as the *Didache* (c. first century A.D.). The *Didache* or *Teaching of the Twelve Apostles* is an ancient statement of Christian principles. Among its proscriptions are: "You shall not slay a child by abortion. You shall not kill what is generated" (*Didache* 2:2).

For some of the early philosophers and some of the early theologians, the questions of the determination of the humanity of an entity were answered in terms of the kind of soul – the ψυχή (psyche) – that was the source of the observed activities of the entity, that is, the soul was understood as the principle of its life. Ensoulment was not a narrow theological question. It was an account of the internal source for the variety of activities manifested in the life of the entity. The move was from observed activities, the phenomena, to the intrinsic principle, the source, of those activities. Nutritive activities, such as living, growing, and developing, offered evidence of the presence of a vegetative soul. The activity of motion suggested the presence of a sentient soul, which as a higher level soul, subsumed the lower level activities, that is, the nutritive. Rational activities indicated the presence of the rational soul, a soul that has the capacity to think, to understand, to reason, to choose, and to decide. The rational soul, as a higher level soul, subsumed the vegetative and sentient activities. The discussion of ensoulment, although part of the mid-twentieth-century debate on abortion and an interesting philosophical exercise in its own right, has for the most part disappeared. Nonetheless, because soul theory sometimes reenters the debate, it will be examined in Section D-4-h of this chapter.

(C) The Object of the Act of Abortion

In the contemporary world, the abortion debate is embedded in a matrix which is defined by limits which range from the most subjective claims to the barest objective claims. Included in these elements on the subjective side or the justification of abortion is the claim of the right of women to abortion as the necessity of absolute control over reproductive processes in order that women be free to develop their potential. Some social planners have offered abortion as an aid to families in circumstances of social and/or economic distress and others have offered abortion as a humane solution to the problems of deformed, battered, and disabled children. On a global level, abortion has been suggested as a significant contribution to the solution of population problems. In addition, the contemporary culture is rife with a particular kind of liberalism which canonizes autonomy and makes personal choice as decisional liberty the essential criterion for the determination of the rightness of an action. Choice has become the trump card in the culture; human beings are considered autonomous rights-bearing individuals whose obligations are only those freely chosen. To raise the question of what is chosen or to suggest that human beings exist in real relations that define obligations is considered an interference with individual personal liberty.

On the objective side or the "what" side lie the questions of the beginning of human life, the nature of the *conceptus* – the conceived but not yet born human being – and the question of personhood or the value of a human life. Because the objective question must be answered first in order to be able to weigh the adequacy of the subjective determinants, it is appropriate to start there. The empirical sciences, especially embryology, fetology, and developmental psychology are the sources of the empirical facts describing the developmental stages of human life. They serve as the sources of information regarding the ontogenetic beginning and unfolding of an individual human life from its beginning. It is important to attend to the findings of these sciences, if the claim to practice from empirically based evidence is to be honored.

(1) The Science of the "What"

In those sciences which study human development, the occurrence that marks the beginning of the process that is the life and development of an individual human being is fertilization. The process begins when the ovum, containing in its pronucleus the species kind and half of the species number of chromosomes, is penetrated by the sperm, which contains in its pronucleus a similar complement. This penetration marks the binding of the egg and sperm to each other and the fusion of their membranes to form the zygote – a *new organism* with a unique material composition and a particular developmental sequence. As an organism, the zygote, "acts in an interdependent and coordinated manner . . . directed towards . . .[a] higher level of organization" (Condic, 2008, p. 6). With the completion of this fusion, a new level of metabolic activity begins in the single-cell organism. This new level of activity is not limited to the nuclear activity as evidenced by the gravitation of the cytoplasm which establishes a polarity most likely in a direction following the penetration by the sperm. The activity of the new being is directed to its survival and appropriate development. It generates barriers to its being penetrated by additional sperm. With time and further development beyond the single cell stage, it generates barriers directed to preventing its implantation in an inappropriate environment; and when it arrives in a suitable environment, it generates those initial structures to nurture and support its continued existence and growth.

The occurrence of sperm/egg fusion in the resultant zygote marks a locus of simultaneous convergence and divergence. The convergence is the coming together of the genetic donation of both parents and that of their ancestors. Here, the continuity of life is maintained. The divergence is not simply the discontinuity between parent and offspring because of genetic uniqueness but also discontinuity because of inner unity and separateness from others of the *de novo* being. Once the zygote is constituted there is a new developing organism. The coming to be of the zygote is appropriately designated the ontogenetic zero point of development. The ontogenetic zero point of development is to be distinguished from the later emergence of the ontogenetic zero point of behavior.

The ontogenetic zero point of *development* for an individual human being is defined as that point on the continuum of development that marks the beginning of the development of a new individual. Prior to this point, the individual, and also the particular continuum used to delineate its existence, did not exist. From this point forward, the individual exists, develops, and expresses or actualizes the potentialities that are its genetic endowment until some point in time when, because of exogenous or endogenous factors, the individual ceases to exist.

The ontogenetic zero point of *behavior* requires significant neural and muscular development. With the commencement of neuromuscular activity, behavior follows. This beginning of behavior is dependent upon prior structural growth which is genetically determined. The structural growth is such that it may be said to anticipate and determine the subsequent behavioral expression. According to Carmichael's Law of Anticipatory Function, behavior matures in a direction following organ maturation and behavior functions to reinforce and to refine organic capacities. Development is continuous and is organized in a specific and forward direction. While various stages of development are designated by name for reference and for convenience, one stage merges into another with appropriate physical, psychological, and social markers as is the case from infant to toddler to child to adolescent and so on.

The following is a summary of the biological process. Morphological growth and subsequent behavioral development are products of genetic encoding at work in an environment that is normal for the species of organism. Basic self-generating developmental stages succeed one another in a genetically determined manner.[3] The phenotype (apparitional characteristics) of the individual which was identical to the genotype (assemblage of genes) at the completion of zygote formation now emerges as the expression of the particularities of the genetic constitution in the process of a continuously changing environment. From this point forward until death, the genetic code continues to influence and to determine growth and behavior, provided the presence of a suitable environment and the achievement of the proper stage of development. The present reality of the human being from its ontogenetic zero point of development onward, that is, from zygote to preimplantation embryo, to embryo, fetus, neonate, child, adolescent, and adult, is marked by an upper directed dynamism toward an ever fuller realization of being until the onset of decline, senescence, and death. Each lower stage lays down the conditions for the emergence of the next higher stage and each lower stage is the necessary condition for the possibility of the becoming of the next higher stage.

The self-actualization of the human being is not limited to its biological determinations. The life of the individual is a process that presses toward the actualization of psychological and intellectual potentialities that are inherent in the constitution of the individual human being. Abraham Maslow described this process of self-actualization in the following:

> Man is ultimately not moulded or shaped into humanness or taught to be human. The role of the environment is ultimately to permit him or to help him actualize his own potentialities, not its potentialities. The environment does not give him his potentialities, he has them in inchoate or embryonic form, just exactly as he has embryonic arms and legs. And creativeness, spontaneity, selfhood, authenticity, caring for others, being able to love, yearning for truth are embryonic potentialities belonging to his species membership just as much as are his arms and legs and brain and eyes.
>
> (Maslow, p. 8)

Maslow is making at least two important points here. One of these is that what a human being is – as constituted in his nature – determines what a human being may become. The second point is that neither culture nor history nor socialization creates human beings. Environmental factors, including psychological and biological, may inhibit or encourage the actualization of psychological potentialities. For Maslow, what a human being is and what a human being could be exist simultaneously. He says, "Potentialities not only will be or could be; they also are" (Maslow, p. 8). The existential reality of the being at its earliest stages of development is that of a being in whom the perfections, whether bodily or behavioral or psychological, exist as an unachieved state of affairs. The existential reality of the adult human being is that of a being in whom some of these perfections exist in a relatively more or less achieved state of affairs. The possibility of self-actualization requires the continuous existence of a being with the capacity for these perfections and the existence of that human being in its normal environment. Removal from the normal environment or destruction of the normal environment renders impossible the actualization of the capacities of the individual.

(2) *The Metaphysics of the "What"*

Since much of the philosophical discussion about the ontological status of the *conceptus* has centered on the notion of its potentiality, that issue will be addressed next. The rich philosophical notions of potency (potentiality) and act (actuality) were coined by the Greeks to describe the phenomenon of development – both change and stability – in the same entity. This account allowed a more adequate response to the phenomena than that offered by either Parmenides (being only) or Heraclitus (change only). These notions of act and potency, when sufficiently developed, provide distinctions adequate for describing the developing life of a human being. The description of the present reality at any developmental stage in the life of an individual human being must convey the fact neither of nothing nor of a completed being. The *conceptus* exists as a present reality – in act – with potentialities directed toward a particular perfection the goal established by the genotype. The *conceptus* is a human being in act. Within that act resides the active natural potentiality to become a more fully developed human being. Explication of this complex notion of potentiality requires attendance to its differentiations as active/passive, constitution/tendency, natural/specific, and remote/proximate.

In active potency, a being goes from not acting to acting and is also the agent of the action. For example, in the exercise of active potentiality, the human being, by its intrinsic agency, develops or moves, whether remotely or proximately, from being not conscious to being conscious. The sleeping human being can upon waking fully engage in conscious activity. The proximate active potentiality for conscious activity permits this transition. The remote active potentiality for conscious behavior must be present in the genetic encoding within the zygote. The subsequent expression is directed intrinsically by this encoding if there is to be conscious activity in the future. So in the earliest stages of development, the potentiality for conscious activity is active and remote, that is, the organism's ability, its own ability, to exercise its power lies in the future. In passive potency, a human being has the capacity to receive a modification but the agency of the modification is an external agent. For example, a presidential candidate may actually become president by the agency of the voters. The candidate received the office – a passive reception – from a set of extrinsic agents. The key for present purposes is this: the present reality of the *conceptus* in relation to the adult human being is not that of passive potentiality which requires extrinsic agency for actualization. In the act that is the *conceptus*, there resides the active potentiality to become a more fully developed human being.

There are two distinct factors that make up the notion of active potentiality. One is constitution or nature and the other is tendency. Constitution is the underlying manifold which determines the direction of the tendency. It is that which tendency by its dispositive thrust urges to completion. Tendency is the drive to action. The *conceptus* is, by its constitution – its genotype – determined as a human being and is, by tendency – an inner dynamism – determined to become and to become in a fashion prefixed by its constitution rather than not become. Since the tendency of the *conceptus* in regard to fuller human development proceeds in a completely determined manner and since it cannot become something other than what the constitution determines it to be and since it cannot of itself not become, it may be said that the potentiality of the fetus for more fully developed human life is an active potency.

Active potentialities are designated either natural or specific. In the accomplishment of an active specific potency, such as the choice of a particular food to satisfy hunger, the agent has a degree of freedom in the actualization of the potency. The agent may specify the manner in which to actualize the potency. Active natural potencies, such as the formation of the cerebral cortex, are accomplished in a completely determined manner. The agent is not free to choose whether or not to actualize the potency. Tendency determines that the potentiality will be actualized and constitution determines the manner of actualization. In addition, the agent is not free to specify the manner in which to actualize the potency. For the actualization of an active natural potency, assuming its normal environment, nothing is needed on the side of the agent beyond its constitution and the tendency to realize that constitution. Factors external to the agent, such as chemical destruction or surgical removal from its normal environment, may bring about its destruction and hence inhibit the actualization but the agent itself cannot inhibit the actualization.

A further distinction is made between those potentialities which may be designated remote and those which may be designated proximate. This distinction is a function of time and development. The presence of the proximate potentiality allows the possibility of immediate realization. The presence of the remote potentiality allows the possibility of future activity and future realization. However, the remote precedes the proximate and is the necessary condition for the existence of the proximate in terms of both constitution and tendency. The proximate is the further developmental specification of the remote. In regard to specific functions characteristic of more developed stages, there exist in the *conceptus*, the remote potentialities which specify the proximate potentialities which proximate potentialities are necessary for action. For example, in the genetic encoding in the chromosomal material, in a relatively unachieved state of affairs, there is that which is necessary for the becoming of the neocortex which, when more fully expressed and developed, serves as the basis of the proximate potency for the higher thought processes.

In summary, the existential reality of the *conceptus* is that of a human being in act. It expresses that being as a unified whole, unified in itself, and distinguished from others. That it is living is indicated by its growth and its ability to utilize materials from its environment to sustain its existence. Its individuality and uniqueness derive from its genetic constitution. It is human and in it reside not only the biological potentialities but all the potentialities that are distinctive of human existence. A brief, but precise, account is contained in the following: "The complexity of the whole human body is contained in some real way in its first cell" (Granfield, p. 28).

From the facts of biological and psychological development and from the translation of these facts into metaphysical terms, a minimal notion of the life of the human being emerges. A human being is an open, unfinished being who begins its existence with the union of the egg and sperm to form the zygote – the ontogenetic zero point of development – and who becomes what it is by developing its potentialities. The becoming which is described in various stages is a time-conditioned unfolding of the possibilities given at fertilization. The existential reality at each stage of development is different only in degree of actualization. What exists in the more fully developed human being in a relatively achieved state existed in the zygote in a relatively unachieved state. If there is to be intellectual development, there must be prior neural development. If there is to be neural development, there must be prior organic development. Each prior stage is the necessary condition for the emergence of each successive stage, and each prior stage anticipates in its development the specifications of the next higher stage. It is the same human being who begins in existence, who develops, matures, declines, and dies. The adult human being cannot be more than the reality contained in the zygote. The existential reality of the adult is that of a being who is in action the fulfillment of the existential reality of the zygote in whose act the sum of the potentialities of that being reside. The zygote is the living human being at a particular stage of its development. It is what the human being should be at that age. The embryo is the living human being at a particular stage of its development. It is what every human being should be at that age. It is the same individual who develops organically, neurologically, psychically, and intellectually from fetus, to neonate to toddler through maturity to senescence. And if this is so, then abortion destroys a developing human being along with all the possibilities represented in that life.

(D) The Contemporary Debate

If the position developed here is correct, then abortion is an act which takes the life of a living developing human being, and hence it is a kind of homicide, that is, the killing of a human being. This position is not without opposition and the opposing views are powerfully represented in the contemporary culture. Some opponents frame their arguments in terms of compassion – compassion for women, for families, and for children with disabilities. Now there is no denying that these arguments deeply touch the wellsprings of human emotion, but compassion unchecked by reason is a dangerous guide. Others frame their position in terms of women's rights. Some embed their arguments in a contemporary postmodern philosophical position that is marked by an extreme and elite Western individualism that lacks an adequate epistemology that results in an incomplete metaphysics which yields a defective ethics. In the presence of these philosophical controversies, both sides look to the law for a resolution. Others develop their position in terms of a distinction between human persons and human nonpersons and, by placing the *conceptus* in the human nonperson category, its destruction is defended. Still others make autonomy the sole criterion in choice. In 1973 and again in 1992, the Supreme Court stepped in and engineered what it considered a socially appropriate settling of the issue in its finding that abortion is a fundamental right, first as a privacy right (*Roe*, 1973) and then as a liberty interest (*Casey*, 1992), of a pregnant woman. In the early twenty-first century, the Supreme Court overturned the *Roe* and *Casey* rulings (*Dobbs*, 2022) and returned the issue to the states.

Responses to (1) the claims of feminism, (2) the claims that arise from within the philosophical position that canonizes autonomy and individualism, and (3) the Court decisions will be framed. In addition, (4) specific responses will be offered to significant arguments that have been presented in support of the discontinuity of development claims and the resultant distinction of the human person from the human nonperson.

(1) *Feminism*

Feminism had three distinctive moments in the twentieth century. The first moment was marked by the suffragette movement. Women demonstrated their rights as active and determining participants in the polity – first as voters and then as lawmakers. They pressed for these goals and were successful in achieving them. The suffragettes, however, were mindful of the fact that women get pregnant and men do not, so they sought appropriate protections for pregnant women.

The second moment in the feminist movement was born during the Civil Rights Movement of the 1960s. At first, feminists voiced the rightful claim to full participation in the goods of society, that is, to education, to work, and to appropriate compensation. Technological developments emancipated them from some of the physical labor of housework and advances in conception control freed them from the uncertainties of their fertility cycles. Women claimed places in medical schools, in law schools, in business schools, and in universities and, after that, places in the hospital, in the firm, in the corporation, and in the academy. These are laudable goals, each and every one. While women physicians, attorneys, CEOs, and professors are not yet at the top of their professions in proportional numbers, they are also no longer considered novelties.

In the midst of the success of second moment of the feminist movement, however, a division occurred. The two factions that emerged have been designated gender equity feminism and gender equality feminism. Both continued to hold many of the important values of feminism, namely, the rights of women to be full participants in the polity; the rights of women to education; the rights of women, essentially to be persons with a set of interests and talents and, as well, the freedom to act on them. The gender equity feminists acknowledge that there are real differences between men and women. These differences are material differences. They are differences in biology, chemistry, and anatomy, and consequently, there result differences in psychic and emotional characteristics and interests which influence actions as well as judgments. These differences must be acknowledged and respected. Gender equity feminists recognize too that it is still the case that arbitrary barriers have been in place that impede the advancement of women, but that there have been substantial gains in breaking down the artificial barriers.

The gender equality feminists pressed the claim that gender differences are social constructs and they pressed for social reform to acknowledge these oppressive constructs and political reform to dismantle the constructs and to ensure the recognition of gender equality. For equality feminists, the fact that women become pregnant and men do not became a particularly oppressive obstacle to the advancement of women. Pregnancy, they claimed, sidelined women from the rise to the top. So if men are free from the burden of pregnancy, women too must have that freedom. The equality feminists sought to advance the claim of a right to abortion as a fundamental right – a necessary right to ensure that women might have absolute control over their reproductive finality and, hence, absolute control over the trajectory of their lives. Only this freedom, they claim, would allow women a place on the playing field equal to the place of men. These feminists articulated the defense of the absolute right to abortion through appeals to the following constellation of ideas: (a) the right of her control over her body; (b) the necessity of autonomy and choice in the attainment of personal responsibility; (c) the moral right of women to full social equality; (d) the right of women to self-determination; (e) the very American sounding "freedom to choose"; and finally (f) a restriction – no man has a right to enter the discussion.

All of the claims articulated here are framed in the language of absolute claims and violate the claims of ordered liberty that limit our rights in the presence of the rights and claims of others. To the claim of right over one's body, there are two responses appropriate here. The first has to do with the claim of absolute right over one's body; the second acknowledges that there are two bodies involved in every abortion decision. In regard to the latter, the human being developing within the woman has its own body which is genetically distinct from the body of the woman within whom it is developing and upon whom it is dependent to sustain it in its normal environment. The right of the woman to her body is limited by the right of the nascent human being to the integrity of its body. Furthermore, the appropriate human response to human dependence is care, not power to destroy. Hans Jonas, one of the pioneers in modern medical ethics, suggested that the appropriate human response to total dependence is total care, that is, "utter helplessness demands utter protection" (Jonas, 1980b, p. 128). He designated this as an inflexible principle.

In regard to the former, the right over one's body is a limited right as recognized in law, in medicine, and in the Catholic religious tradition that frames these chapters. In the law, the right to control one's body is limited by the interests of the state in exercising its *parens patriae*[4] obligations. Among the most significant of the *parens patriae* obligations are the preservation of life, protection from undue influence, and protection of the integrity of the medical profession. The famous and often quoted words of Mr. Justice Cardoza are frequently rendered in support of an absolute right to one's body. Cardoza wrote in 1891,

> No right is held more sacred or is more carefully guarded, than the common law right, the right of every individual to the possession and control

> of his own person, free of all restraint or interference from others, *unless by clear and unquestionable authority of law*. [emphasis added]

Note carefully, the "authority of law" (*Union Pacific Railway* Company, 1891). Those who claim the authority of Cardoza more often than not disregard the authority of law and the derivative authority of ethics of the medical profession. The range of application of the authority of law may be limited, nonetheless, the authority remains. The law internal to the practice of medicine limits the ministrations of medicine between the prescription to use the art of medicine to heal and the proscription to do no harm. Abortions performed where there is no medical indication violate both the prescription and the proscription.

Within the religious tradition that informs these chapters, there can be as well no claims to absolute autonomy. Human beings are creatures who are radically dependent on God for their existence and the continuation of their existence. The patience of God with His creatures should serve as the paradigm for the patience of creatures, including the patience of pregnant women, with each other. The religious tradition recognizes the body as a gift and temple of the Holy Spirit. The gift is to be used in the service of human life and with reverence for the author of human life.

On the common sense level, the claim of absolute autonomy fails. A simple analysis of experience reveals the fact that human beings are radically dependent on each other. Consider the act of purchasing a box of cereal. There must be a store to have the cereal in stock so the supply chain must be effective. The store must have employees and an employer. Someone had to grow the corn and someone must have manufactured the cornflakes on machines built by someone else. Then there is the car, the fuel, and the roads. Moreover, there is the maintenance of peace locally, nationally, and internationally. The list of interconnectivity and interdependence is endless, all for a box of cereal.

Women's rights, claimed as interests that the government should protect, ought to be grounded in an adequate account of the nature of woman as distinguished from the nature of man. While there are certain equalities of man as human and woman as human that the law ought to protect, there are certain material differences – which have their source in chromosomal differences and in hormonal differences and in subsequent differences in anatomical structure and function – of man as male and woman as female. As a consequence, of these material differences women, as a matter of fact, bear and give birth to children; men do not. Recognition of these real material differences requires discrimination, in the sense of making distinctions (treating different things differently), not in the sense of unjust discrimination (treating different things the same, or the same things differently). The law has the capacity to make such distinctions. The law ought to be able to recognize this material difference and to fashion appropriate protections for women in the exercise of this role. When a woman is pregnant, she retains "her ability to stand in relationship to man, society, and the state as an independent, self-sustaining, equal citizen," (Ginsburg, p. 383) and, in addition, she carries a new human being within her body that has claims on her, on the father, on society, and on the state. In the failure to make appropriate distinctions, the law is susceptible to do foolish or harmful things that diminish respect for the law and interfere with the good that the law seeks to accomplish.

In regard to the claim of absolute autonomy, the postmodern period has indeed witnessed both the expansion of the notion and the expansion of its role in medical ethical decision-making. Some feminists have embraced the absolutization of autonomy. The philosophical notion of autonomy has been torn from its position as an integral part of morality and has become the whole of morality. The philosophical notion of autonomy traces its modern parentage to Kant's search for the axiom of morality. Within Kant's moral theory, it functions to provide the account of the direct experience of the rational creature of the categorical imperative as duty, that is, the absolute command of practical reason. Because the command of duty comes directly from the self as legislating morality, rather than another, it is experienced as self-rule – autonomy – rather than other rule – heteronomy. According to Kant, it is the will as practical reason issuing commands, not as bare commands but as imperatives, that are capable of universalization and that are compatible with membership in the possible Kingdom of Ends.[5] Kant says in his account of the will of every rational creature as a will giving universal law, "[t]hus the principle of every will as a will giving universal laws in all its maxims is very well adapted to being a categorical imperative, *provided it is otherwise correct*" [emphasis added] (Kant, p. 206). In the expansion of this notion, Kant says,

> [t]he concept of each rational being as a being must regard itself as giving universal law through the maxims of its will, so that it may judge itself and its actions from this standpoint leads to a very fruitful concept, namely that of a *realm of ends* . . . a systematic union of different rational beings through common laws.
>
> (Kant, p. 207)

Thus, for Kant, autonomy is not the right to do as one pleases, but rather the obligation to do what one ought. And one ought to do those things which are capable of being universalized and those things which treat others as ends and never as means only. The nascent human being as a possible member of a possible kingdom of ends exercises a limiting function over the autonomous claims of the mother.

The final claim, which demands the removal of all men from the abortion decision, at least in the case of pregnancy resulting from consensual acts of men and women, violates the rights of men as full participants in the community and as full participants in the lives of children. This is an erroneous claim and is counterproductive in a feminism that avers and desires equal rights and equal responsibilities. Rather than dismissing the role of men in the procreation and education of children, it would be better to ask men to step up to the plate and take on the obligations and responsibilities that come with these sets of relationships – their relationships with the mothers of their children and their relationships to their children.

(2) *Postmodern Philosophy*

The present moment in the history of philosophy and of the culture, at least in the English-speaking Western world, has been described as post-religious (particularly as post-Judeo-Christian), post-scientific, and post-humanist. This position exercises significant influence on morality, medicine, public policy, and law as well as the intersection of these disciplines. The central notions in this postmodern philosophy are (a) a content-full secular morality cannot be discovered; (b) we are moral strangers; (c) peaceful negotiation is the only possible way to secure a general moral framework; and (d) only human beings who are autonomous, that is, fully developed, rational, and self-conscious are persons, that is, (i) personhood is a matter of accomplishment; (ii) only persons are bearers of rights in the strict sense; and (iii) as a consequence, human nonpersons are vulnerable.

In brief, the responses to (a), (b), and (c) of this postmodern position are: while a content-full secular morality cannot be discovered, reason is not paralyzed. Reason discovers some things and reason constructs others. What reason discovers allows for the affirmation of an understanding that is supported by the preponderance of evidence. Reason is appropriately constrained in its constructing by that which reason discovers. There are specific markers in the human community that can be discovered by reason that place limits on and give direction to moral theory. Two critical markers are (1) human beings, although retaining their individuality, live as related beings and from these relationships concrete duties arise and roles are defined and (2) human beings begin their lives in radical dependency; live much of their lives in varying degrees of dependency; achieve autonomy, if at all, relatively late in life and for a limited time; and return to endure dependence in their decline. Hence, human beings are neither absolute moral strangers nor absolutely autonomous individuals. Inasmuch as human beings live in concrete relationships with each other, concrete duties arise that ought not be subject to negotiation. Human relations vary, but the individuals who make up these relationships do not exhaust their reality in these relationships. Some of the more obvious relationships are those of husband and wife, mother and *conceptus*, parent(s) and children, family and community, citizen and nation, physician and patient, professor and student, and attorney and client. It is existence as related that is the source of our traditions of community and hospitality, of mutual respect, and of liberty as ordered. These relationships constitute the links in the web of sociality. This understanding of human life as woven in relationships gives direction, even substance, to obligations and to the negotiations in and for a peaceable community.

Pregnancy provides an example of human lives embedded in a relationship. It is a temporary relationship between two whole human beings – one immature and the other more mature. This temporary physical union is also a moral union. Neither of the human beings who constitute the relationship is determined to accomplish the totality of existence within this relationship. The woman is a relatively autonomous being. Her life is characterized by a set of ends that extend beyond pregnancy. For the duration of the pregnancy, the *conceptus* is a radically dependent being. While the growth and development of the *conceptus* is intrinsically directed, its continued existence is possible only within the nurturing environment of the body of the woman. The accomplishment of the ends of the *conceptus* which lie outside the pregnancy requires the cooperation of the woman to allow it to endure through the pregnancy. The care that a woman exercises toward this temporally radically dependent being might serve as the paradigm of care for building a peaceful society – a society marked by a people who know they are loved by a providential God and who are called to love and out of that love care for each other in their dependencies. This particular relationship is more fully developed in Chapter 8.

(3) The Law

The 1973 Supreme Court decisions, *Roe v. Wade* and *Doe v. Bolton*, locate the pivotal point for discussion of abortion as law in the contemporary era. This account of the decisions and the legal context will present (a) a sketch of the legal landscape leading up to the decisions, (b) a summary of the essential points of the decisions and their sequelae including *Casey*, and (c) an account of the changed legal landscape with the 2022 *Dobbs* decision.

(a) Legal Landscape

While the rise of feminism and the power of the regnant philosophy contributed to the framing of the 1973 abortion decisions, developments in prior law prepared the path. Among the significant developments were (i) an alteration in law in the understanding of the nature and permissibility of abortion; (ii) the articulation of a zone of privacy which included reproductive autonomy; and (iii) the separation of the legal order from the natural order.

With respect to (a-i): Prior to 1973, the laws of all 50 states of the United States, in recognition of the scientific facts of human development, proscribed abortion in varying degrees.[6] The early modern history of abortion legislation in the United States begins in the middle of the nineteenth century at about the time of the American Civil War. The reasons were multiple. Some reasons were simply professional guild promotion and protection. Notwithstanding these personal professional interests, the law sought the protection of women from the risks attendant upon a surgical procedure without the advances of antibiotics and without the skills and technology of contemporary medicine. The law included also the recognition, at least by the contemporaneous medical profession, that when a woman is pregnant, she is with child. These state laws were included in the legal statutes dealing with crimes against persons. Abortion was forbidden in the law with the exception of a threat to the life, and sometimes the health of the woman. The life of the woman exception was universally present in the laws of all the States. There were no provisions for the prosecution of the woman in the laws. The abortion provider, however, could be prosecuted.

A century later, the change in culture initiated a change in the law. In 1962, the American Law Institute proposed a model law draft which would continue to incriminate abortion as a felony of the second or third degree except in those instances when abortion was considered justifiable (Model Penal Code §230.3 Proposed Official Draft, 1962). Justifiable abortions were determined to be those which were deemed, by a licensed physician, to be medically necessary because (a) the continuation of the pregnancy would endanger the life of the woman or (b) the continuation of the pregnancy would seriously and permanently injure her health or (c) the possibility that the child would be born with a grave, permanent, and irremediable mental or physical defect or (d) the pregnancy resulted from rape or incest or statutory rape. Throughout the next decade, several states modified their laws on abortion in accordance with the Model Law.

New York State provides a case in point. Until 1968, the law of New York State proscribed abortion and considered it a kind of homicide except when the life of the mother was at risk. Pressure to align New York Law with the Model Law of the American Law Institute resulted in the legislature's changing the law. The new law expanded the justifiable reasons for abortion to include the health of the mother, serious fetal defect, and the permissibility of abortion if the pregnancy resulted from rape or incest. It held, however, that abortion after the 26th week of pregnancy would remain a crime. In the face of an uproar over this new law and the immediate experience in New York of the failure to restrict abortion to the specified serious reasons claimed by supporters of the new law, the legislature was forced to change the law in the very next session and revert to the previous law. The Governor, Nelson A. Rockefeller, thwarted the action of the legislature by vetoing the reversion to the previous law.

By the early 1970s, more than a dozen states had adopted the American Law Institute's Model Law provisions into their statutes. But, many states resisted changing their laws and in this resistance reaffirmed, by way of referenda or legislative action, the prohibition of abortion except to save the life of the mother. This resistance to abortion, without a sufficient and proportionate reason, was effectuated by educational programs developed by physicians, attorneys, university professors, nurses, and ordinary citizens that had sprung up across the nation. An essential part of this educational program was the observation of the results in the states that had adopted the Model Law of the American Law Institute. The vast majority of abortions procured in the wake of the new law were performed for nonmedically indicated reasons. The remaining states continued the prohibition of abortion unless the life of the woman was at risk.

With respect to (a-ii) Zone of Privacy: An expansion of the notion of a protected zone of privacy was affirmed in a series of Court decisions which would in time affect the choice of abortion. Among the Court decisions which fashioned an evolving zone of privacy were *Griswold v. Connecticut* and *Eisenstadt v. Baird*. In *Griswold v. Connecticut* (381U.S. 479 1965), the Court fashioned a zone of personal privacy and reproductive autonomy for married couples that protected their use of contraceptives from interference from the state. *Eisenstadt v. Baird* (405 U.S. 438 1972) extended *Griswold* by overturning state statutes which prohibited the sale of contraceptives to the unmarried. What had heretofore been considered behavior appropriate to marriage, that is, sexual intercourse as a right of the marriage bond wherein the goods of marriage might be accomplished and protected, now appeared to be permissible to the unmarried with the assistance of state approval of prescription contraceptives. There are two significant points to be noted in these rulings. The first to note is that the purpose of the use of contraceptives and the permission granted by the legal rulings were intended to prevent conception not to destroy what was already conceived. This difference, while later lost sight of, is significant. The second is the failure of the Court in *Baird*, operating within the context of the sexual revolution of the sixties, to attend to the real difference between the appropriate activities of the natural state of the married and those who are single. *Baird* attempted to provide protection for single women to be free of one of the possible complications of sexual intercourse, namely offspring, and at the same time set them and their sexual partners free from the benefits of the marriage union. This expansion of the zone of privacy and articulation of reproductive autonomy prepared the ground for elective abortion.

With respect to (a-iii) Separation of the Legal Order from the Natural Order: In the separation of the notion of person from that of human being, there can be seen the explicit separation of positive law from the natural order. It is important to note, however, that not all law is grounded in nature. Some law is convention and is the creation of reason to facilitate the effective operation of society. Nonetheless, some law has a foundation in human nature and failure to attend to that nature causes error in the law. From the earliest moments in the contemporary abortion controversy, a clash of jurisprudence was evident in this distinction of person and human being. In 1971, Robert Byrn, a law professor at Fordham University, was appointed guardian *ad litem* for the unborn in the womb in order to protect their right to life in the face of impending abortion. Judge Robert Brietel granted that the unborn in the womb are human and unquestionably alive but they are not persons. "It is not true," Brietel said, "that the legal order corresponds to the natural order" (*Byrn v. New York City Health and Hospitals Corp.*, 31 N.Y. 2d 194, 286 N.E. 2d 889 (1972)); appeal dismissed, 410 U.S. 940 (1973). Judge Adrian Burke argued the opposing position. Judge Burke averred that inalienable liberties precede the state and arise from a source superior to the state. Burke continued maintaining that the state cannot deny these by classifying a "group of living human beings as fit subjects for annihilation" (*Byrn v. New York City Health and Hospitals Corp.*, 1973, at 893). This latter position, articulated by Judge Burke, affirms that the rights granted constitutional protection are rooted in and premised on our humanity; that is rights flow from human nature. The former, Brietel's position, roots constitutional protection in the government as the granter of legal status. Brietel's position would prevail that day and would signal a transition and the immediate future direction of the abortion jurisprudence.

(b) A Changed Legal Landscape

The legal landscape changed in 1973 when women in the United States were accorded as a fundamental right the right to abortion in a set of decisions, *Roe v. Wade* and *Doe v. Bolton,* which were issued from the United States Supreme Court. The Court, in this set of 7–2 decisions, not only overturned the laws of Texas and Georgia but also overturned the laws regulating abortion in all 50 states. The holdings of the Supreme Court decisions, *Roe v. Wade* and *Doe v. Bolton* fashioned a regime of abortion on demand by proclaiming abortion as a woman's fundamental right and by denying the *conceptus* the protection of the law rendered to persons.[7] These decisions skewed the relationship between mother and her developing child. Subsequent decisions and related decisions altered the relationship between wife and husband and between parent and minor child when the decision to abort was at hand.

The focus of *Roe* was the Texas law, which originated in the 1854 statute (1854, C. 49 §1). In this 1854 statute, whose passage was urged by the newly formed Medical Association, the Texas legislature accorded legal recognition of the status of the developing unborn human being and had afforded it the protection of the law. The law permitted abortion only when the life of the mother was at risk. The Georgia law, which was the focus of *Doe*, followed the American Law Institute Model Law provisions. Neither law was held acceptable in the contemporaneous judicial culture. Two points are of particular interest here. The first is that the litigant in *Roe v. Wade* later revealed that she had falsified the claim that her pregnancy, the issue central to the litigation, had resulted from rape. The second is that the litigants in *Doe v. Bolton* were a married couple, who not wanting children, desired access to abortion as a possible backup for failed contraception.

Justice Blackmun, in both decisions, affirmed and amplified the position of Brietel in the New York case by rendering the conceived unborn as the object of a theory of life, a merely potential human life, and, hence, a non-person. Having negated the reality of the conceived unborn, except in as much as its existence has to be acknowledged for the performance of surgery or the application of abortifacient pharmaceuticals, Justice Blackmun proclaimed a right and a liberty for the carrier of the conceived unborn to abortion and turned the attention of the state solely to her protection. Legal theory was set adrift from its moorings in human nature. The state once conceived as the protector of rights held by human beings prior to government, became the determiner of personhood which now made possible the exclusion of a class of human beings and rendered them susceptible to being killed.

The opinion of the Court was claimed to be derived from the Constitution and from previous Court decisions. In summary, the critical holdings of the Court are (1) the right of privacy, whether it be found in the Fourteenth Amendment's concept of personal liberty and restrictions upon state action or . . . in the Ninth Amendment's reservation of rights to the people is broad enough to encompass a woman's decision whether or not to terminate her pregnancy. (*Roe v. Wade,* 410 U.S. 113, 1973 at 726–32) (2) this "right to privacy" is a fundamental right and regulation to limit it can be justified only by a "compelling state interest" (Roe at 728); (3) "the word 'person' as used in the Fourteenth Amendment, does not include the unborn" (Roe at 729); (4) that while it has been argued that "life begins at conception and that the State has a compelling interest in protecting life from conception," (Roe at 730) the Court "need not resolve the difficult question of when life begins" (Roe at 730); (5) the State does have an important and legitimate interest in preserving and protecting the health of the pregnant woman . . . the State may regulate the abortion procedure to the extent that the regulation reasonably relates to the preservation and protection of maternal health. (Roe at 731) and (6) the health of the mother – which is to be protected even at the cost of the life of the child – was defined to include "all factors – physical, emotional, psychological, familial, and the women's age – relevant to the well-being of the patient" (*Doe v. Bolton* 410 U.S. 179, 1973 at 747). This Court chose to remain silent with respect to the rights of fathers or to the rights of parents of pregnant minor daughters (Id. at 733). The constitutional guarantees that the Court claimed are the right of a woman to abortion as rooted in the concept of personal liberty provided in the due process clause of the Fourteenth Amendment and in the reservation of rights to the people provided by Ninth Amendment protection. The Court found the right of a woman to abortion as a privacy claim – personal, marital, familial, and sexual – protected in the Bill of Rights or in its penumbras and in cases previously decided by the Court. Here, the Court looked to *Griswold v. Connecticut* and *Eisenstadt v. Baird* whose subjects were, respectively, the legal permissibility for the purchase of contraceptives for the married and then that same permissibility for all those desiring sexual intercourse free of the consequence of pregnancy and the encumbrances of marriage.

As if to accord some recognition and protection to the new life developing within the body of the women, the Court fashioned a trimester structure within which it claimed to offer increasing protection for the conceived yet unborn. The trimester structure is as follows:

First trimester: "The abortion decision and its effectuation must be left to the medical judgment of the pregnant woman's attending physician."

Second trimester: "The State, in promoting its interest in the health of the mother may . . . regulate the abortion procedure in ways that are reasonably related to maternal health."

Third trimester: "The State in promoting its interest in the potentiality of human life, may . . . regulate, and even proscribe, abortion except where it is necessary, in appropriate medical judgment, for the preservation of the life or health of the mother."

(*Roe v. Wade* 410 U.S. 113, 1973, pp. 163–165)

Of course inasmuch as the *conceptus* was declared a nonperson in these legal decisions, it has no standing in the law and since the health of the mother is broadly defined as her physical, mental, social, economic, and familial well-being, there is little the State can do to protect the life of the *conceptus*.

Subsequent to *Roe v. Wade* and *Doe v. Bolton* decisions of 1973, all challenges from the states and from Congress to the abortion decisions failed to reverse the Court's claim of the fundamental right of a woman to abortion. Each Court decision affirmed the right to abortion as constitutionally grounded, affirmed its reach, and permitted the crafting of only some minor limitations. Court decisions would determine that the father has no rights in the abortion decision and that the rights of parents of a minor pregnant daughter are limited to notification of one with the consent of the minor daughter. In regard to the former, *Planned Parenthood of Central Missouri v. Danforth* (428 U.S. 52, 1976) ruled that a woman may obtain an abortion without her husband's consent or even without his knowledge. This was reaffirmed in the *Planned Parenthood of Southeastern Pennsylvania v. Casey* (505 U.S. 833, 1992) decision which offered the following: "It cannot be claimed that the father's interest in the fetus's welfare is equal to the mother's protected liberty."

The findings in *Planned Parenthood v. Casey* (1992) provide a convenient summary of subsequent Court findings. The findings reveal the strength of the original holding and as well some modest modifications. The Court affirmed a woman's right to abortion as a liberty right as well as a privacy right. The Court rejected the trimester structure of *Roe* in favor of a viability standard. The modifications permitted by the Court were limited by (1) the caveat of an "undue burden" analysis for the woman and (2) the possibility of medical emergency. The Court permitted the provision of information about the developing *conceptus* so that the woman might exercise a measure of informed consent to guide her decision. The Court upheld a 24-hour waiting period before she might act on her decision. This same decision addressed the issue of parental involvement in the decision of a minor daughter in regard to an abortion. The Court permitted the consent of one parent provided that the consultation with the parent does not constitute an undue burden for the daughter. A judicial bypass was put into place if the minor daughter cannot obtain or does not want her parent's consent. The relationship of the pregnant woman or pregnant girl to the state now supersedes, respectively, her relationship to the father of her child, even if he is her husband, or her parents. The Court repeated the rejection of any role for the putative spouse in the decision or action. The putative father need not even be informed. The Court permitted the gathering and reporting of data by the abortion provider to the state regulatory agencies. In its understanding of liberty, the Court crafted the following: "At the heart of liberty is the right to define one's own concept of existence, of meaning, of the universe, and of the mystery of human life" (505 U.S. 833, 1992). This capacious understanding of liberty appears boundless.[8]

In the almost 50-year presence of *Roe, Doe,* and *Casey,* three persistent questions continued to be raised about the legalization of abortion. They are (1) Were the 1973 decisions of the Court in the abortion cases and subsequent decisions derived from those cases rightly decided? (2) Did the Court decision and the subsequent derivative decisions settle the issue? and (3) What lies in the future as the debate goes forward in the States? To the question of whether these cases were rightly decided, there are several issues of concern. For the approximately one million women who undergo the procedure each year, the response might be *yes*. The legalization of abortion provided them, for the most part, with a technically safe procedure. The procedure is not, however, safe for the *conceptus*. This last highlights an egregious error on the part of the Court and that error imputes the rightness of the judgment of the Court. That error is the unwillingness of the Court to attend the reality of the *conceptus*. The Court claimed ignorance about the beginning of human life and, out of that learned ignorance, decreed that the *conceptus* is not a person and can thus be destroyed. The notion of person as a juristic construct determines whether an entity is a bearer of rights and of what rights. In the U.S.A., the history of the application of the term person to human beings has been expansive. At the founding of the nation, only male white property owners were persons, that is, had standing in the law. Over time, other classes of human beings – African American males, the indigenous Native Americans, and women – have been included within the ambit of this juristic concept and have been accorded standing in the law. Furthermore, a distinctive feature of rights in the juristic sense is that while individual human beings (and other entities whose activities mimic human action) are bearers of rights, the law protects the exercise of rights at various stages. Before the law, rights are a function of the capacities of human beings. For example, the right to consummate a contract receives legal approbation when a human being has the present capacity to exercise that right. The right to marry and establish a family is accorded legal protection when a human being has the present capacity to exercise that right. Since a human being begins its existence as an organism with the sperm/egg fusion and the resultant zygote, its right to life should be accorded legal protection at that time.

Other holdings of the Court are similarly problematic. In the words of the *Roe* decision, the Court decrees that "the abortion decision and its effectuation must be left to the medical judgment of the pregnant woman's attending physician." On its face, this would seem to require that there are some medical indications for abortion and that the physician is the appropriate judge of the medical necessity of this procedure. Data collected from abortion providers reveal that most abortions are elective and motivated by social reasons rather than medical reasons. This renders the role of the physician as merely the most qualified technician to perform a procedure to serve the wishes of the woman. This last raises an important question in regard to the goals and limits of medicine.[9] Finally, the *Roe v. Wade* and *Doe v. Bolton* decisions not only cut short the debate that was going on in the states but also rendered unenforceable the abortion laws of all 50 states.

To the question of whether the decisions settled the issue for the nation, the answer is *no* by all parties to the debate. Many state legislatures regularly attempt to limit the reach of these federal court decisions even as they are hindered by the notion that abortion is a woman's fundamental right guaranteed in the constitutional provisions of privacy and liberty. The position of abortion has become a litmus test for the appointment of judges and as well every seeker of political office who is required to articulate a position on the issue. Finally, the annual Washington protests by thousands on both sides of the issue and the numerous articles in scholarly and popular journals offer concrete evidence that the issue is not settled.

(c) The Current Legal Landscape

In 2022, the legal landscape changed once again with the *Dobbs v. Jackson Women's Health Organization* decision (hereinafter *Dobbs*) of the United States Supreme Court. The Court held (6–3) that the Gestational Age Act of Mississippi is constitutional. The Mississippi Act prohibited abortion after the 15th week of pregnancy except in two instances, namely, (a) threat to the life or health of the mother and (2) severe fetal deformity. In addition, a majority of the Court (5–4) ruled that *Roe v. Wade* and the *Casey* Court decision subsequent to *Roe* have no basis in the Constitution. In the presence of the apparent conflict between *Roe* and *Casey* and *Dobbs*, the majority reasoned that affirming *Dobbs* required negating *Roe* and *Casey*. Justice Alito who wrote the Majority decision reported that the Solicitor General, in his role as respondent for the federal government, and other respondents in their opposition to *Dobbs* claimed that the Court cannot affirm the Mississippi law without the reversal of *Roe* and *Casey*. Alito wrote:

> [R]espondents and the Solicitor General ask us to reaffirm *Roe* and *Casey*, and they contend that the Mississippi law cannot stand if we do so. Allowing Mississippi to prohibit abortions after 15 weeks of pregnancy, they argue, "would be no different than overruling *Roe* and *Casey* entirely" (Brief for Respondents 43). They contend that "no half-measures" are available and that we must either reaffirm or overrule *Roe* and *Casey*. Brief for Respondents 50.
>
> (*Dobbs v. Jackson Women's Health Organization*, No. 19–1392, 597 U.S. ___ (2022), "Opinion of the Court," pp. 4–5)

The Majority (5–4) agreed with the Solicitor General and the respondents and held that *Roe* and *Casey* be overruled in the following:

> We hold that *Roe* and *Casey* must be overruled. The Constitution makes no reference to abortion, and no such right is implicitly protected by any constitutional provision, including the one on which the defenders of *Roe* and *Casey* now chiefly rely – the Due Process Clause of the Fourteenth Amendment. That provision has been held to guarantee some rights that are not mentioned in the Constitution, but any such right must be "deeply rooted in this Nation's history and tradition" and "implicit in the concept of ordered liberty."
>
> *Washington* v. *Glucksberg*, 521 U. S. 702, 721 (1997, p. 5)

In a separate concurring opinion, which affirmed the validity of the Mississippi Law, Chief Justice Roberts claimed that the judgment in favor of Mississippi's law did not "require the Court to overturn *Roe v. Wade*" (*Dobbs*, 1997, Roberts, C.J., Concurring in Judgment). The Chief Justice, while he agreed that there are issues with *Roe* and *Casey*, accused his colleagues of a failure of judicial restraint inasmuch as they should have limited their decision to the case at hand. The Chief Justice maintained that the right at issue is the right of a woman to terminate her pregnancy. He suggested the following: "That right should therefore extend far enough to ensure a reasonable opportunity, but need not extend any further – certainly not all the way to viability" (Roberts, C.J., Concurring in Judgment).

The major holdings in *Dobbs* are (1) there is no right to abortion either explicitly in the Constitution or implicitly protected by any Constitutional provision including the due process clause of the 14th Amendment[10]; (2) the due process clause protects only those unarticulated rights deeply rooted in the Nation's history and traditions and implicit in the concept of ordered liberty; and (3) there is no right to obtain an abortion as part of a broader entrenched right that is supported by other precedents as an application of the doctrine of *stare decisis*.[11] An examination of the Nation's history and traditions reveals that for 185 years from the adoption of the Constitution (1788) until *Roe* and *Doe* (1973) both in statutory provisions and common law, abortion was prohibited by laws, particular to the individual states, except under compelling medical indications. The most compelling circumstance is the life of the mother which was protected in all 50 states prior to *Roe*.[12] While other non-enumerated rights such as the right to contraception for the married (*Griswold*, 1965) and the unmarried (*Eisenstadt*, 1972), the right to intimate sexual relations (*Lawrence*, 2003), and the right to same-sex marriage (*Obergefell*, 2015) have been recognized by previous decisions of the Court, these rights are significantly different from the right to abortion. The claimed right to abortion disregards the object of abortion, that is, what is destroyed in the procedure. *Dobbs* indicates this difference in several places throughout the ruling. Two significant iterations are found in the following:

> The abortion right is also critically different from any other right that this Court has held to fall within the Fourteenth Amendment's protection of "liberty." *Roe*'s defenders characterize the abortion right as similar to the rights recognized in past decisions involving matters such as intimate sexual relations, contraception, and marriage, but abortion is fundamentally different, as both *Roe* and *Casey* acknowledged, because it destroys what those decisions called "fetal life" and what the law now before us describes as an "unborn human being" (*Dobbs*, 2022, p. 5).
>
> "[A]bortion is a unique act" because it terminates "life or potential life."505 U.S., at 852: see also *Roe*, 410 U. S., at 159 (abortion is "inherently different from Marital intimacy," "marriage," or "procreation"). And to ensure that our decision is not misunderstood or mischaracterized, we emphasize that our decision concerns the constitutional right to abortion and no other right. Nothing in this opinion should be understood to cast doubt on precedents that do not concern abortion.
>
> (*Dobbs*, 2022, p. 66.)

The concept of ordered liberty would require acknowledging and balancing the interests of what *Roe* and *Casey* call "potential life" and "fetal life" (*Roe v. Wade,* 410 U.S. 113, 163 (1973) and what the Mississippi law describes as an "unborn human being" (Miss. Code Ann §41–41–191(4)(b) (2018)) as well as the interests of the woman. Both count. The Breyer, Sotomayor, and Kagan dissent to *Dobbs* focuses singularly on the interests of the woman as her privacy, her liberty, her autonomy, her full equality, and her body. These rights are claimed more than 70 times in a document of only 60 pages. The *Dissent* while making occasional reference to fetal life or potential life is silent on the interests of the conceived unborn human being even as it remains the possible object of a medical intervention. The only exception can be found in footnote 7 with the suggestion that the proposition that a fetus might be a constitutionally protected person is a revolutionary proposition.[13]

Finally, the *Dobbs* decision of the Court dismissed the *Stare decisis* claims of the minority to secure a fundamental right to abortion. The minority maintained that the Court should stand by its previous decisions in *Roe* and *Casey* and dismiss the challenge presented by the Mississippi Act. The majority presented evidence of the Court's overturning of previous decisions of the Court in a long list of cases including *Plessy*, *Lochner*, and *Barnette*. A decision of the Court is not settled until it is rightfully settled. Claiming that a wrongfully decided case cannot serve as a precedent, that is, *Roe* cannot serve as a precedent for *Casey* and *Casey* cannot serve as a precedent upon precedent in support of *Dobbs*, Justice Alito wrote in *Dobbs:*

> *Roe* was egregiously wrong from the start. Its reasoning was exceptionally weak, and the decision has had damaging consequences. And far from bringing about a national settlement of the abortion issue, *Roe* and *Casey* have enflamed debate and deepened division.
>
> (*Dobbs*, 2022, p. 6.)

Having found no explicit or implicit right in the Constitution to abortion, no right to abortion in the Nation's history and traditions, no right to abortion implicit in the concept of ordered liberty which would invoke the protection of the due process clause of the 14th Amendment, and no worthy precedent to require *stare decisis* privilege, the *Dobbs* majority, recognizing the profound moral issue of abortion, returns the issue of abortion to the citizens and their elected representatives.

As the *Dobbs* decision moved toward its conclusion, the Court considered the standards to govern state abortion regulations (*Dobbs*, 2022, pp. 77–78). The standard of review is to be a rational basis review, that is, "the States may regulate abortion for legitimate reasons and when such regulations are challenged under the Constitution, courts cannot 'substitute their social and economic beliefs' for the judgment of legislative bodies" (*Dobbs*, 2022, p. 77). Further a law "regulating abortion, like other health and welfare laws, is entitled to a 'strong presumption of validity'" (*Dobbs*, 2022). Included in legitimate state interests are the following: (1) protection of maternal health and safety; (2) respect for and preservation of prenatal life at all stages of development; (3) the elimination of particularly gruesome or barbaric medical procedures; (4) the preservation of the integrity of the medical profession; (5) the mitigation of fetal pain; and (6) the prevention of discrimination on the basis of race, sex, or disability (*Dobbs*, 2022, p. 78).

In his conclusion, Justice Alito wrote:

> We end this opinion where we began. Abortion presents a profound moral question. The Constitution does not prohibit the citizens of each State from regulating or prohibiting abortion. *Roe* and *Casey* arrogated that authority. We now overrule those decisions and return that authority to the people and their elected representatives.
>
> (*Dobbs*, 2022, p. 79)

(4) *Discontinuity Arguments: The Status of the* Conceptus *and Responses*

In the early days of the abortion debate, a series of arguments was presented to challenge the claim that human life is continuous from the union of the gametes. While these arguments have been displaced by the solitary emphasis on the rights of the woman – her right to privacy, her liberty, and her right to be free of the burdens of pregnancy and a child – it is instructive to examine them.[14] These arguments, for the most part, are directed to the ontological status of the *conceptus* and they maintain that the *conceptus* is not fully human. The arguments are usually framed in terms of discontinuity between human biological life and human personal life with the subsequent distinction of the human nonperson and the human person. Some limit the discontinuity claim to the early *conceptus,* that is, prior to 14 days; others are more expansive in choosing the emergence of a particular feature as the basis for protection in the law. Those who attempt such a separation frame a variety of arguments. Among the most frequently recurring arguments are (a) brain death criteria; (b) the ordinary use of referential language; (c) the consideration of potentiality (the notion of potentiality was developed more fully in Section C-2 of this chapter) in the transition from being an animal to being a human; (d) the distinction between abstract potentialities and concrete potentialities; (e) the related issue of vulnerability and probability; (f) unity of organization; (g) the related issues of totipotentiality and twinning; and, finally (h) ensoulment. These arguments, varying in degrees of credibility, will each be addressed.

(a) In regard to the current use of brain death criteria, it is important to note that in the medical notion of brain death, and in the ensuing disjunction between personal life and biological life, the potentiality for the activities of the higher level nervous system no longer exists in the human being who is designated dead by such criteria. In the *conceptus*, on the other hand, there exists from the beginning, in its very act, the remote potentiality for the activities of the higher central nervous system. The remote potentiality is the source and the necessary condition for the emergence of the proximate potentiality, which is the source of the here-and-now higher brain activities.

(b) It is often noted that in the ordinary use of language, the *conceptus* is referred to as "it" and because of this use, the social status and the ontological status of the *conceptus* are diminished. The denotation of the *conceptus* as "it," rather than as "she" or "he," is a defect on the part of the observer rather than a defect on the part of the *conceptus*. The ordinary observer may not know the sex of the *conceptus*, but the trained observer, the cell biologist, the geneticist, and the embryologist, can make that determination.

(c) Some who argue discontinuity use the language of potentiality to frame their arguments and to dismiss the *conceptus* from the category of personhood. One such argument describes the *conceptus* as "an animal with great promise of becoming more than just an animal," that is, a human person. The claim here is that while there is material continuity, there is substantial change. The substantial development has its source in and from the material that existed at the beginning. The appropriate response is that the *conceptus* by virtue of its active natural potency, which is a guarantee of its future development, will develop itself (tendency) into the adult human (constitution) unless *otherwise interrupted*. (It could be interrupted in a number of ways. It could be removed from its natural environment; it could be infected by a virus; its natural environment might prove insufficient for its continuation; it could be dismembered by surgical instruments, and so forth.) That guarantee, which is present from the beginning, is more than just a promise.

(d) Another argument makes a distinction between concrete potentiality for human activities and abstract potentiality for human activities. The *conceptus* is described as possessing abstract potentiality and is contrasted with the person who possesses concrete potentiality. As found in the literature, this is a strange set of distinctions. On the one hand, it seems to embody a distinction used in medical practice in problems such as those that arise in the allocation of scarce medical resources when a decision has to be made between the patient that the physician knows and has treated and the similarly situated set of patients whom the physician does not know and has not treated. The physician perceives the former patient as concrete and the latter set of patients as abstract. On the other hand, the concrete/abstract distinction seems to be rooted in the person/personal consciousness distinction, that is, one is a person so long as one is conscious of oneself. From the perspective of the first distinction, the reality of each patient is the same; the difference lies in the relation of the physician to each of the patients. From the perspective of the second distinction, the person is reduced to personal consciousness. Personal consciousness is an attribute of a person; it is not the whole person. Human beings have the capacity to be conscious; they cannot be reduced to consciousness. Human beings are (1) sometimes conscious and aware of self as subject; (2) sometimes conscious with the awareness of self as object; (3) sometimes in act with a potentiality for consciousness that is remote or proximate as in the *conceptus*, or the person under anesthesia, or the person asleep; and (4) sometimes in action but so immersed in a problem or an activity or an encounter that the awareness of self is lost. These different states of consciousness are states of one being who continues throughout these states.[15]

(e) In the discussion of probability as it relates to the possibility of the eventual birth of the *conceptus*, the claim has been made that because only 40% (or whatever percentage is offered) of human zygotes survive to become fully developed self-conscious rational human beings, it is more appropriate to consider the human zygote a 0.4 probable person. Here, there is confusion of predictions of the future with descriptions of present states of existence and a failure to distinguish classical laws from statistical laws. Classical laws describe regularities, a one-to-one causal relationship, and other things being equal. There is the anticipation of invariance. The example of a classical law in operation is fertilization, that is, the union of the egg and the sperm and the restoration of the diploid number of chromosomes that marks the beginning of a new life. Statistical laws, on the other hand, relate to probabilities, that is, assessments based on relative actual frequencies. The statement that only 40% of embryos survive to be born can be used to formulate a probability statement, that is, a statistical assessment of the likelihood that a fertilized ovum will survive to be born. It says nothing about the nature of the surviving being. What might be concluded from this probability statement is that the continuation of existence is precarious at this period in the life of a human being. At the other end of the continuum of life, it may be the case that only 40% of those human beings who reach the age of 75 survive to be 80. This does not make those who are now 75 only 40% persons. It simply means that those who have reached the age of 75 are rather vulnerable in a statistical sense.

Three additional particular issues are brought forward to cast doubt on the claim that the *conceptus* is a continuous, individual developing human being. These are (f) the lack of unity of organization as evidenced by general appearance and as evidenced by the specific time-limited capacity of totipotentiality of the blastomeres, (g) the possibility of monozygous twinning, and (h) the controversies over theories of ensoulment. In regard to

(f) the unity of organization, this so-called aggregate of loosely associated blastomeres has an immediately apparent unity as an individual organism in its containment within the *zona pellucida* and within the *corona radiata*. Each of the blastomeres has specific functions in the survival of the new individual. In addition, the individual blastomeres, even at this earliest stage, while giving a superficial appearance of loose association, are in constant and intense interaction as the organism, through its genetically determined internal dynamism, continues its self-development. As early as the eight-cell stage, the process of the compaction of the blastomeres takes place. This compaction has at least two functions. The first function is to protect the *conceptus* – here in the preimplantation embryonic stage – from the influence of outside fluids which might be damaging to its integrity. The second function is to couple the blastomeres to permit ion exchange and molecular exchange from each blastomere to the next. The point here is that the "aggregate of loosely associated blastomeres" is actually a highly organized and self-organizing cohesive entity.

The blastomeres do indeed have a time-limited capacity for totipotentiality. Totipotentiality is the ability of a cell to be the source of an entire organism. Rather than considering totipotentiality as a suggestion of lack of individuality, it might be considered a particular strength of the human being at this particularly vulnerable stage of development. Because this stage of human development is particularly vulnerable, the earliest blastomeres have the capacity to repair, by means of the biological process designated regulation, damage to the individual developing human being. The individual cells at this early stage of development have a prospective potency, that is, the capacity to form many types of cells (pluripotent) or a new organism (totipotent), which is greater than its prospective fate, that is, the capacity to form the types of cells it normally does, if in the course of development, it is not disturbed (Patten, p. 173). After this stage in human development, there is a subsequent decline in human potentialities. This is true of human development in general. As certain potentialities are actualized, others are lost.

(g) As to the lack of unity as evidenced by the occasional occurrence of monozygous twinning, it is appropriate to indicate (1) that the occurrence is infrequent and (2) that very little is known about the etiology of the process. Monozygous or identical twins occur in approximately 0.35% of human births. The frequency of occurrence of monozygous twins increases to approximately 2% in the process of assisted reproduction (ART) (Condic, 2020, p. 42). This significant increase in the frequency of monozygous twinning in the ART process suggests the influence of environmental factors. While the exact mechanism for the occurrence of monozygous twins remains unknown, there have been several possible accounts offered.

Among them are (1) monozygous twinning may be caused by an environmental change such as a precipitous drop in oxygen level; (2) monozygous twinning may be caused by genetic mutation such as a mutation on a chromosome during mitosis; (3) monozygous twinning understood as a type of regulation process, that is, healing made possible by the latent totipotentiality of the earliest blastomeres with the ability to produce the inner cell mass and the trophectoderm necessary for the generation of a new organism and called into operation on the occasion of significant damage to the developing entity; and (4) monozygous twinning may occur with structural changes occasioned by disruption during the hatching process when the embryo emerges from the *zona pellucida*. Both the infrequency of the occurrence and its possible random occurrence, by environmental alteration or structural damage, suggest that monozygous twinning is a departure from the norm. A summary of monozygotic twinning has been offered in the following:

> Monozygotic twinning most closely resembles regeneration or wound healing of an injured human organism; development proceeds without pause along the trajectory initially established by the zygote, indicating that one of the two twins produced by splitting is ontologically identical to the original zygote.
>
> (Condic, 102)

Despite the lack of knowledge about the mechanism of the occurrence of monozygous twins, the rare occurrence of monozygous twins is a fact. This occurrence has called into question the developmental individuality of the *conceptus* at the earliest stages of development. While continuing to recognize the genetic individuality from the zygote forward, the possibility of twinning suggests lack of developmental identity for the early embryo. The separation of developmental individuality from genetic individuality generated what has become known as the 14-day rule. The claim here is that with the appearance of the primitive streak on the 14th day, monozygous twinning is no longer possible. Therefore, since the 14th day marks both genetic and developmental individuality, the entity, sometimes designated the pre-embryo, that exists before that day need not be considered a human being requiring respect and protection. It may be manipulated and used for putative scientific or medical progress. An appropriate and parsimonious account, consistent with scientific observations of various occurrences in the natural order, is that the completion of the process of fertilization normally establishes genetic and developmental individuality directed toward the emergence of an integrated and single human being. Rarely, but occasionally, this process is interrupted. This interruption most likely occurs at hatching with the emergence of the blastocysy from the *zona pellucida* when part of the emerging organism separates. In the interruption, the original zygote remains. The new entity, if it is equipped with essential structures such as the inner cell mass and the trophectoderm intact, emerges and begins its trajectory as an integrated and single human being who is the genetic twin and sibling of the original zygote. As each twin matures its interaction, both natural and social, with its environment will occasion subtle differences. None of this, however, should have an effect on the legal protection of the *conceptus*. To say there two human beings might develop, does not allow it to be said that there are no human beings there. A similar situation is described in the following: "Creating an identical twin of a mature human by removing a skin cell and using it to clone a new embryonic human would not raise any questions about the individuality of the adult skin-cell donor" (Condic, 26).

(h) Finally, theories of ensoulment have been brought forth to add to the mix of issues in the determination of when human life begins and whether or not human life is continuous from zygote forward. The two most significant theories are that of (1) immediate animation and immediate ensoulment and that of (2) immediate animation and delayed ensoulment. A defense of the theory of ensoulment must be its adequacy as an appropriate understanding of the phenomena of the development of the being.

Ensoulment theories have been conceived of differently in different historical periods. In ancient and medieval philosophy, ensoulment theories were tied to scientific theories of the origin of human life and to concerns about the proper disposition and organization of matter to receive the soul. In the contemporary era, they are framed in response to claims of discontinuity or continuity of development from biological life to human life.

Theories of immediate animation and immediate ensoulment or immediate animation and delayed ensoulment are tied to the acceptance of a particular biological understanding of the development of human life. In the period in which preformation theories, such as the homunculus, held biological prominence, the prevailing view was that of immediate animation and immediate ensoulment. The human being, termed the homunculus, was completely present in the seed. When the seed was sown in appropriate matter, the new human being simply grew bigger. Animation and ensoulment were thus immediate.

Those who argue for immediate animation but delayed human ensoulment include Aristotle in the ancient world, Thomas Aquinas in the medieval world, and, in the twentieth century, with some modifications, Joseph Donceel. They argue from a particular biological perspective which understands that the human being is present when its formation has been completed, that is, 40 days for a male and 80 days for a female. The essential elements in that position are presented in the following: (1) the soul is the substantial form of the human being; (2) a substantial form requires matter capable of receiving it; and (3) in the case of the human being, this means that the human soul can exist only in a highly organized body. What is being presented here is a theory of serial ensoulment, that is, first a vegetative soul, then a sentient soul, and finally a rational soul. The animation of the new being is immediate at fertilization. But, the soul that animates the body is commensurate with the kind of life lived by the body and the degree of organization of the body. So in the early stages, the body of the human being is animated by a vegetative soul which organizes the operations of nutrition and growth, that is, vegetative activities. As the new being develops in complexity and activities, such as sensation a new soul, an animal soul, replaces the vegetative soul. As the development in complexity of the being continues and as the development of sense organs and nervous system progresses, another threshold is crossed. When the material substratum is sufficiently disposed, the rational soul appears and the human being as rational being is constituted. The significant points in the theory of serial ensoulment are the following. First, because the soul is the substantial form of the body, the rational soul cannot be present until there is a body present that is significantly complex and organized to receive the soul. Second, a formal cause is present only in a finished product. An actual human soul cannot be united with a virtual human body. Third, there is no human body in the zygote. Fourth, inasmuch as all the positive features of the human body derive from the soul, until the soul is present, there is no human being.

The responses are as follows. The first point is insufficiently aware of the high degree of organization and the high degree of complexity of activity and development. From the zygote stage forward the *conceptus* contains billions of atoms, and thousands of molecules all organized for its survival and growth. To the second point: inasmuch as the genotype fixes the goal and inasmuch as the adult human being cannot be more than what it is determined to be in the zygote, there is a very real sense in which the human being is fully formed in the zygote stage. The ultimate stage from a natural perspective is the adult human being who is the becoming of the initial stage. To the third point: the human body is really present in the zygote stage. It is present in the active natural potentiality of the zygote. It is not a fully developed body in the sense of a completed adult body. It is, however, a fully developed body in terms of what is to be expected of the normal body at this stage of development. It might be appropriate to say, "It is an actual human person with a body whose full development is already in dynamic process" (Mangan, p. 24). To the fourth point: the human body does derive all its positive features from its rational soul.

However, all the potentialities of the human being are established, that is, are in act as active natural potentialities at the zygote stage. It seems more appropriate to maintain that the rational soul is present at that time. A more economical theory of ensoulment, one that applies the principle of parsimony, is as follows. There is one soul present from the beginning. At first, the rational soul, which subsumes the sentient and vegetative powers, is active at its lowest levels and is anticipating the higher levels of human activity similar to the manner in which organ development anticipates subsequent behavioral expression. In the early stages of human development, the rational soul may be said to be present and to be exercising its vegetative powers as it does in a comatose human being. At a later stage of development, the rational soul may be said to be present and to be exercising its vegetative and sentient powers as it does in the sleeping human being. At a still later stage of development, it may be said to be present and to be exercising its vegetative, sentient, and rational powers as it does in the fullest expression of rational human life.

(E) Afterword

If the position developed earlier, that is, that human life is a continuum from the union of the gametes until the occurrence of death, rests on a sufficiently solid foundation and if the responses to the counter-positions are adequate, then it appears appropriate to claim that abortion is an act that takes the life of a human being. Abortion, then, is a species of homicide. The ethical injunctions that apply to the destruction of human life apply similarly to abortion.

A feminism which claims as its core value a philosophy of care would reject abortion as violence to the *conceptus* and exploitation of vulnerable women. A more robust feminism, one that understands that all human life is lived in relationships, that the more powerful are obliged to care for the more vulnerable, and that eschews killing, might serve as a corrective for the fiction found in the holding of contemporaneous philosophy that human beings are autonomous rights-bearing individuals whose choices are right simply because they are freely chosen. Moreover, the prohibition of abortion by law, except in those instances where the life of the mother is at issue and those instances where the *conceptus* represents a material aggression on the life of the woman, is commensurate with the legal code of a society that aspires to liberty ordered by solidarity and subsidiarity.

However, these conclusions and their defense in the public square are but pieces, albeit essential pieces, in the possible transformation of culture that appears to embrace abortion as an acceptable choice for women and girls. Another essential piece is the creation of the conditions that make the consideration and provision of abortion unnecessary. To build this culture requires that children, their mothers, and their families have the requisite goods, through appropriate institutions that operate in adherence to principles of solidarity and subsidiarity, to facilitate their flourishing. Because the fundamental institution of human flourishing is the family, additional essential realities must be reclaimed. They are (1) children should be born within marriage in order to facilitate their flourishing; (2) the exercise of sexual intercourse should be held an act appropriate only in marriage; (3) appropriate care be given to mothers during and after pregnancy so that their children may flourish; and (4) fathers recognize and claim their roles in protecting the life and well-being of mothers and children. Absent the creation of these and other conditions to foster respect for human life, the prevalence of abortion in the culture will go unabated.

Another part of the task in the essential work of building the culture of life requires our engagement in the intellectual controversies of our time. If we think we hold the truth, we ought to fear no pursuit of knowledge. To build this culture requires our participation in the deliberations of the democracy and in its political processes. Catholics have a right in the public square as citizens and an obligation to be in the public square as Catholics. The former is a guarantee of the First Amendment and the latter the command of Christ that we "render to Caesar the things that are Caesar's." To build that culture finally requires that we make abortion unthinkable because it is unnecessary.

Questions for Reflection

1. In the assessment of the morality of an act, the object, intention, and circumstances must be considered. What is the object of the act of abortion? Why is it important to know what the object of a proposed act is?
2. What do *you* think is the pivotal point in the abortion debate? What do you observe that *others* hold to be the pivotal point in the abortion debate? How would you argue that one point or another is the *pivotal* point?
3. In what ways might the Catholic Church be able to *change* the terms of the debate? Where is the appropriate place for the Catholic Church to enter the abortion issue?
4. What are some good examples of the distinction between potency and act?
5. What are some important examples of how human life is characterized by dependence and interdependence (rather than solely by independence)?

6. What would society look like if it took care of the vulnerable and dependent rather than claiming that the vulnerable and dependent are nonpersons?
7. What are various ways in history that some have judged others to be "nonpersons"? What have been the consequences?
8. What do you think is the right way to construe the relationship between *human law* and *human nature*?
9. Abortion as an elective procedure was unknown until contemporary medical practice. What do you think is the best way to conceive of the role of the physician vis-à-vis the wishes of the patient?
10. The notion of autonomy is a powerful notion in the contemporary culture. Present and assess its implications for the culture.

Notes

1 The term *conceptus* will be used in this chapter to designate human life from the beginning – the zygote – through the embryo and through fetal development. Its use provides an economy of words and an appropriate reference, as well as a respect not normally accorded by reference to this human being as a "blob of tissue" or a "mere fetus" as if to suggest it is a prehuman life form.

2 Note that Plato showed the short distance and natural link between abortion and infanticide.

3 Note that this still leaves room for further specification due to epigenetic factors.

4 *Parens patriae* literally means "parent of the nation." It is a legal term that delineates interests worthy of state protection. Examples include (1) the authority of the state to take care of those who are unable to take care of themselves, for example, when Child Protective Services steps in to remove a child from an abusive household; (2) the involuntary commitment of a person with mental illness to a treatment facility; (3) the ability of the state to bring a lawsuit on behalf of its citizens, to protect them; (4) the protection of the professions in the exercise of their special functions; and (5) protection from suicide.

5 The notion Kingdom of Ends referenced here is found in the *Foundations of the Metaphysics of Morals* by Immanuel Kant. A kingdom of ends would be a community of rational beings whose lives are directed by adherence to the categorical imperative. The categorical imperative commands that one be self-legislating (the command comes from within the self as autonomous and not from outside as heteronomous) in the realm of morality in a manner in which one never acts in such a way that one cannot will one's maxim to be a universal law, that one always acts in such a way that one can will one's maxim to be a universal law, and that one always treats humanity whether in yourself or in another always as an end and never as a means only.

6 The *Dobbs* (*Dobbs v. Jackson Women's Health Organization*, No. 19–1392, 597 U.S. ___ (2022)) decision provides two appendices delineating the laws of the states from mid-nineteenth century until *Roe v. Wade* (410 U.S. 113, 1973).

7 Students of history and students of law should not overlook the parallel between this aspect of the decision and the ruling in *Dred Scott*.

8 In fact, it is difficult to see how *any* law can stand, on the basis of this principle.

9 Farr Curlin and Christopher Tollefsen in *The way of medicine: Ethics and the healing professions*. University of Notre Dame Press, 2021 provide an account of medical practice that challenges the provider of services model that is operative in contemporary medicine. They argue that the end of medicine is the preservation and restoration of health. Reclaiming this end is good for patients, physicians, and the profession.

10 Fourteenth Amendment Section 1:

> All persons born or naturalized in the United States, and subject to the jurisdiction thereof, are citizens of the United States and of the State wherein they reside. No State shall make or enforce any law which shall abridge the privileges or immunities of citizens of the United States; nor shall any State deprive any person of life, liberty, or property, without due process of law; nor deny to any person within its jurisdiction the equal protection of the laws.

11 *Stare decisis* literally means "to stand by things decided." In the law, it refers to the practice of the Court to accept previous decisions as precedents for the case before the Court. Here, the respondents claim *Roe* and *Casey* as precedents for *Dobbs*. Justice Alito wrote that inasmuch as *Roe* was an abuse of judicial authority the Court is not required to adhere to *Roe*.

12 The *Appendices* to *Dobbs* list in *Appendix A* the statutes criminalizing abortion in the States in existence in 1868 and in *Appendix B* the statutes criminalizing abortion in each of the territories that became states and in the District of Columbia. It is important to note the almost universal protection of the life of the woman and the universal lack of criminalization of the woman.

13 In their dissent of in *Dobbs Justices Breyer, Sotomayor and Kagan wrote*,

> Indulge a few more words about this point. The majority had a choice of two different ways to overrule *Roe* and *Casey*. It could claim that those cases underrated the State's interest in fetal life. Or it could claim that they overrated a woman's constitutional liberty interest in choosing an abortion. (Or both.) The majority here rejects the first path, and we can see why. Taking that route would have prevented the majority from claiming that it means only to leave this issue to the democratic process – that it does not have a dog in the fight. See ante, at 38–39, 65. And indeed, doing so might have suggested a revolutionary proposition: that the fetus is itself a constitutionally protected 'person,' such that an abortion ban is constitutionally mandated. The majority therefore chooses the second path, arguing that the Fourteenth Amendment does not conceive of the abortion decision as implicating liberty, because the law in the 19th century gave that choice no protection. The trouble is that the chosen path – which is, again, the solitary rationale for the Court's decision – provides no way to distinguish between the right to choose an abortion and a range of other rights, including contraception.
>
> (*Dobbs*, Dissent)

14 The argument for discontinuity would allow abortion prior to the determination that a human being was present. If a human being is not present, there is no homicide. Among significant scholars who argued for discontinuity were the early Tristram Engelhardt, H. (1974, April). The ontology of abortion. *Ethics*, *84*(3), 217–234) and McCormick, S. J., Richard A. (1991). Who or what is the preembryo. *Kennedy Institute of Ethics Journal*, *1*(1), 1–15. Callahan, D. (1970). *Abortion: Law, choice, and morality*. Macmillan Publishing Co. made a distinction between a human being and a person; a person is one who has standing

in the law. He claimed that the fetus is not a person, hence, it can be aborted if the woman so chooses. Others such as Peter Singer, Mary Anne Warren, and Michael Tooley accepted continuity of development of the fetus as a human being but denied the fetus (or infant) the status of a person. Because the fetus is not a person, the permissibility of abortion remains as the choice of the woman. Warren's list provides an example of characteristics required for personhood in the following:

> 1. consciousness . . . and in particular the capacity to feel pain; 2. reasoning (the developed capacity to solve new and relatively complex problems); 3. self-motivated activity (activity which is relatively independent of either genetic or direct external control); 4. the capacity to communicate, by whatever means, messages of an indefinite variety of types . . .; 5. the presence of self-concepts, and self-awareness.
>
> (Warren, p. 55)

Tooley argued for the acceptance of infanticide for children born without particular capacities. His list is similar to those listed by Warren.

15 Think of this as a principle that rules some beings "in" as persons, and other beings "out" as persons. If "personal consciousness" marks the dividing line, then the conceptus is ruled out – but so are many other beings who are obviously persons. That means "personal consciousness" is not a good differential principle.

5 The Reproductive Finality

The Scriptures are replete with passages noting the joy of the gift of children. The Psalmist wrote,

> Fatherhood itself is the Lord's gift, the fruitful womb is a reward that comes from him. Crown of thy youth, children are like arrows in a warrior's quiver. Happy, whose quiver is well filled with these; their cause will not be set aside when they plead against their enemies at the gate.
>
> (*Psalms* 127:3–5)

Luke records an experience that is a privilege unique to women, namely, the joy of a mother as she experiences the first movements of her child within her body. In his Gospel, Luke wrote,

> Why, as soon as ever the voice of thy greeting sounded in my ears, the child in my womb leaped for joy. Blessed art thou for thy believing; the message that was brought to thee from the Lord shall have fulfillment.
>
> (Luke 1:44–45)

The notion of children as joyful gift from the Lord to mothers and fathers, notwithstanding the allusion of the Psalmist to arrows, seems to accord with much human experience.[1]

Nonetheless, human history presents a more complex understanding of this gift. Most often, the gift is understood as a natural occurrence and children are welcomed as a renewal of the human family. Sometimes, however, it seems that the reproductive finality is superabundant and children are experienced as a burden. At other times, the accomplishment of reproduction seems lacking and medical/technical intervention is desired. Yet, at other times still, as a stiff-necked people, the gift is refused or accepted only reluctantly.

The growth of modern science and the growth of modern technology have had a significant impact on understanding and controlling human

DOI: 10.4324/9781003627197-5

reproduction. Modern science, from the mid-nineteenth century forward, contributed to the understanding of human reproduction as the union of the female and male gametes. The simultaneous growth of modern technology has had significant impact on understanding the mechanism of reproduction and on the control of human reproduction whether that control be an aid in the accomplishment of reproduction or an aid in the avoidance of that end. Both the accomplishment and avoidance of reproduction can be human goods if they contribute to human flourishing in morally acceptable ways. The moral acceptability of an act requires an understanding of the integral human act, that is, it must be right in its object, intention, and circumstances. Moreover, the analysis, within this tradition, of any act must take place under the guidance of both reason and revelation.

From the outset, it is appropriate to acknowledge that the existence of a child is a good. Children are among the goods toward which marriage inclines. The accomplishment of children as one of the ends of marriage must intend the good of the child as well as the good of the parents and the good of the family. It is also appropriate to acknowledge that sometimes it is both necessary and prudential to avoid having children or more children. Furthermore, it is sometimes both necessary and prudential to seek the assistance of medical technology to remedy material deficiencies that interfere with the accomplishment of reproduction.

The focus of this chapter will be the accomplishment and avoidance of reproduction understood as sexual, that is, of conception understood as the union of egg and sperm or the avoidance of conception understood as the prevention of the union of egg and sperm. Human reproduction by way of asexual means, that is, cloning as somatic cell nuclear transfer, is treated separately in Chapter 6. Abortion as a means of preventing offspring by the destruction of the young human being, whether embryo or fetus, is treated as a separate issue in Chapter 4. This chapter will proceed in the following order:

(A) Introduction: framing the issue;
(B) Advances in reproductive technology to ameliorate infertility and to accomplish conception;
(C) Advances in understanding of the reproductive process and cycle to prevent conception;
(D) The development of the teaching of the Catholic tradition as it guides the reproductive finality;
(E) The examination of particular ethical and practical issues embedded in the contemporary practices of reproductive science;
(F) Afterword: challenges facing forward.

(A) Framing the Issue

All issues regarding reproduction, whether to have children or to avoid having children, are to be addressed within the understanding of marriage in the Catholic tradition as a natural social institution as well as a sacrament. Marriage is understood in this tradition to have an essential nature.[2] That nature is the source of the several finalities or goals to be accomplished within marriage. Moreover, this understanding exercises governance over the accomplishment of the goals, including the reproductive finality, within marriage. In brief, the tradition holds that sexual intercourse is the marriage act. It is not to be exercised outside of marriage. Its expression is reserved for marriage and is limited to the partners of the marriage. Conjugal intercourse serves the goods of (1) the satisfaction of the sexual inclinations, (2) the accomplishment and nurturing of children, if there are to be children of this marriage, and (3) the nourishing of the indissoluble, sacramental bond of marriage. The tradition holds these claims in its understanding of human beings as physical, rational, and spiritual beings and of marriage as the natural social institution within which human flourishing as physical, rational, and spiritual is to be accomplished. The physical pleasures experienced and properly ordered in conjugal intercourse dispose, refresh, and replenish the friendship of husband and wife and, moreover, are dispositive to their spiritual development as the joy of their union prefigures the joy of union with God. The movement is from *eros* through *philia* to *agape*. This movement is one of the ways that marriage reflects God's love in and for the world.

The delineation of this account of the tradition begins with understanding the physical as the essential fundamental aspect of sexual intercourse, then moves to higher levels, that is, the more excellent level as rational of the human experience, and then to the level of grace, that is, the transcendental level. On the physical level, conjugal intercourse is an intimate act accompanied by intense and exquisite pleasure of two people in the marriage relationship. This same act, which nourishes their relationship, may also result in the generation of offspring. On a rational level, practical reason intervenes and exercises control. The satisfaction of this pleasure is to be reasonable, that is, appropriate to the persons and circumstances. It is to be reasonable and responsible in the face of the possibility of the generation of offspring and, as well, their care and education. It is to be reasonable in the continuation of the marital relationship in order to serve the good of the persons engaged in the act. Thus far, this understanding is grounded in natural law as a set of claims including (1) there is human nature that can be understood by human reason; (2) the ends – the goods – of human nature can be experienced as inclinations pressing for fulfillment; and (3) these ends ought to be accomplished under the direction of reason. However, the human person is more than physical and rational; the human person exists as a unified totality – physical, rational, and spiritual. Hence, the tradition has recourse to revelation and magisterial teaching to complete and augment its position. The tradition will be more fully developed in Section D.

(B) Reproductive Technology to Ameliorate Infertility

To set the real-world context for technological assistance in reproduction, it is important to understand the need for such technology. Studies of human infertility report statistics that range from 7% to 18% for the frequency of infertility in couples in the developed world. The Center for Disease Control (CDC) in the United States reports that 12% of women of childbearing age suffer from infertility or impaired fecundity (cdc.gov/nchs/fastats/infertility.htm). It is in response to this need that assisted reproductive technologies were developed. At first, the technology was limited to married couples whose desire to have children led them to invest a great deal of time, energy, money, and love to conceive a child. But of course, with the development and success of the technology, it was not long before what had been developed to serve a real human *need*, became the object of human *desire* as another service to be purchased. Hence, the demand for the technology expanded. In the contemporary era, the desire by unmarried women for children, for unmarried women to experience pregnancy and childbirth, for women who have been widowed prior to the opportunity to have a child with their husband, and for persons of homosexual inclinations to have children have fueled the press for more and better technology.

Causes of infertility are varied. Some are structural, some are chemical, and some are related to gamete production. If the organs of reproduction are intact in the male and the female, infertility may be caused by the quality of the egg or the sperm. If that is the case, then treatment focuses on the germ cells. If the egg and the sperm are mature and are adequate and available, infertility may be caused by structural or chemical problems in the reproductive system. Among those problems for women are: the occlusion of the fallopian tube, a condition sometimes caused by scarring subsequent to infection, or endometriosis unresponsive to medical or surgical therapy or the production of vaginal secretions that are inimical to sperm survival. For the male, the structural impediments include blockages or varicoceles or abnormalities of the ejaculatory ducts or injury to or surgery on the reproductive organs. For both men and women, an unfortunate side effect of chemotherapy and/or radiation is the destruction of gametes and the subsequent loss of fertility. Finally, it is generally acknowledged that the increased incidence of sexually transmitted disease brought on by casual sex is one of the factors contributing to the increased rate of infertility.

In the contemporary culture, the practices common to accomplish the reproductive finality outside of sexual intercourse are generally grouped together under the title – ARTs – for Assisted Reproductive Technologies. Included among these are artificial insemination, *in vitro* fertilization and embryo transfer, gamete intrafallopian transfer, zygote intrafallopian transfer, intracytoplasmic sperm injection, embryo micromanipulation, embryo hatching, and surrogacy. Because of the speed of the growth of the assisted reproductive technology industry and because of the deliberate cultural ambiguity in regard to abortion, these industries remain, for the most part, unregulated and outside of professional oversight. This lack of regulation in a quasi-medical process aimed at the production of children is startling when compared to the difficult and burdensome regulatory procedures in place for the adoption of children.[3]

The following is a brief description of the different types of ART as a means to accomplish the end of reproduction, moving from the simplest to the more complex of available technologies.[4] If infertility is caused by the inability of the woman to produce mature eggs and her husband is able to produce mature and motile sperm, fertility drugs will be administered to the woman to stimulate the development of multiple follicles and multiple mature eggs. Ovarian hyper-stimulation, more often than not, produces multiple mature eggs. If that is the only infertility remedy attempted and if normal intercourse follows, the risk of multiple pregnancies is a real possibility and many such pregnancies have been reported. Hence, great care must be exercised in limiting the number of eggs released.

In artificial insemination, the sperm of the potential father or of a donor are injected, usually by a technician, into the cervix of a woman. Insemination with the spousal sperm is designated homologous; insemination with donor sperm is designated heterologous. The sperm travel up through the fallopian tube to fertilize a mature oocyte at the distal end of the fallopian tube. If all goes well, the fertilized ovum, the zygote, begins development as it proceeds down the fallopian tube to a uterus that should be a receptive and appropriate host for the implantation of what is now the embryo.

In vitro fertilization is a laboratory process. Sperm from the potential father or the donor is placed in proximity to an oocyte(s) from the mother or a donor in a laboratory dish. The oocytes are produced by hormonal hyper-stimulation of the ovaries of the egg donor. The eggs are then harvested by either laparoscopy surgery or ultrasound-guided follicular puncture. Because of the high rate of failure of both the fertilization and implantation processes, multiple oocytes are typically used and fertilized. If the attempt at fertilization is successful, that is, if sperm and egg fuse to form a zygote, then organized cell division commences and embryos are produced. The embryos are transferred in a timely manner to an appropriately prepared uterus, either of the mother or of the surrogate, for implantation there. The usual procedure, again because of high rate of failure, is to transfer multiple embryos to the uterus and to freeze other embryos for future use, if necessary. The freezing and storing process, and occasional embryo destruction, of additional embryos carries with it moral implications for the use of this technology.

Gamete intrafallopian transfer (GIFT) is a process which transfers sperm and eggs in a special catheter, which keeps the sperm and eggs separated, to the distal end of the fallopian tube, where fertilization takes place. In the GIFT procedure, fertilization takes place within the body of the woman who intends to be the mother and, generally, the sperm of the spouse of the woman is placed in the fallopian tube. The greater success of the GIFT procedure is attributed to the fact that it more closely mimics the natural process of conception. Zygote intrafallopian transfer (ZIFT) is similar to GIFT. ZIFT is the transfer of the zygote, the fertilized ovum, to the fallopian tube through which it should traverse into the uterus.

Intracytoplasmic sperm injection (ICSI) is the injection of a single sperm directly into the cytoplasm of the egg. This procedure is done when the concentration of sperm is low or when the sperm evidence poor motility or when sperm supply is limited such as is the case in men who, on account of illness or medical treatment, have stored sperm for use in generating biologically related children. The availability of the ICSI procedure reduces the need for multiple donor sperm and makes possible the maintenance of the biological tie of the father to the offspring.

Gamete micromanipulation is a process in which the sperm and/or the egg are manipulated through microscopic procedures that enhance the quality of the sperm or the egg to increase the probability of fertilization. Embryo micromanipulation or assisted hatching is a procedure that modifies the *zona pellucida*, the membrane which surrounds the egg, by opening the membrane or thinning the membrane to facilitate embryo hatching and the subsequent implantation of the embryo into the wall of the uterus.

To all of these possible manipulations of egg and sperm and embryo, the possibility of surrogacy must be added. As methods of reproductive technology have expanded, so too have the methods of surrogacy. Now the idea of surrogate motherhood is not new. Recall Abram and Sarah and Hagar and recall too the problems which followed. Biblical surrogacy, though, required sexual intercourse. The new technologies render sexual intercourse unnecessary for surrogacy. For completeness of treatment, there is a distinction made between two types of surrogacy. In traditional surrogacy, a woman is inseminated by sperm for the purpose of conceiving and bearing a child for someone else. The woman is the donor of the egg and, therefore, she is, by that genetic material, biologically related to the child. Once the child is born, the child is given over to the commissioning couple or the commissioning person to be reared by that couple or person.

In gestational surrogacy, the child is not conceived in the body of the woman who will carry the pregnancy forward and give birth. The child may be conceived in any of the many ways described in the assisted reproductive technologies and transferred to the body of a female for gestation. This makes possible a variety of different relationships. The child may be genetically related to either or both of the commission parties, or to none or neither of the commissioning parties. This complexity leaves open the possibility that a single child may be related to an egg donor, a sperm donor, a gestational woman, and a rearing person or persons.

(C) Understanding the Reproductive Cycle to Prevent Conception

Fifty years ago or so, the central concern of many couples was to prevent conception. Over time, with the development of new technologies, that question appears less pressing. As a matter of fact, with the change in sexual mores since the 1960s, there is now greater concern with the inability to procreate. Nonetheless, for many who live within the Catholic tradition, there remains a commitment to limit reproduction within the teaching of the tradition. Furthermore, for some outside the Catholic tradition, there is an interest in preventing conception in a manner more consistent with natural means. Among the means of preventing conception are the following: (1) abstinence throughout the marriage; (2) periodic continence; (3) incompletion or interruption of the act of conjugal intercourse; and (4) sterilization of the act by (a) barrier method or (b) medication or (c) surgery. Following a brief account of (1) and (3), this section will focus on (2) and (4).

The first, abstinence from conjugal intercourse throughout marriage, can be understood as heroic or deeply spiritual when undertaken for a sufficient reason. The husband and wife must have the capacity (*potentia coeundi*) to have conjugal intercourse and to form a physical union, but choose to forego that right. The spouses would be committed to form the bond of friendship and the spiritual bond of their marital union without the nourishing upward dispositive effects of the pleasure of the physical union. The marriage of Mary and Joseph would seem to exemplify this understanding. In the twentieth century, it was reported that Jacques and Raïssa Maritain made this commitment to celibacy as well as a commitment to marriage as friendship and spiritual companionship to complete what they understood as their work on earth as ordered to their salvation.[5]

The third option, incompletion or interruption of the act of conjugal intercourse is the conscious effort to prevent conception by withdrawal of the penis prior to the ejaculation of the sperm into the vagina. If ejaculation follows withdrawal, the act is designated *coitus interruptus*; if no ejaculation follows, the act is designated *amplexus reservatus*.

The second, periodic continence – often referred to as Natural Family Planning – is the attempt to avoid conception by refraining from conjugal intercourse at those times within the ovulatory cycle of the woman when the egg is susceptible to fertilization. Its development began in the early twentieth century with the realization that women ovulate once a menstrual cycle and that menstruation, in a normal cycle, generally occurs 14 days after ovulation. This understanding of the cycle served first as an aid to accomplish conception and, then later, this understanding of the cycle was used as an aid to avoid conception by limiting conjugal intercourse to those times in the cycle when a woman is infertile. This regularity of cycles as ordering conjugal intercourse became known as the Rhythm Method.

Over time more accurate methods – symptom-based as well as additional calendar-based methods – were developed. These symptom-based methods include the Billings Method, the Creighton Model, and the ClearBlue Easy Fertility Monitor developed at Marquette University. Georgetown University Medical Center developed an adaption of the counting days in the cycle. The Billings Method relies on daily observation and charting of the quality and sensation of the cervical secretions as they discharge from the vulva. The Creighton method trademarked as CREIGHTON MODEL FertilityCare System (CrMS) is similarly based on observation and charting of the appearance and viscosity of the mucosal discharge. Marquette's ClearBlue Easy Fertility Monitoring Method utilizes a device to measure levels of luteinizing hormone and estrogen in the urine. The Institute for Reproductive Health at Georgetown University Medical Center developed the Standard Days Method (SDM) utilizing its patented CycleBeads. The ring of beads facilitates counting and sorting of days in the woman's fertility cycle to locate the days on which conception might occur. The success of each of these methods depends on the accuracy of the observations and the commitment of the users to adhere to the observations and avoid intercourse on the days indicated.

The Billings Ovulation Method has been repeatedly tested, including an extended study of its use in China. Its site, Billings.Life, reports that "the method-related" pregnancy rate was zero. The method-related rate reports the occurrence of pregnancy when couples correctly follow all the instructions for the method of birth control. The use-related pregnancy rate was 0.5%. The use-related rate includes couples who misunderstood or did not comply with all the instructions. These results make the Billings Ovulation Method™ as effective as the Pill, and substantially more effective than IUDs, condoms, and diaphragms. The Creighton Model reports similar findings at its site, CreightonModel. com. The site reports that the

> range of effectiveness to avoid pregnancy at the 12th ordinal month to be 98.7 to 99.8 (with five-study composite 99.5). The use effectiveness to avoid pregnancy for the same time period ranged from 94.6 to 97.9 and was shown to continually improve over the 14 years of the study (five-study composite was 96.8).

The Natural Family Planning site at Marquette University, which developed the ClearBlue Easy Fertility Monitor (MM), reported "a 97–98% efficacy of the MM in avoiding pregnancy when taught by a qualified teacher and correctly applied."[6]

Contraceptive intercourse may be facilitated by barrier method, medication, or surgery. The barrier methods to reduce the probability of pregnancy include condoms, diaphragms, cervical caps, sponges, and spermicides. Each functions to prevent the sperm from reaching and fertilizing the ovum. Manufacturers of condoms report results in avoiding pregnancy that range from 98% with perfect use to 82% with typical use.

Hormonal medications are also used to prevent pregnancy. They usually contain a combination of estrogen and progestogen. They may be taken by mouth, or implanted into the body tissue, or injected under the skin, or absorbed from a patch, or placed into the vagina. Most of these medications function to prevent ovulation and/or to prevent sperm from fertilizing the egg. A few render the uterine wall inhospitable for implantation. This last is considered abortifacient if the fertilized ovum enters into a uterus whose normal environment has been destroyed. Manufacturers of these drugs report results that range from 99.7% with perfect usage and 91% with typical usage in avoiding pregnancy.

The most common surgeries for contraception are vasectomy for men and tubal ligation for women. In traditional vasectomy, the vas deferens is cut and the ends sealed; thereby preventing the entry of sperm into the seminal fluid. More recently, a procedure for clipping the vas deferens closed has been developed in order to increase the possibility of reversal. In tubal ligation, the fallopian tubes are severed and sealed. This prevents the egg from reaching the uterus and prevents sperm from reaching the egg. More recently, a procedure, which inserts a coil into the fallopian tubes, has been attempted to ensure temporary sterility. Hysterectomy, that is, the removal of the uterus, also renders a woman sterile. While these surgical methods are considered permanent means of contraception, there has been some success with surgical reversal of vasectomy and tubal ligation with the result of the accomplishment of reproduction.

(D) The Teaching of the Catholic Tradition on Reproduction

Within the Catholic tradition, regulation of reproduction and the accomplishment of the goods of marriage are governed by the tradition's understanding of the essential nature of marriage. Knowledge about the nature of marriage resides in many sources. Among those sources are (1) the Scriptures; (2) natural law; (3) the two signs of marriage; and (4) the teachings of the Magisterium as the tradition applies the wisdom drawn from these sources in the presence of the advancements of science and medicine.

(1) The Scriptures address marriage in the very first book, *Genesis*, and they end with marriage in the feast of the Lamb in the *Book of Revelation*. The divine institution of marriage was "from the beginning" in God's creation of man and woman, in God's image and likeness, for each other (*Genesis* 1:26). This account of God's creation of man and woman from man signifies their marital union. In marriage, they become one again as they were once one (*Genesis* 2:18, 22–23). Moreover, God commands that they "Be fruitful and multiply; fill the earth and subdue it" (*Genesis* 1:27–28). What is affirmed here is that (a) marriage has as its essential nature the union of one man and one woman; (b) human beings are to exercise providential creative power; (c) children are understood as a good of marriage; and (d) marriage, as a creation of God, is good.

The Scriptural treatment of marriage is not limited to *Genesis*. Marriage is addressed throughout the Old Testament, especially in the prophets who speak of the relationship between God and Israel in terms of a marriage.[7] This description carries over into the New Testament, and helps to explain why Jesus refers to himself as the Bridegroom.[8] The reference might seem mysterious. But if the relationship between God and Israel is understood on the pattern of the relationship between husband and wife, and if Jesus is the God of Israel in the flesh, then of course he is the Bridegroom of his people.

In addition, Jesus explicitly confirms the teaching of the Old Testament on the nature of marriage in New Testament passages including *Matthew*: 19, 1–9 and *Mark*: 10, 2–9. The text from *Matthew* reads, in part, the following:

> Have you not read that from the beginning the Creator 'made them male and female' and said 'For this reason a man shall leave his father and mother and be joined to his wife, and the two shall become one flesh'? Therefore, what God has joined together, no human being must separate.
>
> (Matthew, 19: 4–6)[9]

While the book of Genesis is a key touchstone for the Catholic understanding of marriage, it does not stand alone as the grounding of that teaching. Understanding the nature of marriage unfolds gradually over the course of salvation history.

(2) Natural law principles are a legacy of ancient Stoicism to moral reasoning and this legacy continues to exercise influence in the contemporary era. The central claims are (a) there is order – law – in the universe; (b) the realities in the universe have natures; (c) these natures can be experienced and can be known by human reason; and (d) knowledge of these natures is action-guiding. Marriage, understood as a natural social institution,

has an essential nature that can be known by human reason. While the understanding of the nature of marriage develops over time, the reality of marriage does not change.[10] The proximate source of the precepts – the commands – of natural law regarding human sexual behavior lies in the direct experience of the demands of human nature to engage in sexual intercourse and to nurture children. Human reason grasps these demands and apprehends them as good. Practical reason commands that these drives be fulfilled under its direction as a way of accomplishing human flourishing. Marriage is the natural social institution within which it is reasonable to engage in sexual intercourse and within which it is reasonable to have and nurture children.

In his *Summa Theologiae,* Thomas Aquinas, whose philosophy is foundational for the tradition, developed an outline of the generation of the precepts of natural law and an ordered specification of three levels of precepts from more general to more specific. They are (a) those which arise from inclinations humans have in common with all substances; (b) those which arise from inclinations humans have in common with animals; and (c) those inclinations that are specific to humans as rational beings. Aquinas claims that human sexual activity has its source in

> [A]n inclination toward certain more specific [goods] with respect to the nature that he shares in common with the other animals. Accordingly, those things are said to belong to the natural law which nature teaches all the animals, i.e., the union of male and female, the education of offspring.
>
> (*Summa Theologiae,* I-II, Q. 94, a.2)

Aquinas designated the procreative end as primary and the union as secondary. Aquinas indicates that by primary, he means that which is accomplished by man as an animal; by secondary that which is accomplished by man as man (*Summa Theologiae,* I-II, q. 65, a. 1).

Within the natural law tradition, the following can be observed. The bodies of men and women are both like and unlike each other. In their similarities, each normally has a brain, heart, lungs, liver, and intestines, which function similarly in men and women even while having some differences such as brain size. In their dissimilarities, each has a set of organs that makes them complementary. The physical complementarity between men and women is such that the two can form a "one flesh union." In conjugal intercourse, this union is made real. Moreover, the coming together of this one flesh union establishes a reproductive system. It is the same kind of act that is unitive and that, under certain conditions, is reproductive. Whether or not the act of marital intercourse results in a new life is another question. However, any other type of union is, by its nature, incapable of reproduction.

(3) *The Two Signs of Marriage*

The Catholic tradition maintains that there are two signs of marriage. They are (a) the love of Christ for His Church and (b) the act of conjugal intercourse itself. Thomas Aquinas developed the theology of the two signs in the *Summa Theologiae* (Aquinas, 1994, Supplement, q. 42, a.1 ad 4 and ad 5). The love of Christ for His bride the Church is the sign which *signifies* the reality of marriage. Aquinas says, "The union of Christ with the Church is not the reality contained in this sacrament, but is the reality signified but not contained" (Aquinas, 1994, ad 4). Marital intercourse is the sign which both *signifies and contains* the reality that is marriage. Aquinas says, "[T]he acts externally apparent are the sacrament only; the bond between husband and wife resulting from those acts is reality and sacrament" (Aquinas, 1994, ad 5). Aquinas characterizes the bond in two ways. It is a union of purpose and it is a union in being. Among its many ends as a union of purpose is the good of procreation. Its end as a unity in being is to be found in the metaphysics of marriage as the husband and wife are the two principles of this new being – the marriage bond as reality and sacrament. It is important to note that it is this bond that has juridical standing before the marriage tribunals of the Church in those instances where the theological and practical questions of annulment are at issue. There is, then, a correspondence between the knowledge of the nature of the act of marital intercourse and the understanding of the nature of marriage. Moreover, on natural law principles, there is a claim that the understanding of both is the same. Hence, a more complete understanding of marital intercourse leads to a more complete understanding of marriage; a more complete understanding of the nature of marriage directs the activity of marital intercourse.

(4) *Magisterial Teachings*

The modern treatment of the nature of marriage and the ordering of its ends begins with *Casti connubii* of Pope Pius XI (1922–1939) and moves forward through the writings of the various popes, Pius XII (1939–1958), John XXIII (1958–1963), Paul VI (1963–1978), John Paul II (1978–2005), Benedict XVI (2005–2013) to the present Pope Francis (2013). While it is not possible to present in full the teaching of the Church and the development of the teachings on marriage, it is appropriate to present the essential elements of the teaching and their development as they relate to reproduction, and as well, to indicate elements of the continuing debate.

(a) *Casti connubii* is the pivotal document for the contemporary treatment of marriage and its ends. This encyclical was issued in 1930 in the presence of four specific pressures. The first pressure was the Lambeth Conference Resolution 15, which permitted the use of material/artificial contraceptives within a framework of responsible parenthood and Christian moral principles.[11] The second was the pressure of some scientists, academics, and physicians who encouraged the use of contraceptives not only to limit reproduction in marriage but also as public policies directed to population control and eugenics. The third pressure lays in the pastoral realm, that is, the concern over whether priests understood and clearly articulated the position of the Church in their teaching and in confessional practices. The fourth pressure was the technological development of artificial means and relatively safe surgical procedures to control reproduction.

Casti connubii summarizes the history of the tradition and sets forth the foundation from which the tradition continues its development. In its summary of the tradition, the following themes are present: "the Hebrew emphasis on procreation, the anti-gnostic teaching of Timothy, the Augustinian doctrine of marital goods (*fides*, *proles, sacramentum)*, the Thomistic view of the nature of the coital act, the nineteenth-century theology of the sin of Onan" (Noonan, 1986, p. 427).

In setting down the nature of marriage, *Casti connubii* maintains that marriage is a divine institution; marriage is a sacrament; and marriage has multiple ends – goods – including procreation, the cultivation of love, the satisfaction of sexual inclinations, and the formation of an intimate union between husband and wife. As divinely instituted, marriage has a specific nature. Inasmuch as marriage has a nature, men and women are not free to define what marriage is. Men and women are at liberty to enter into marriage with a particular person by a free will decision, but not to choose to define the nature of marriage. Marriage as a sacrament is claimed to be "the principle and foundation of domestic society" and "a truly great sacrament of the New Law" (Pius XI, 1930, §1). To consider marriage as a sacrament is to recognize it as a graced state in which the grace of the sacrament perfects the natural condition of marriage in order to direct the spouses to the attainment of their proper supernatural end.

Procreation and the education of children is designated the primary end of marriage "[t]he primary end of marriage is the procreation and the education of children" (Pius XI, 1930, §17).[12] From its sacramental character flow the indissolubility and firmness of marriage and the sanctification – the interior formation – of husband and wife. The intimate union of husband

and wife in matrimony is a joining of souls and bodies, "the souls of the contracting parties are joined together more directly and more intimately than their bodies" (Pius XI, 1930, §7). What is being maintained here is that marriage involves not just a bodily union but the union of two persons brought together by a free, firm, deliberate act of their wills. Moreover, *Casti connubii* maintains that this blending of life as a whole is "[t]he chief reason and purpose" of the sacrament of matrimony.

> This mutual molding of husband and wife, this determined effort to perfect each other, can in a very real sense, as the Roman Catechism teaches, be said to be the chief reason and purpose of matrimony, provided matrimony be looked at not in the restricted sense as instituted for the proper conception and education of the child, but more widely as the blending of life as a whole and the mutual interchange and sharing thereof.
>
> (Pius XI, 1930, §24)

Note here that the procreative end is designated as following from a restrictive understanding of the nature of marriage. The blending of the lives of the spouses is described as a broader "more widely" understanding. Secondary ends such as "mutual aid, the cultivating of mutual love, and the quieting of concupiscence [are permissible] so long as they are subordinated to the primary end and so long as the intrinsic nature of the act is preserved" (Pius XI, 1930, §59).

Casti connubii presents a layered treatment of the goods of marriage.[13] It does not limit the specification to the physical good but adds the layer of rational and spiritual good. Moreover, it does not stop with a natural good but adds the layer of the supernatural good. Physical, rational, and spiritual are held together as related and appropriately dispositive to human formation and human dignity. The natural and the supernatural are similarly held together as dispositive and perfective. This integration is important to the articulation of the essential nature of marriage in *Casti connubii*. The good of children is claimed as the primary end of marriage. This claim is not limited to the physical existence of children but to their nurturing including their religious and spiritual development. The good of the faithful relationship between husband and wife includes the physical union, mutual affection, and their advance in grace.

The operant understanding of marriage in *Casti connubii* remains that of marriage as a procreative institution, that is, as an institution in which the partners accept their role as cooperators with God in the task of procreation. Sexual relations are permissible as a means of cultivating friendship and love. While Pius XI continues to speak of the human good in terms of the good of the body, the notion of marriage as an intimate personal union in which the husband and wife perfect themselves, each other, and their marriage – "the blending of life as a whole and the mutual interchange and sharing thereof" – appears in inchoate form in *Casti connubii*.

In response to the questions at hand, *Casti connubii* maintains that conjugal intercourse is the marriage act; it has an intrinsic nature which directs and sets limits to its engagement. It is not to be engaged in outside of marriage even to attain the procreative good. That would violate the faithful union of the spouses. The primary end of conjugal intercourse is procreation and education of children. It is permissible to avoid procreation by abstinence from or continence in sexual relations between husband and wife. The use of artificial contraceptives in marriage is impermissible as a violation of the procreative end of marriage. Every act of conjugal intercourse must respect the "intrinsic nature of the act" understood primarily as procreative. The understanding of the conjugal act as necessarily unitive has limited application here.

(b) The explication of the nature of marriage during the long pontificate of Pope Pius XII (1939–1958) is presented, for the most part, in his Allocutions.[14] While there is considerable continuity in the tradition from Pius XI to Pius XII, there is also development of the tradition as new issues came to the fore and as advances in medical knowledge and technology continued. In statements from early in his pontificate, there is simple continuity with the tradition. Marriage is regarded as a procreative institution, and conjugal intercourse is regarded as primarily a procreative act. This is consistent with the 1917 Code of Canon Law. There is recognition that there are two ends of conjugal intercourse, a procreative end and a unitive, but the procreative end is treated as primary and controlling. In his 1951 *Address to the Midwives*, he reiterated his decree of 1944 and offered the following:

> [T]he appeal of certain modern writers who deny that the procreation and education of the child is the primary end of marriage, or teach that secondary ends are not essentially subordinate to the primary end, but rather are of equal value and are independent of it, cannot be admitted.
>
> (Pius XII, October 29, 1951a, Address to the Midwives)

The scientific and medical development of artificial insemination and *in vitro* fertilization presented a new issue. In as much as this new technology serves the procreative end of marriage, perhaps approval might be possible. Upon analysis, however, Pius XII concluded that it violated the unitive dimension of marriage and of conjugal intercourse. Here, the essential nature of marriage as a union is determinative. In his address to the Congress of Italian Urologists, he offered the following:

> But the Church has likewise rejected the opposite attitude which would pretend to separate, in generation, the biological activity in the personal relation of the married couple. The child is the fruit of the conjugal union when that union finds its full expression by bringing into play the organic functions, the associated sensible emotions, and the spirited and disinterested love which animates the union. It is in the unity of the human act that we should consider the biological conditions of generation. Never is it permitted to separate these various aspects to the positive exclusion either of the procreative intention or of the conjugal relationship.
>
> (Pius XII, September 30, 1954, Address to the 26th Congress of the Italian Society of Urologists)

The fullest expression of conjugal intercourse is understood to include the realization of all its ends as appropriate of complex humans as physical, rational, and spiritual beings. Note the multiple goods specified here, namely, "sensible emotions and spiritual and disinterested love which animates the union" and "the child as fruit of the conjugal union." While artificial insemination intends the good of procreation, the good is accomplished outside the act of conjugal intercourse which unites the spouses. Furthermore, if the source of the gametes is other than the spouses, the act, even while procreative, violates the marital union itself. Artificial insemination was assessed by the Pontiff as an evil; it was found to violate the personalist, relational, unitive aspects of marriage.

Another question that arose during the pontificate of Pius XII regarded sterilization that resulted from procedures such as hysterectomy or orchiectomy. The moral question was whether these medical procedures were simply to be regarded as forms of direct mutilation, and therefore morally impermissible, or whether there were certain circumstances under which they could be permitted as indirect mutilation with the application of the principle of totality and the principle of double effect.[15] In the presence of diseased organs where their continued presence in the body posed a lethal threat to the person, the straight forward application of the principle of totality would apply. These medical questions, including that of cosmetic surgery, lobotomy, and organ transplantation – both live and cadaveric – brought Pius XII to a more careful consideration of the different circumstances under which the principle of totality does and does not apply.

In the developing trend in the thought of Pius XII, there is an increasingly clear articulation of marriage as a procreative union. Conjugal intercourse, the marriage act, is both procreative and unitive. Procreation outside the marital union is not morally permissible. At this point, it becomes increasingly clear that both ends are morally governing. Throughout his pontificate, Pius XII, in addressing the notion of the human good, spoke repeatedly and explicitly of the good of the whole person. The nature of the whole person – physical, rational, and spiritual – rather than simply the biology of the body came to be regarded as governing. There are occasional references to marriage as a special kind of human relationship and marriage begins to be considered a procreative union with two distinct ends, procreation and union. The development of his thoughts on marriage, articulated within the background of advancing science and technology which required further moral consideration, provides an example of the development of Church teaching.

(c) The question of the nature of marriage was revisited in the Second Vatican Council convened by Pope John XXIII (1958–1963) in 1962. While the Council did address the essential nature of marriage in *Gaudium et Spes*, the Holy Father removed from conciliar deliberations specific questions about the regulation of reproduction in the presence of new technologies such as oral contraceptives. A period of intense discussion of the nature of marriage, its goods, and the regulation of its goods followed. This section addresses first the appointment of the Commission established by John XXIII in 1963, then the document *Gaudium et Spes* issued by the Council in 1965, and finally the two reports of the Papal Commission sent to Pope Paul VI in 1966.

(c-i) Work of the Commission: Pope John

Pope John XXIII delegated the special questions about the regulation of reproduction in the presence of new technologies to a special commission – The Pontifical Commission for the Study of Problems of the Family, Population, and Birth Rate – appointed by him in March of 1963. The new Commission had just six members. Their first meetings were held on October 12–13, 1963 just four months after the death of John XXIII on June 3, 1963. Cardinal Montini succeeded as Pope Paul VI on June 21, 1963. He continued the work of the Commission. The Commission met five times over a period of three years from 1963 until 1966. Over that period, the membership of the Commission grew from the original 6 members appointed by Pope John XXIII to 72 members. From the beginning, there were lay members as well as clergy. Among the clergy were cardinals, bishops, and priests. By profession, the membership included theologians, physicians, sociologists, demographers, diplomats, professors, pastors, and administrators. While the overwhelming majority of members were male, there were several women members, two of whom joined their husbands on the Commission. For the final meetings in June 1966, a group of 16 members of the hierarchy – cardinals and bishops – were appointed as official members of the Commission. The function of the lay members remained advisory.

(c-ii) The Work of Vatican II:

On December 7, 1965, Pope Paul VI (1963–1978) promulgated the conciliar document *Gaudium et Spes* – the Pastoral Constitution on the Church in the Modern World. This major document of the Council, while not addressing the question of the regulation of birth, did address marriage. *Gaudium et Spes* reiterates the claim that marriage has an essential nature with a specific set of ends as procreative, unitive, and sacramental. However, there is an explicit emphasis on the essence of marriage as an intimate partnership of marital life and love rather than considering marriage primarily as a procreative institution. Among the significant teachings of *Gaudium et spes*, the following are included: (1) the essential nature of marriage, (2) the specific ends of marriage, (3) the role of conjugal intercourse, (4) responsible parenthood, and (5) respect for the tradition. In regard to the first, the claim that marriage has an essential nature persists. However, there is explicit emphasis on the essence of marriage as an intimate partnership of marital life and love, rather than the consideration of marriage, exclusively, as a procreative institution. Marriage is described as a covenant between two persons in which there is a mutual giving and accepting of persons. The human person, not the body, is offered and received. The claim that the conjugal union that is a particular marriage persists even when there are no children echoes the similar claim of *Casti connubii* and is consistent with other teachings in the tradition. In regard to the second, union and procreation continue to be acknowledged as the ends of marriage. However, the ends and purposes of marriage are no longer designated as primary or secondary. There appears no hierarchical structure of values and no subordination of ends and purposes. In regard to the third, conjugal intercourse as an expression of marital love is valued in itself. Conjugal intercourse does not need a special motive beyond that of marital love, such as procreation or remediation of concupiscence, to give it moral character. In addition, there is an explicit recognition of the role of conjugal intercourse in the nurturing of the marital union. Fidelity and indissolubility appear as requirements and characteristics of the marriage considered as an intimate union in which the perfection of the partners is to be realized, rather than as a requirement of marriage as a procreative union. Understood in this latter sense, marriage would seem to require only a relative indissolubility, lasting as long as the children remain children, that is, they are dependent. In regard to the fourth, the opportunity to procreate, which emphasizes human creative power, is characterized as an act in collaboration with God. Procreation and education are acts marked by special dignity. In procreation and education, the parents are carriers and imitators of the love of God. However, this opportunity carries with it the obligation that it be exercised consciously, responsibly, and generously. The decision regarding the number of children is, ultimately, the prudential judgment of the parents. Finally, the teachings of the tradition exercise a limiting function on the manner of exercising control of the number of children.

(c-iii) Completion of the Work of the Pontifical Commission for the Study of the Problems of Population, Family, and Births: Pope Paul

Pope Paul VI continued to examine the teaching of the tradition in regard to the nature of marriage and the accomplishment of its ends. He continued the work of the Commission appointed by his predecessor and he expanded its membership. The expanded Pontifical Commission continued its deliberations through 1966. At the final meeting on June 24, 1966, the official members[16] – the 15 members of the hierarchy present and voting – of the Commission addressed three questions: (1) Is contraception intrinsically evil? (2) Is contraception in basic continuity with the tradition? and (3) Should the magisterium speak on this question? To the first question – the intrinsic evil of contraception – nine bishops (Doepfner, Suenens, Lefebvre, Dearden, Dupuy, Pulido-Méndez, Shehan, Zoa, and Ruess) voted no, that is, contraception is not an intrinsically evil act; three bishops (Ottaviani, Colombo, and Morris) voted yes, that is, contraception is an intrinsically evil act (one with reservations); and three (Heenan, Gracias, and Binz) abstained. Cardinal Wojtyla, having been refused permission from the Polish government to travel to the meetings of the Commission, did not vote. To the second question, that of continuity with the tradition, the reported vote was nine yes, five no, and one abstention. To the third question, that of the magisterium's addressing the question, the reported vote was 14 yes and 1 no. At this final meeting, the majority of bishops and cardinals who constituted the official commission were reported as having given assent to the report, now designated the Majority Report, of the Commission. On June 28, 1966, the Holy Father received the Majority Report of the Pontifical Commission.[17] On July 1, 1966, the Holy Father received the Minority Report of the Commission.[18]

(d) On July 25, 1968, Pope Paul VI issued the encyclical *Humanae vitae*. The encyclical begins by acknowledging key components of the historical situation such as population growth, the scarcity of resources, the dignity of women, and the growth of human control over various aspects of life. The encyclical reiterated the claim of the two essential aspects of marriage as procreation and union and it reaffirmed the essential act of marriage as conjugal intercourse. It speaks of marriage as a union of spouses, as a union bringing forth new life, and as a representation of the union of Christ and the Church. Married love is described as having four characteristics: it is free; it is total; it is fruitful; it is faithful (Paul VI, 1968, §9). The language of primary and secondary ends is not found in *Humanae vitae*. The central position of the Holy Father is set forth in the claim that there is an indissoluble connection between the unitive signification and the procreative signification of the conjugal act. *Humanae vitae* offers the following:

> The Church, nevertheless, in urging men to the observance of the precepts of the natural law, which it interprets by its constant doctrine, teaches that each and every marital act must of necessity retain its intrinsic relationship to the procreation of human life.
>
> This particular doctrine, often expounded by the magisterium of the Church, is based on the inseparable connection, established by God, which man on his own initiative may not break, between the unitive significance and the procreative significance which are both inherent to the marriage act.
>
> (Paul VI, 1968, §11–12)

Here is the rejection of the claim proffered by the Majority Report that the ends of marriage are to be accomplished from within the totality of marriage rather than in every act of conjugal intercourse. This indissoluble connection is so binding that its deliberate sundering is forbidden. Every act of conjugal intercourse must convey unitive and procreative significance. "Similarly excluded is any action which either before, at the moment of, or after sexual intercourse, is specifically intended to prevent procreation – whether as an end or as a means" (Paul VI, 1968, §14).

While the Holy Father did not give an extended treatment to the rejection of the claim of the Commission that the two ends of marriage were to be accomplished over the totality of the marriage rather than in every single act of conjugal intercourse, he gestured to the development of the principle of totality as found in Note 3 of Pius XII's address *To Participants In The VIII Congress Of The World Medical Association* on September 30, 1954. (Chapter 2, D-7 develops the principle of totality.) The apothegm no conception without intercourse and no intercourse without conception became the repetitive summary of *Humanae vitae*.

(e) Post *Humanae vitae*: Following *Humanae vitae*, there was a period of both intense significant dissent from the teaching of the document and as well intense significant support for the claims of *Humanae vitae*. The dissent continues, as scholarly debate[19] – both in the larger Catholic community and here between the theologian author and the philosopher author – and in the practical realm of the lives of married Catholics. The dissent has been well documented and, while noted, will not be treated here. The most significant support of *Humanae vitae* came from Pope John Paul II, who in a series of homilies (from 1979 through 1984) on marriage, offered an enrichment of the teaching on marriage rooted in Scripture and natural law by tying it to the central mysteries of the tradition. Those mysteries are the Trinity, the Cross, the Eucharist, and salvation history. This work has become known as his *Theology of the Body.* A brief essay by the theologian author of this book on the *Theology of the Body* is appended here in Endnote 20.[20] The position of the philosopher author can be found in Endnote 29 and in her book, *Marriage as a Relationship: Real and Rational,* which presents the position that the marital union as itself a union in being and hence the relevant ethical entity.

(f) The 1987 Instruction *Donum vitae*: *The Instruction on Respect for Human Life in Its Origin and on the Dignity of Procreation* was prepared by the Congregation for the Doctrine of the Faith under the direction of its prefect, Joseph Cardinal Ratzinger (later Pope Benedict XVI). The primary purpose of *Donum vitae* was to apply the principle of inseparability to new technologies, such as *in vitro* fertilization and embryo transfer, surrogacy, and gamete intrafallopian transfer. Significant conclusions of *Donum vitae* in regard to reproduction are the following. First, heterologous artificial insemination is forbidden. Second, surrogate motherhood is forbidden. Both of these involve third-party intrusion into the union constituted by the marriage partners. Third, the procedure of homologous artificial fertilization and embryo transfer (IVF-ET) is forbidden. IVF-ET is claimed (a) to be an instance of third-party intrusion – here the doctors and scientists – into the marriage; (b) it is accomplished outside the bodies of the marriage partners; (c) it violates the inseparability principle; (d) it is an instance in which technology dominates rather than serves the human good; and (e) it is violative of the special dignity of the transmission of human life. Fourth, some forms of assistance, such as gamete intrafallopian transfer (GIFT), are permissible provided that the procedure is one that facilitates the accomplishment of the inseparable goods of union and procreation of the marriage. The defense of the inseparability principle, that is reproduction as inseparable from marriage and as inseparable from every instance of conjugal intercourse of the couple,[21] is rooted in the dignity of the parents and the child. In regard to the benefits of the inseparability of reproduction from marriage, *Donum vitae* says,

> The fidelity of the spouses in the unity of marriage involves reciprocal respect of their right to become a father and a mother only through each other. The child has the right to be conceived, carried in the womb, brought into the world and brought up within marriage: it is through the secure and recognized relationship to his own parents that the child

> can discover his own identity and achieve his own proper human development. The parents find in their child a confirmation and completion of their reciprocal self-giving: the child is the living image of their love, the permanent sign of their conjugal union, the living and indissoluble concrete expression of their paternity and maternity. (35) By reason of the vocation and social responsibilities of the person, the good of the children and of the parents contributes to the good of civil society; the vitality and stability of society require that children come into the world within a family and that the family be firmly based on marriage. The tradition of the Church and anthropological reflection recognize in marriage and in its indissoluble unity the only setting worthy of truly responsible procreation.
>
> (*Donum vitae*, 1987, §II, A, 1)

In regard to the inseparable connection of the goods of procreation and union in each act of conjugal intercourse, *Donum vitae* says,

> The moral value of the intimate link between the goods of marriage and between the meanings of the conjugal act is based upon the unity of the human being, a unity involving body and spiritual soul. (42) Spouses mutually express their personal love in the "language of the body", which clearly involves both "spousal meanings" and parental ones. (43) The conjugal act by which the couple mutually express their self-gift at the same time expresses openness to the gift of life. It is an act that is inseparably corporal and spiritual. It is in their bodies and through their bodies that the spouses consummate their marriage and are able to become father and mother. In order to respect the language of their bodies and their natural generosity, the conjugal union must take place with respect for its openness to procreation; and the procreation of a person must be the fruit and the result of married love. The origin of the human being thus follows from a procreation that is "linked to the union, not only biological but also spiritual, of the parents, made one by the bond of marriage". (44) Fertilization achieved outside the bodies of the couple remains by this very fact deprived of the meanings and the values which are expressed in the language of the body and in the union of human persons.
>
> (*Donum vitae*, 1987, §II, B4b)

(g) Pope John Paul II: In all of his writings on marriage and the family, Pope John Paul II maintained the focus on the family as grounded in marriage as a *consortium totius vitae* – a partnership of the whole of life. Family and marriage, love and life are inseparable. In 1981 in the Apostolic

Exhortation *Familiaris consortio*, John Paul II wrote that conjugal love "does not end with the couple . . . The couple in giving themselves to one another, give not just themselves, but also the reality of children" (*Fc*, 1981, §96). The gift of self in love has spousal meaning and parental responsibility. This meaning requires respect for the biological laws inscribed in the persons of the spouses. Here, the Holy Father repeated the claim of the inseparability of procreation and union in every conjugal act. He wrote:

> When couples, by means of recourse to contraception, separate these two meanings that God the Creator has inscribed in the being of man and woman and in the dynamism of their sexual communion, they act as 'arbiters' of the Divine plan and they 'manipulate' and degrade human sexuality – and with it themselves and their married partner – by altering its value of 'total' self-giving. Thus the innate language that expresses the total reciprocal self-giving of husband and wife is overlaid, through contraception, by an objectively contradictory language, namely, that of not giving oneself totally to the other. This leads not only to a positive refusal to be open to life but also to a falsification of the inner truth of conjugal love, which is called upon to give itself in personal totality.
> (*Familiaris consortio*, 1981, §32)

This claim remains a persistent theme throughout his papacy. In his encyclical *Evangelium vitae,* John Paul II states that contraception "contradicts the full truth of the sexual act as the proper expression of conjugal love" (*Ev*, 1995, §13). He also repeats the claim of the connection between contraception and abortion that appeared in the Minority Report that followed the work of the Pontifical Commission for the Study of the Problems of Population, Family, and Births.[22] Here, the Holy Father says that despite the differences in both the nature and the moral gravity of abortion and contraception, they,

> [A]re often closely connected, as fruits of the same tree. It is true that in many cases contraception and even abortion are practised under the pressure of real-life difficulties, which nonetheless can never exonerate from striving to observe God's law fully. Still, in very many other instances such practices are rooted in a hedonistic mentality unwilling to accept responsibility in matters of sexuality, and they imply a self-centered concept of freedom, which regards procreation as an obstacle to personal fulfilment. The life which could result from a sexual encounter thus becomes an enemy to be avoided at all costs, and abortion becomes the only possible decisive response to failed contraception.
> (*Evangelium vitae*, 1995, §13)

As a consequence, all procedures, whether to accomplish or avoid the reproductive purpose, that are (a) inconsistent with respect for life and bodily integrity; (b) inconsistent with respect for the family and respect for the origin of the child; or (c) inconsistent with respect for the integrity of human sexuality are not morally acceptable.

(h) Pope Benedict XVI: In 2008, during the pontificate of Pope Benedict XVI, the Congregation for the Doctrine of the Faith issued *Dignitas personae*, an instruction on certain questions that had arisen as a consequence of new technologies that had been developed to assist reproduction. From within the matrix of the teaching of the tradition on marriage, *Dignitas personae* maintained that aid to the conjugal act to achieve reproduction is permitted and surgeries to remove obstacles in the anatomical structures that are required to accomplish conception are permitted. Among the interventions that are forbidden as violative, the understanding of marriage and the respect for human life are the following: (a) heterologous artificial insemination as a violation of the marital union; (b) homologous artificial insemination in those instances in which technology replaces the conjugal act; (c) *in vitro* fertilization as violative of the integral unity of the marriage act and embryo freezing or destruction as violative of the respect owed to the human embryos; (d) intracytoplasmic sperm injection as the separation of procreation from a discrete conjugal act and as the interjection and domination of technology; (e) freezing of oocytes; (f) embryo reduction is understood as a killing of a human being; and (g) cloning as somatic cell nuclear transfer.

In his 2009, encyclical *Caritas in veritate*, Pope Benedict XVI, while focusing on evangelization propelled by the gospel of love as the vehicle for the linked advancement of the society and the individual, briefly alludes to the essential role of marriage as understood in the encyclical *Humanae vitae* of Pope Paul VI. Benedict acknowledges that marriage between a man and a woman is the foundational institution for the flourishing of society. He reiterates the traditional understanding of the unitive and procreative meaning of marriage in which "the married couple, man and woman, who accept one another mutually, in distinction and in complementarity: a couple, therefore, that is open to life" (*Caritas in veritate*, 2009, §15).

(i) Pope Francis: In his 2016 apostolic exhortation, *Amoris laetitia*, Pope Francis presents an extended reflection on the essential nature of marriage and as well a pastoral reflection on the good and the struggles of marriage. In that reflection, he presents an understanding of marriage as an icon of the Trinity – "an image of God, who is a communion of persons" (*Amoris laetitia*, 2016, §71) and again in the mystery of marriage, "God makes of the two spouses one single existence" (*Amoris laetitia*, 2016, §121). The isomorphism between the reality of the Trinity and its replication in marriage is conveyed in two distinct understandings. One is the father, mother, and their child; the other is the husband and wife and their union of love, friendship, and grace. In regard to the former, the fecundity of marriage is realized in the child; in regard to the latter, the fruitfulness of marriage is realized in the union – the marriage bond as reality and sacrament. In his treatment of the goods of marriage, the Holy Father reiterates the teaching set forth in the work of the Second Vatican Council in its Pastoral Constitution on the Church in the Modern World, *Gaudium et Spes,* that conjugal intercourse is

> 'ordered to procreation by its very nature'. . . the child who is born 'does not come from outside as something added on to the mutual love of the spouses, but springs from the very heart of that mutual giving, as its fruit and fulfillment.'
>
> (*Amoris laetitia*, 2016, §80)

He also repeats here the claim that appeared in the 1968 encyclical *Humanae vitae* in these words: "no genital act of husband and wife can refuse this meaning [procreation], even when for various reasons it may not always in fact beget a new life" (*Amoris laetitia*, 2016).

In this expansive understanding, the Holy Father also repeats the position set forth in *Gaudium et Spes*, "marriage was not instituted solely for the procreation of children . . . marriage still retains its character of being a whole manner and communion of life and preserves its value and indissolubility" (*Amoris laetitia*, 2016,§125, §178). In his treatment of marriage as a union, the Holy Father writes of the affection, the tenderness, the friendship, the passion, and the all-encompassing love of the spouses for each other. Again returning to *Gaudium et Spes,* the Holy Father maintains that conjugal love

> embraces the good of the whole person; it can enrich the sentiments of the spirit and their physical expression with a unique dignity and ennoble them as the special features and manifestation of the friendship proper to marriage . . . love lacking either pleasure or passion is insufficient to symbolize the union of the human heart with God.
>
> (*Amoris laetitia*, 2016, §142)

In *Amoris laetitia*, Pope Francis also has a special eye on the struggles that people experience as they try to live this teaching on marriage and family life. Picking up on the pastoral dimensions of *Familiaris consortio*, Pope Francis constantly reiterates the relation between (a) the fullness of Church teaching, (b) the complex situations in which people – living in a world marked by sin – find themselves, and (c) the path from those complex situations into the fullness that the Lord intends for marriage and family life.[23] As he draws near to the end of the letter, the Holy Father draws his thoughts together in this way:

> In order to avoid all misunderstanding, I would point out that in no way must the Church desist from proposing the full ideal of marriage, God's plan in all its grandeur . . . To show understanding in the face of exceptional situations never implies dimming the light of the fuller ideal, or proposing less than what Jesus offers to the human being . . . At the same time, from our awareness of the weight of mitigating circumstances – psychological, historical and even biological – it follows that "without detracting from the evangelical ideal, there is a need to accompany with mercy and patience the eventual stages of personal growth as these progressively appear.
>
> (*Amoris laetitia*, 2016, §307, §308)

In summary, the essential elements in the tradition as developed from Pope Pius XI to Pope Francis are (1) marriage is an intimate partnership of love and life; (2) the essential act of marriage is conjugal intercourse; it is the sign which signifies and contains the reality that is marriage; (3) there are two essential aspects of marriage – procreation and union; (4) there is an indissoluble connection between the unitive signification and the procreative signification in the conjugal act; (5) reproduction is to be accomplished only within marriage and only within an individual act of conjugal intercourse; and (6) every act of conjugal intercourse must signify procreation and union.

To provide Catholic institutions, health care providers and, as well, Catholic people in the United States with a set of guidelines to govern the reproductive finality, as well as the whole series of contemporary medical issues as noted throughout this book, the United States Conference of Catholic Bishops examined the issues in *Ethical and Religious Directives for Catholic Health Care Services*. The document was framed from within the magisterial understanding of the nature of marriage as developed in the documents of the tradition. The sixth iteration was issued in 2018; Directives 38–42 focus on issues of assisted reproduction.

> 38. When the marital act of sexual intercourse is not able to attain its procreative purpose, assistance that does not separate the unitive and procreative ends of the act, and does not substitute for the marital act itself, may be used to help married couples conceive.
> 39. Those techniques of assisted conception that respect the unitive and procreative meanings of sexual intercourse and do not involve

the destruction of human embryos, or their deliberate generation in such numbers that it is clearly envisaged that all cannot implant and some are simply being used to maximize the chances of others implanting, may be used as therapies for infertility.

40. Heterologous fertilization (that is, any technique used to achieve conception by the use of gametes coming from at least one donor other than the spouses) is prohibited because it is contrary to the covenant of marriage, the unity of the spouses, and the dignity proper to parents and the child.
41. Homologous artificial fertilization (that is, any technique used to achieve conception using the gametes of the two spouses joined in marriage) is prohibited when it separates procreation from the marital act in its unitive significance (e.g., any technique used to achieve extracorporeal conception).
42. Because of the dignity of the child and of marriage, and because of the uniqueness of the mother–child relationship, participation in contracts or arrangements for surrogate motherhood is not permitted. Moreover, the commercialization of such surrogacy denigrates the dignity of women, especially the poor.

Assistance to married couples in attaining the reproductive finality of marriage is permitted so long as the assistance respects the inseparable bond between the procreative end of marriage and the unitive end of marriage (Directive 38). The nature of marriage, as a union between one man and one woman and a union within which children are to be born, requires that the gametes must be the gametes of the couple who are united in a specific marriage act (Directives 40–42). Heterologous fertilization of any sort is forbidden as a violation of the unity of marriage. Directive 40 forbids heterologous fertilization as "contrary to the covenant of marriage, the unity of the spouses, and the dignity proper to parents and the child." The directives, recognizing the human embryo as a living, developing human being, proscribe any reproductive assistance that involves the direct destruction of embryos. The intentional destruction of the embryo is regarded as the direct taking of human life and, hence, a species of homicide. In addition, the directives forbid the use of any reproductive techniques that involve the production of embryos without the intention of implanting the embryos. Surrogacy is forbidden as violative of the unity of marriage. Surrogacy is assessed as third-party intrusion by the gestational mother and by technicians and as violative of the unique relationship of mother and child. Commercial surrogacy is viewed as violative of the dignity of women especially of poor women inasmuch as it views women as objects for reproduction and as it presents an occasion for poor women to exchange the use of their bodies for money (Directive 42).

(E) Particular Ethical and Practical Issues

In addition to the violation of religious principles of the Catholic tradition, there are other harms, some potential and some real, as the accomplishment or avoidance of reproduction is pursued in the contemporary culture which accepts scientific progress and human desires as the only significant criteria in limiting human behavior.

The legalization of elective abortion in the United States, from 1973 to 2022, and its continuation in many States as a means of birth control has resulted in the destruction of, on average, a million conceived and developing human lives per year – the total now exceeds 60 million. The rise in the use of ultrasound technology for pregnant women and the consequent increased awareness of the reality of the life developing within her body have brought about a slight decline in the total number of elective abortions, but an increase in the number of elective abortions for specific conditions such as Down syndrome. Notwithstanding its legalization, elective abortion remains a solution of a human problem by killing another human being without sufficient proportionate reason. While some women view this access to abortion as a means of personal liberation, others carry emotional scars that last a lifetime.[24]

The easy access to contraceptive devices has, on the one hand, permitted married couples the ability to regulate conception with greater certainty, but on the other hand, has spawned a culture of casual sex and sexual intercourse outside of marriage. The visible consequences of the latter include the increase in sexually transmitted diseases, children born outside of marriage, and the phenomenon of the single-parent family. The less visible effects include (1) the objectification of both men and women as merely means to satisfy the sexual appetites of others, (2) the emotional damage to the used men and women, and (3) the stunting of development of the higher human faculties as the pursuit of sexual pleasure takes control.

While there have been significant advances in the practices and the success of artificial reproductive technologies (ARTs) toward the goal of pregnancy and live birth, there remain serious concerns about these practices. The concerns include risks to the intended offspring, to the women involved in the procedures, to the family, and to the society.

Since the regulation of ART procedures remains, for the most part, under the auspices of the medical profession, it has been assumed that the standards of the medical profession guide these practices. The Society for Assisted Reproductive Technology (SART) and the American Society for Reproductive Medicine (ASRM) represent the efforts of the profession to ensure safe, successful, and ethical practices. The SART site reports that 80% of fertility clinics are associated with the organization. The federal government through the office of the Food and Drug Agency (FDA) at 21CFR884 lists a set of regulations governing the use of devices and accessories associated with the process. The federal government through the Center for Disease Control (CDC) assisted by the American Society for Reproductive Medicine (ASRM) and the Society for Assisted Reproductive Technology (SART) collects data that are submitted by facilities that are associated with those professional associations. In its 2017 report of data collected in 2014, SART reported the percentages of children born as a percentage of cycles attempted rather than patient numbers at term, preterm, and very preterm across the various procedures available for women at specific age ranges at its member clinics. The percentage of preterm and very preterm infants born as a result of assisted reproductive technologies was significantly greater than the national average for all premature births reported by the CDC at 10% in 2014 with a slight increase in 2015. Premature births of less than 37 weeks gestation coupled with low birth weights of less than 2,500 grams show a high correlation as predictors of developmental delays. The CDC in its *Child Health USA 2104* Report offered the following:

> Babies born preterm (before 37 completed weeks of gestation) or at low birth weight (less than 2,500 grams or 5.5 pounds) are at increased risk of immediate life-threatening health problems as well as long-term complications and developmental delays. Complications that can occur during the newborn period include respiratory distress, jaundice, anemia, and infection. Long-term complications can include learning and behavioral problems, cerebral palsy, lung problems, and vision and hearing loss.
>
> (https://mchb.hrsa.gov/chusa14/health-status-behaviors/infants/preterm-birth-low-birth.html)

The same CDC Report estimated that there is a heavy societal toll attached to the incidence of preterm birth and low birth weight with "the annual economic burden related to preterm birth estimated to exceed $26 billion, including costs for medical care and early intervention as well as lost productivity due to disabling conditions" (https://mchb.hrsa.gov/chusa14/health-status-behaviors/infants/preterm-birth-low-birth.html). Neither the CDC nor SART studies short-term or long-term effects including any cognitive, developmental, or physical impairments or delays for children produced by the assisted reproductive processes.

Among the problems that arise in *in vitro* fertilization and embryo transfer, in addition to the possible physical harm to the individual embryo produced, are the possibility of multiple fetuses and ectopic pregnancies.

Both of these present serious survival complications for the fetus and potential serious medical complications for the mother. In addition, a significant issue arises in the processes which involve the union of egg and sperm and multiple embryo production in the laboratory. If the embryo is a living, developing human being, then it is not surplus material to be frozen, to be donated, to be sold, to be destroyed, or to be the subject of an experiment. It is a human subject with all the same rights and protections as other human subjects. The embryo, then, must be accorded the same respect given to all other human beings. Chapter 4, on the beginning of life, developed and supported the position that the embryo is a living developing human being. Inasmuch as that is the case, the embryo may not be destroyed or sold or given away. In the early days of IVF-ET, principled fertility centers limited the availability of assisted reproductive technologies to marriages deemed reasonably stable; they limited the production of embryos to the number that might be safely implanted and carried to term; and, because they recognized the embryo as a living developing human being, they implanted all the embryos produced. There were no surplus or spare embryos.

The use of hormonal hyper-stimulation of the ovaries of women and the possibility of the production of multiple fetuses presents another significant problem both for mother and for fetus. If too many fetuses result, the life of the mother may be at risk. There have been reported cases of pregnancies involving five or more fetuses. In the recent past, reproductive centers aimed for two pregnancies and recommended fetal reduction, if more than two pregnancies occur. At present, because of potential risks associated with twin births, reproductive centers are inclining toward the conception of one child. The very neutral language of fetal reduction tends to hide the fact that fetal reduction is the killing of a fetus usually by a chemical injection. The process in which one fetus is selected and killed sometimes causes miscarriage with the unintended and undesired effect of the death of all the fetuses. In multiple pregnancies, the fetus is at risk of direct destruction or of unintentional death if the uterus of the woman is incapable of carrying the fetuses to term or, perhaps, at risk for impairment of this new life which may be physical or cognitive if the womb is unable to be a sufficiently suitable environment for all the fetuses.

Finally, there are the social justice issues. There is a natural inclination – a real and deep longing – to want children and to desire children of one's own family line. But, if natural conception is not possible, is the use of reproductive technologies the only answer? Is it the best answer? The use of reproductive technologies represents a considerable economic investment. The costs vary as the process is more complicated and as multiple procedures are required. The cost of oocytes may be as much as $25,000.

Sperm, because they are more easily retrieved and more numerous, are relatively cheap. So the cost to produce "my child" may exceed $100,000 and the money may be spent without success. Most fertility clinics report a less than 20% success rate where success is defined as delivery of a child. In a first world country where so many children are hungry and abused, in a developing world where so many children are dying from malnutrition and from diseases no longer present in the developed world, and in a world where the number of children orphaned by disease, desertion, and violence, including the violence of war, increases daily, might the time and energy, as well as financial and emotional resources, expended by couples to have children be directed more broadly toward rescuing one or more of these children? Might this better serve to witness the scriptural exhortation to care for "the least of these?"

Further, in a world in which there must be choices among the goods to be pursued including the good of the development of medical technology – what ends ought technology serve? When a significant percentage of physicians develop specialties tied to substantial remuneration to serve human desires rather than human needs and when significant resources of the medical community are enlisted to serve those specialties, are there pressing human needs that will remain unmet? How does a society direct its resources, including the resource of medicine? Where should the line be drawn between needs and desires?

The use of assisted reproductive technologies is not without risk even within the confines of the tradition. There are risks to both the marriage and the new human being. Children must be conceived from within the body of the marriage. There must be no third-party material assistance whether of germ material or place of maturation. The intimacy of marriage, of necessity, becomes open to the presence of technicians and scientists who have the expertise to assist the couple to attain the good of procreation. Couples must be made aware of this intrusion and take appropriate means to protect their intimacy and to protect each other. Technicians and scientists who will assist the couple must be sensitive both to the dignity of the couple and the sacredness of the new lives whose existence they, with their special technical skills, are privileged to serve.

(F) Afterword

These teachings of the tradition come under scrutiny quite regularly in their articulation and their practices by both those outside and those within the tradition. Notwithstanding the richness of the tradition, which operates from within a presumption in favor of fulfilling all the ends of conjugal intercourse in every act of conjugal intercourse, there remain challenges. Marriage is the work of a lifetime and is completed, that is consummated, only in death. Pope Francis offers the following:

> Each marriage is a kind of "salvation history," which from fragile beginnings – thanks to God's gift and a creative and generous response on our part – grows over time into something precious and enduring. . . Love is thus a kind of craftsmanship . . . At every new stage, they can keep "forming" one another. Love makes each wait for the other with the patience of a craftsman, a patience which comes from God.
>
> (*Amoris laetitia*, §211)

While the Holy Father articulates a developmental vision of marriage, he wonders if just articulating that vision is sufficient. He presents his own critique here: "[w]e have long thought that simply by stressing doctrinal, bioethical and moral issues, without encouraging openness to grace, we were providing sufficient support to families, strengthening the marriage bond and giving meaning to marital life" (*Amoris laetitia,* §37).

Among the challenges to the tradition are the following: (1) those who find that articulation peculiarly particular; (2) those who find that the application of the tradition hampers the accomplishment of important goods; (3) those who in witnessing the scandalous practices of some Catholics, even those in high office, claim that the tradition does not and cannot hold; and (4) those within the tradition who, while they affirm many of its claims in regard to the reproductive good of marriage, find the explication of the tradition incomplete.

(1) The first challenge can be found in the claim that the Roman Catholic tradition has a quite particular, even peculiar, understanding of the nature of marriage that cannot be sustained in general secular terms. Now this statement is partially right and partially wrong. Some of what the tradition has to say about marriage and the appropriate exercise of sexual intercourse can be understood as natural law claims and hence understood as human reason apprehends human nature, its goods as ends, and the reasonable accomplishment of those goods. These truths are open to reason as *recta ratio*. On the other hand, the documents of the tradition itself often speak of offering to human reason the light of Revelation. It is important to recognize that reason has its proper task and Revelation has its proper task. Once human reason has completed its work, revelation functions to inform understanding and enrich the results of reason. Moreover, if the adherents to the tradition actually live the tradition, their lives should provide powerful public witness to the soundness of its beliefs and practices.

(2) The second challenge is that the application of the tradition hampers the accomplishment of important goods. Here, critics of the tradition claim that (a) it fails to engage in practices that might prevent disease and (b) it forbids ART practices that might accomplish the good of procreation in difficult circumstances for the married couple. The first (a) is most often raised in the presence of the AIDS epidemic caused by the transmission of the HIV virus through sexual intercourse.[25] It is the case that the tradition proscribes the use of condoms prophylactically in the presence of the possibility of the transmission of potentially fatal diseases that can be spread through sexual intercourse. While on its face, this seems a hard teaching, the deeper issue is (i) the concern on the practical level for the appropriate engagement of the sexual appetite and (ii) the concern on a pedagogical level for the possibility of transforming an evil, even a lesser evil, into a good. The tradition acknowledges that the sexual appetite is good, but that appetite is to be fulfilled in an appropriately human manner, that is, as directed by reason. It is only within the faithful relationship of marriage that the fulfillment of that appetite is accomplished in a way that recognizes the human and spiritual dimensions of sexuality and the dignity of the human person. The contemporary obsession with the right to orgasm whenever, wherever, and with whomever, renders sexual intercourse banal. The widespread distribution of condoms contributes to a coarsening and routinization of sex. Recent Pontiffs have addressed this issue.[26] The proscription by the tradition found in challenge (b) in regard to the harvesting and storing of ovum and sperm for possible future procreation, understood as the primary end of marriage, in the presence of illness and treatment of those illnesses that resulted in the destruction of the gametes of one of the partners of a marriage appears harsh, especially to those couples so afflicted. While no one and no marriage can claim the right to a child, the longing for a child of one's family line is not only a strong desire but also a natural inclination whose fulfillment within marriage seems worthy of study.[27]

(3) Another challenge is rooted in the scandalous practices of some who claim to be members of and advocates for the tradition while at the same time violating the tradition. It is a valid and painful accusation against those, both lay and clerical Catholics, involved in the sexual abuses committed against vulnerable populations. These remain sinful, in some instances criminal, and in all instances a scandal perpetrated by those whose actions sully the tradition and a rebuke to those whose inaction permits the continuation of these sins and crimes. These actions diminish the possible witness of the goodness of the teaching of the tradition, but they do not change the truth of the tradition. In his assessment of the magnitude of the scandal, American Church

historian Gerald P. Fogarty, S.J. observed that he was unaware of any similar crisis in the history of the Church in America (personal communication from Fr. Fogarty to MMH).

(4) The fourth challenge is internal to the tradition and the focus here is both the affirmation and the development of the tradition. The challenge questions whether the relationship between the unitive and procreative dimensions of conjugal intercourse has been adequately rendered. Within the explicit teaching of the tradition from *Casti connubii* to the present, the claim persists that reproduction is limited to the single acts of a married couple and in every act of conjugal intercourse the possibility, the meaning, the significance, the dimension of reproduction is to be respected. Now, if this is a true understanding of the nature of marriage, that is, the correct and complete response, then assistance in reproduction is very limited, perhaps only to the GIFT procedure, and avoidance of reproduction is limited to abstinence of varying durations. This question requires repeated attention to the explication of the nature of marriage by the magisterium and theologians and, as well, concern for the proper development of doctrine.[28] Furthermore, attending this question seems an appropriate response to the renewal called for by Vatican II that the tradition be nourished by Scripture and linked to dogma, but also scientifically and philosophically grounded. While attending this question in detail would require movement beyond the scope of the expressed purpose of this text, it is appropriate to acknowledge the ongoing challenge this understanding.[29]

So while acknowledgment of the goodness of the tradition remains, there remain also the many challenges presented in the four critiques. There is no doubt that the reservation of sexual intercourse to marriage and to the partners of the marriage contributes to human flourishing for the individual, for the family, and for society. Study of the regulation of conjugal intercourse, in the presence of the magisterial teaching in the modern period, that is, from *Casti connubii* to the present, and in the presence of the practices of many contemporary Catholics, requires humility, courage, listening, and prayer.

Questions for Reflection

1. What are the significant pressures that have influenced medical science to develop assisted reproductive technologies?
2. What are the essential elements of the Catholic tradition regarding marriage that serve to guide the accomplishment or the avoidance of the reproductive finality?

3. If the claim of the inseparability of the procreative and unitive ends of conjugal intercourse is correct, what is the proper moral evaluation of the reproductive technologies listed here?

    a. Ovarian hyperstimulation
    b. Homologous insemination
    c. Heterologous insemination
    d. *In vivo* fertilization
    e. *In vitro* fertilization
    f. Gamete intrafollopian transfer (GIFT)
    g. Zygote intrafallopian transfer (ZIFT)
    h. Intracytoplasmic sperm injection (ICSI)
    i. Embryo micromanipulation
    j. Assisted hatching
    k. Traditional surrogacy
    l. Gestational surrogacy

4. Within the Catholic tradition what is the sign that signifies the meaning of marriage? What is the sign that signifies and contains the reality of marriage? What is to be understood from these signs?
5. What are the essential elements in the Catholic teaching on marriage from *Casti connubii* of Pope Pius XI to *Amoris laetitia* of Pope Francis?
6. Read Directives 38–42 in Part Four, "Issues in Care for the Beginning of Life" of the *Ethical and Religious Directives for Catholic Health Care Services*. What guidelines are set down there for married couples in accomplishing the reproductive finality of marriage?
7. What are the significant potential harms for offspring, for women, for the family, and for society in the use of ART processes?
8. What social justice issues are pressing in the development and use of ART technologies?
9. What is the best way to understand the relation between *continuity* and *development* in the Church's teaching about marriage?
10. How do the central mysteries of the faith, such as the Trinity, the Cross, and the Eucharist, interact with the natural law and the light of reason when it comes to *other* issues of philosophy and morality? How might these connections need to be made clearer in *other* areas of Catholic medical ethics (i.e., beyond just the reproductive finality)?

Notes

1 While the Psalmist's allusion to children as arrows is meant to be positive, that is children as effective and cooperative agents in a variety of projects, the child as a possible weapon of war, even a just war, is a difficult notion for parents to ponder in their hearts.

2 The delineation of the essential nature of any object, including marriage, is the response to the *Quid sit* question – the "what is" question that propels human inquiry. This method is at least as old as the Socratic elenchus. The response to the "what is" question is the engine that propels the development of understanding. Further development is had as the *An sit* question – the "is it so" question is raised. Think of the development of the understating of matter in its progression from earth, air, fire, and water to the recent account of the standard model of particle physics brought to completion in the experience of the Higgs boson. The dialectic between the *Quid sit* question and the *An sit* question was developed by Bernard Lonergan in his seminal work *Insight*.

3 If the conclusion of Chapter 4 is correct in holding that the *conceptus* is a living developing human being at an early and vulnerable stage, then this entire industry is morally problematic. It is, in essence, a form of human trafficking.

4 Here, a general point needs to be made about means and ends. Both means and ends require moral scrutiny. Some examples may be helpful. Every police officer knows that a person in the midst of the commission of a crime can be stopped by shooting the criminal. That means, in itself, does not justify shooting the criminal. There may be other means to stop the offense. Every military officer knows that when an enemy military unit embeds within a civilian population, that military unit can be defeated by bombing the entire population – combatants and noncombatants alike. Both the death penalty and life in prison are means to punish those convicted of the commission of a capital crime. Each means requires moral assessment.

5 Jacques and Raïssa Maritain. Jacques Maritain was a philosopher noted for his contributions to Catholicism in the twentieth century through his contribution to the recovery of the work of Thomas Aquinas and the development of integral Christian humanism. Raïssa was a poet and philosopher. They were French intellectuals and lay leaders in the Catholic Church in the twentieth century. They met at the Sorbonne where both were students and at a time when both were atheists. They married in 1904 and converted to Catholicism in 1906. There are fine accounts of their lives in *Jacques and Raïssa Maritain: Beggars for heaven* by Jean-Luc Barré. University of Notre Dame Press, 2005, and *We have been friends together* by Raïssa Maritain. Saint Augustine Press, 2016.

6 While all these natural family planning sites report success in their use, the population who utilize these methods is a numerically limited highly motivated group. As reported in the Marquette study, few Catholic couples, perhaps as few as 2–3%, practice natural family planning (Fehring, 177).

7 For example, see Isaiah 54, Jeremiah 2, Ezekiel 16 and 23, Hosea 1 and 2.

8 See, for example, Matthew 9:15.

9 There are similar New Testament confirmations and extensions of the Old Testament understanding of marriage in Matthew 9:15, Matthew 25:1–13, John 3:29, 2 Corinthians 11:2, Revelation 19:7, and Revelation 21:2.

10 The natural law tradition holds that marriage is like any other reality. Understanding the reality at issue develops over time while the underlying reality remains the same. The fundamental elements of the universe remain the same, while understanding of them develops over time.

11 In the summer of 1930, the Anglican Church convened its once-a-decade Lambeth Conference. Among other topics, the 1930 Lambeth Conference took up the question of contraception. In Resolution 15, the conference considered the following proposal:

> Where there is clearly felt moral obligation to limit or avoid parenthood, the method must be decided on Christian principles. The primary and obvious

> method is complete abstinence from intercourse (as far as may be necessary) in a life of discipline and self-control lived in the power of the Holy Spirit. Nevertheless in those cases where there is such a clearly felt moral obligation to limit or avoid parenthood, and where there is a morally sound reason for avoiding complete abstinence, the Conference agrees that other methods may be used, provided that this is done in the light of the same Christian principles. The Conference records its strong condemnation of the use of any methods of conception control from motives of selfishness, luxury, or mere convenience.

When the vote was taken, the final tally stood: 193 in favor and 67 opposed. Within the Anglican Conference that vote was determinative, that is, by means of the vote, Resolution 15 became official Anglican teaching. This was the first time in history that a Christian church formally addressed and approved the use of contraception.

12 The word primary appears in *Casti connubii* four times. In §17, it is used to describe procreation and education of children as the primary end of marriage. In §23, it refers to the expression of the love of husband and wife must have as its primary purpose their interior formation "that they may grow in true love toward God and their neighbor." In §59, it appears as controlling the satisfaction of secondary goods of marriage

> such as mutual aid, the cultivating of mutual love, and the quieting of concupiscence which husband and wife are not forbidden to consider so long as they are subordinated to the primary end and so long as the intrinsic nature of the act is preserved.

In §97, the power of unbridled lust is claimed as an obstacle to man's primary endeavor to subject himself to God.

13 An understanding of the nature of marriage directs the permissibility of the marriage act. Inasmuch as marital intercourse is the sign which signifies and contains the reality of marriage (the union of Christ and His Church signifies but does not contain the reality of marriage), an understanding of marital intercourse contributes to the understanding of the essential nature of marriage. Marriage and marital intercourse have a set of ends as unitive, procreative, and personalist that require actualizing and ordering on appropriate levels. Marital intercourse is always unitive, sometimes procreative, and ought always to be personalist. An understanding of these ends of marriage to be accomplished on horizontal, vertical, and transcendental levels of finality to accomplish goods that are, respectively, essential, excellent, and absolute can be found in "Finality, love, and marriage" by Bernard Lonergan, S.J. in *Collection* Ed. F.E. Crowe, S.J. Herder and Herder, 1967. This work, first published in 1943 was an attempt by Fr. Lonergan to unpack *Casti connubii.* A more recent development of this theme can be found in *Marriage as a relationship: Real and rational* by Margaret Monahan Hogan. Marquette University Press, 2002.

14 These statements did not come in papal encyclicals, which matters for the technical assessment as to the level of authority they occupy in Church teaching. But, as a matter of fact, they were important statements, which can be seen by how often they are cited in the footnotes of *Humanae vitae.*

15 The principle of totality and the principle of double effect are treated, respectively, in Chapter 2 D.5 and D.7. The principle of totality permits the removal of an organ when its presence or functioning is a danger to the organism as a whole. Its application is limited by the determination of the nature of the organism as either a physical or moral organism and the nature of the organ to

be destroyed. The principle of double effect operates in situations where there are two possible ends to a single action in which one end is intended and the other necessarily occurs but is not intended. The removal of a cancerous uterus or cancerous testes is permissible. The coercive removal of healthy organs of reproduction is impermissible. (Recall that forced sterilization for eugenic reasons was still in the historical moment for Pius XII.)

16 The lay members of the Pontifical Commission serve only in advisory roles. The official members of the Commission present at its final meeting were Doepfner, Suenens, Lefebvre, Dearden, Dupuy, Pulido-Méndez, Shehan, Zoa, Ruess, Ottaviani, Colombo, Morris, Heenan, Gracias, and Binz.

17 The Holy Father received the final report of the Pontifical Commission on June 28, 1966. The Majority Report included the assessment that the actualization of the procreative potentiality is to be understood as a requirement of the entire course of the marriage rather than a requirement of every single act of intercourse within marriage. The Report argued that the moral specification of marriage, considered as an act in itself, derives not from particular acts, that is, individual acts of conjugal intercourse, which constitute partial aspects of marriage but from the set of acts throughout the duration of the marriage. The Report claimed that it is the responsibility of married couples together to determine the appropriate size of their family and the appropriate means of birth regulation within their marriage. The Majority Report maintained that there are objective criteria to guide the spouses in the exercise of their conjugal rights. The objective criteria derive from the understanding of marriage as a union of love and life and these same criteria prohibit those activities which are egotistical, hedonistic, violative of the dignity of the spouse, or are directly abortive.

18 On July 1, 1966, a few members of the Commission presented the Pope with their own document which repudiated the findings of the Majority Report. This report, now known as the Minority Report, was presented to the Pope by Cardinal Ottaviani. The Minority Report was essentially a document written by the American Jesuit, Fr. John Ford, who had joined the Commission, along with 42 others, at the time of the fourth meeting in 1965. Ford had submitted this document earlier as a working paper to the Commission. Included among the signatories of the Minority Report were Lestapis, one of the six members of the original Commission of 1963; Visser and Zalba appointed with five others in 1964; and Ford. The Minority Report offered the following: (1) contraception within marriage is an intrinsically evil act – malice, unexcused concupiscence, disorientation; (2) there is an appropriate analogy between homicide and contraception, that is, as human life is inviolable so too is the generative process inviolable as ordered to the good of the species (§D2); (3) the uninterrupted, consistent, and perennial longevity of the teaching; (4) the authority and responsibility of the Church to teach is a power derived from Christ and is necessary to guide the faithful; and (5) the primary end of conjugal intercourse is procreation. In addition, the Minority Report addressed what it considered specific erroneous claims, for example, the meaning of natural claims and the authenticity of the magisterial teaching authority, of the Majority Report.

19 See the two statements written in anticipation of the 50th anniversary of *Humanae vitae*:

(1) Statement of the Wijngaards Institute for Catholic Research. (www.wijngaardsinstitute.com/statement-on-contraceptives) accessed 01/10/2023.

(2) *Affirmation of the Church's Teaching on the Gift of Sexuality.* https://www.catholicculture.org/culture/library/view.cfm?recnum=11380 accessed 01/10/2023.

20 What has become known as the "Theology of the Body" was delivered to 129 Wednesday audiences spread out across five years at the earliest stage of John Paul II's pontificate: (September 5, 1979–November 28, 1984). Clearly, this topic was a priority for the new pope. In some ways, the Theology of the Body was simply something on his heart and mind. In some ways, it was based on a sense that the conclusions of *Humanae Vitae* might have been better received if they were more obviously connected to the central mysteries of the faith.

Rather than giving a thorough explanation of how the Theology of the Body moves (its methodology and its five cycles), four core connections that it draws between the central mysteries of the faith and the nature of marriage are noted.

First, the Theology of the Body draws a connection between the Trinity and marriage. It begins with the biblical notion that human beings are made in the image and likeness of God, but adds that the God in whose image and likeness we are made is the Trinity. This means that relations are at the core of what it means to be human. For example, he notes: "Man became 'the image and likeness' of God not only through his own humanity, but also through the communion of persons which man and woman form from the very beginning" (Audience 9.3). In addition, the Trinity is not only a communion of persons, it is a communion of persons that brings forth life – both in the act of creation and in the life of grace.

On this basis, the Theology of the Body sets up a fundamental parallel: the Trinity is a communion of persons whose union brings forth life, and marriage is meant to be a union of persons whose union brings forth life. Note that John Paul II is not reaching any conclusions that are not already contained in Church teaching. In some ways, this is simply a presentation of the unitive and procreative ends of marriage. Still, he is framing the issues in a radically different way.

Second, the Theology of the Body draws a connection between marriage and the Cross. On the Cross, Jesus makes a complete gift of himself so that we might have eternal life. In marriage, spouses also make a complete gift of themselves to each other, and their self-gift has the capacity to produce new life. This line of thinking is clearly reflected in the following two quotations from *Familiaris consortio* – the apostolic exhortation on the family that John Paul published in 1981, while he was giving the *Theology of the Body* audiences:

> This revelation reaches its definitive fullness in the gift of love which the Word of God makes to humanity in assuming a human nature, and in the sacrifice which Jesus Christ makes of Himself on the Cross for His bride, the Church. In this sacrifice there is entirely revealed that plan which God has imprinted on the humanity of man and woman since their creation; the marriage of baptized persons thus becomes a real symbol of that new and eternal covenant sanctioned in the blood of Christ. The Spirit which the Lord pours forth gives a new heart, and renders man and woman capable of loving one another as Christ has loved us. Conjugal love reaches that fullness to which it is interiorly ordained, conjugal charity, which is the proper and specific way in which the spouses participate in and are called to live the very charity of Christ who gave Himself on the Cross. (*Familiaris consortio*, §13)
>
> Spouses are therefore the permanent reminder to the Church of what happened on the Cross; they are for one another and for the children witnesses

> to the salvation in which the sacrament makes them sharers. (*Familiaris consortio*, §13)

Here, again, John Paul II is not reaching any new conclusions. He is approaching the issue of the unitive and procreative ends of marriage from a new angle. This angle shows more clearly the connection between the nature of marriage, the nature of conjugal intercourse, and the central mysteries of the faith.

Third, the Theology of the Body sets up a connection between marriage and the Eucharist. The basic elements of the connection are fairly simple: the Eucharist is a one-flesh union of persons (between Jesus and the recipient) that is life-giving (in the order of grace), and marriage is a one-flesh union (between husband and wife) that is life-giving (in the order of nature). Pushing the analysis a little further, the Eucharist involves a complete gift of self from one person to another, and when that gift is received it brings forth life. Marriage also involves a complete gift of self from one person to another which has the capacity to bring forth life.

Although this line of analysis originates in John Paul II's Theology of the Body, it was Pope Benedict XVI who summarized this line of thinking most succinctly in his Apostolic Exhortation on the Eucharist, when he said: (1) "For in the most blessed Eucharist is contained the entire spiritual wealth of the Church, namely Christ himself . . . who gives life to humanity through his flesh" (*Sacramentum caritatis*, §16) and (2) "The Eucharist, as the sacrament of charity, has a particular relationship with the love of man and woman united in marriage" (*Sacramentum caritatis*, §27).

Once again, the Theology of the Body is not reaching any conclusions that have not already been stated in Church teaching with respect to the unitive and procreative dimensions of marriage. But, it frames the issues in a new way, with a much deeper and more evident connection with the central mysteries of the faith.

Finally, there is also a historical dimension to the Theology of the Body. John Paul II articulates the historical dimension through his notion of marriage as "primordial sacrament." The idea here unfolds in five steps. (1) There is a mystery hidden in God from all eternity: the mystery of a communion of persons whose union is life-giving. (2) The creation of man and woman takes that eternal mystery and transposes it into a physical dimension. In this way, marriage is "the primordial sacrament" in the sense of taking an invisible reality and making it visible. (3) Building on that physical dimension, the relationship between God and the chosen people in the Old Testament is carried out in terms of the relationship between husband and wife. Thus, a historical dimension is added to the physical dimension. (4) At the culmination of salvation history, Christ comes as the Bridegroom in the flesh, to consummate a spiritual marriage by the gift of his body to his spouse in the Eucharist and on the Cross. (5) Finally, there is an eschatological dimension: the final goal of Christ's self-gift is to allow each person to enter into the wedding feast of the Lamb. This brings the matter full circle, since the entry of the person into the wedding feast of the Lamb is, ultimately, the entry of the creature into the mystery that was hidden from all eternity. It is in this sense that John Paul calls marriage "the primordial sacrament" – the first way in which God expresses his eternal mystery in the dimensions of space and time, and the fundamental building block for all other ways of expressing that mystery.

In light of the Theology of the Body, it is possible to go back and look at the whole discussion about the essential nature of marriage and the normative description of conjugal intercourse in terms of union and procreation, and realize that, for the most part, the discussion was based on Scripture and on a natural law analysis. John Paul II's contribution, with the *Theology of the Body*, is to frame things in more theological terms. The link between natural law, the central mysteries of the faith, and salvation history, begins to be made clear. This is an example of how Church teaching develops; its roots become deeper. Finally, it ought to be noted that this growing depth is reflected in the treatment of marriage in the 1983 Code of Canon Law and the 1997 Catechism of the Catholic Church.

21 Rendered here as "openness to procreation" despite the biological fact that procreation is not possible in a particular act of conjugal intercourse. In other contexts, the act of conjugal intercourse in infertile periods is referred to as having procreative meaning or procreative significance or a procreative dimension.

22 The constant juxtaposition of contraception and abortion presents confusion and a danger to the defense of the unborn. The acts are biologically different and different in moral gravity. While these acts are sometimes connected for some individuals, there is no necessary connection between contraception and abortion.

23 Essentially, Pope Francis is building on the law of gradualness as articulated in *Familiaris consortio*, §34.

24 In addition to taking a stand against abortion, the Catholic Church has developed "Project Rachel" for women and "Project Joseph" for men (More information can be found at: https://hopeafterabortion.com/). These pastoral programs help bring healing to those who carry the emotional and spiritual scars of their involvement in abortion. In addition, the US Bishops have initiated a campaign called "Walking With Moms in Need" to ensure that every woman who feels that abortion is her only option knows that there are other options that will support both her and her child (More information can be found at: https://www.walkingwithmoms.com/).

25 The prophylactic use of condoms to prevent the transmission of disease continues to be discussed by scholars within the Roman Catholic tradition. Christopher Tollefson examines the issue of condom use to prevent HIV transmission between spouses in *The Use of a Condom to prevent HIV among married couples* (Tollefson in "Contemporary controversies in catholic bioethics," Jason T. Eberl, Ed. New York: Springer, 2017, pp. 255–68). Tollefson argues that the use of a condom in sexual intercourse by a serodiscordant married couple is impermissible as a violation of the marriage act understood as requiring the deposit of semen into the vagina. The permissible options available for the couple are abstinence throughout marriage or risk of HIV infection for the noninfected partner. William F. Murphy, Jr. examines the more general issue of the prophylactic use of condoms in *The Disease-Prevention Use of Condoms: Why It Is Not Forbidden According to Catholic Doctrine* (Murphy in "Contemporary controversies in catholic bioethics," Jason T. Eberl, Ed. New York: Springer, 2017, pp. 269–285). Murphy maintains that such use in sexual intercourse by a serodiscordant married couple is permissible within a broader understanding of the nature of marriage and its ends and within an understanding of natural law understood as having its source in reason (ratio) and nature (natura) as reason measures nature as manifested in the inclinations as that which presents to be measured by reason.

26 The Popes, from the time of the onset of the AIDS epidemic in 1980, have taught, clearly and consistently, that the distribution of condoms will not

resolve the epidemic and may contribute to its spread. In addressing this difficult situation in 2010, Pope Benedict XVI, while maintaining the moral prohibition of condom use, recognized at the same time the possibility of the condom use as a step as part of a gradual movement toward sexual responsibility, said the following:

> There may be a basis in the case of some individuals, as perhaps when a male prostitute uses a condom, where this can be a first step in the direction of a moralization, a first assumption of responsibility, on the way toward recovering an awareness that not everything is allowed and that one cannot do whatever one wants. But it is not really the way to deal with the evil of HIV infection. That can really lie only in a humanization of sexuality.
>
> She [the Church] of course does not regard [the use of condoms] as a real or moral solution, but, in this or that case, there can be nonetheless, in the intention of reducing the risk of infection, a first step in a movement toward a different way, a more human way, of living sexuality.
>
> (New York Times November 21, 2010, A 1)

27 See Carlson, J. W. (1989). Donum vitae on homologous interventions. *Journal of Medicine and Philosophy*, *14*(5), 523–540. Carlson suggests that homologous ZIFT (Zygote Intrafallopian Transfer) along with homologous GIFT (Gamete Intrafallopian Transfer) be recognized as acceptable within a marriage.

28 The possibility of development of Church teaching is a matter of historical fact both in the speculative and practical domain. On the speculative side, early attempts to express and to find appropriate language to express the mystery of the Trinity and to express the dignity of Mary serve as two of the clearest examples. Attempts to give an account, using material symbols, of the Trinity failed. The account of the Trinity proffered by Saint Augustine, based on the understanding of the operations of the mind and the procession of the interior words, was more satisfying. The Augustinian account, while not dispelling the mystery, afforded the mind repose. The understanding of the role of Mary has advanced as her role as Mother of God, her Immaculate Conception, and her Assumption have been explicated. This development is a deepening of understanding.

On the practical side of theological development, there is an extensive list of changes including the transitions: (a) from the acceptance of slavery to its condemnation, (b) from the prohibition of interest taking on money to the acceptance of capitalist, but not materialist, principle of the right of the individual to use money to make money, (c) from the indissolubility of marriage to the dissolution of certain marriages for the sake of the faith, and (d) from the requirement of the persecution of heretics and from the teaching that "outside the Church there is no salvation," to the declaration of religious freedom (Noonan (1993). Development in moral doctrine. *Theological Studies*, 662–669). A most recent change is present in the transition from the acceptance of capital punishment as an appropriate societal means of self-defense to the reluctant acceptability of capital punishment in only the rarest of circumstances, that is, circumstances which are "very rare, if in fact they [the circumstances] occur at all" (*Evangelium vitae*, 1995, §56) to the more recent claim of Pope Francis that capital punishment is intrinsically evil.

29 There exists a recurrent but underdeveloped theme in the tradition, that the essential nature of marriage is a union of a particular kind with a set of specifically different but related ends to be accomplished on levels appropriate to the

nature of humans as physical, rational, and spiritual beings. The theme appears as early as *Genesis* 2:24: "so that the two become one flesh" and continues to the present. The notion appears in inchoate form in the recent documents of the tradition from *Casti connubii* forward to *Amoris laetitia* wherein Pope Francis acknowledges its neglect. Examples of significant contributions to this notion can be found in the past in works considered foundational for the tradition. These include the writings of Saint Thomas Aquinas in the thirteenth century and Saint Alphonsus Liguori in the eighteenth century. In his treatment of marriage, Aquinas claims that marriage itself is a reality in the objective order; marriage is an entity constituted in the real relation of subject to subject. The relationship, a union, is established as a nexus or connection between two persons who are, in their nature, mutually ordered to each other. The spouses, as the principles of the relationship, are those whose "to be" precisely as spouses are to be ordered to each other (Aquinas, *Summa Theologiae*, I, q. 28, a. 1). Each acts in the other; each is acted upon by the other. The spouses are the related complementary principles of a new being that is the marriage. The marriage is a being in itself.

Just as the marriage, reified as the marriage bond, is the appropriate juridical entity in canon law, that is, it has privileged standing in the legal order, so too the marriage itself is the appropriate moral entity in the ethical order. Actions of the related principles of the marriage, the spouses, must be evaluated from within the context of the moral entity, the marriage. It is the marriage, not the partners individually, not the reproductive organs in isolation, that has privileged standing in the moral order. As a union, the marriage is a personal relationship, a kind of human friendship between a specific man and a specific woman, each embodying a particular aspect of humanity.

The union of sexually differentiated persons instantiates ontological completeness. The relationship begins on the horizontal plane as a consequence of attraction and desire on the level of sensitive appetite. The essential nature of humanity as male and female includes the inclination of each to desire the other in such a way as to be united with the other. Because humanity, as male and female, has a complex nature, that is, a nature that is physical, appetitive, rational, and spiritual, the union has a similarly complex nature that is physical, appetitive, rational, and spiritual. It is a union of persons. It is a personal union that results in a bond that is more fully a union than a physical union. While the resultant personal unity has characteristics in common with both physical and moral unities, it is, in itself, a unique species of unity.

Aquinas designates conjugal intercourse as the sign which signifies and contains the reality of marriage. The other sign, union of Christ and the Church, is, according to Aquinas, a sign which signifies but does not contain the reality of marriage. In his characterization of the kind of joining that constitutes the union that is marriage, Aquinas describes marriage as a unity of purpose and a unity in being. In regard to a joining of purpose, he says, "By marriage certain persons are directed to one begetting and upbringing of children, and again to one family life in respect of which we speak of husband and wife" (Aquinas, *Summa Theologiae*, I, q. 44, a. 1). In regard to a joining in being, that is the bond, Aquinas maintains that the bond between the spouses is the reality contained in the marriage. He says, "The bond between husband and wife resulting from those acts [conjugal intercourse] is reality and sacrament; and the ultimate reality contained is the effect of the sacrament, while the non-contained reality is that which the Master [Peter Lombard] assigns" (Aquinas, *Summa*

Theologiae, I, q. 42, a. 1, ad 5). The reality signified but not contained in the marriage is the union of Christ with the church. Moreover, Aquinas notes the physical and spiritual aspects of the union which contribute to its constitution as a personal union when he says, "the joining together of bodies and minds is a result of matrimony" (Aquinas, *Summa Theologiae*, I, q. 44, a. 1). And again, in describing the marital union, he says, "for the joining of husband and wife by matrimony is the greatest of all joinings, since it is a joining of soul and body, wherefore it is called a *conjugal* union" (Aquinas, *Summa Theologiae*, I, q. 44, a. 2, ad 3). Because marriage is, in its essence, a joining together, Aquinas maintains that reference to marriage as a conjugal union is appropriate.

Furthermore, in the consideration of marriage as a relation, Aquinas maintains that every relation has a unity in the cause of the relationship and a diversity inasmuch as the subjects that are related in terms of that cause are diverse subjects. Now inasmuch as marriage has a unity of purpose and a unity in being, there is a cause that relates the diverse subjects in the unity of purpose and a cause that relates the subjects in the unity in being. In regard to the unity of purpose, the cause that relates the subjects is procreation. The diverse subjects are the man and the woman as potential parents. In regard to the unity in being, the cause that relates the subjects is the marriage bond. The diverse subjects are the man, as inclined to the woman, and the woman, as inclined to the man, as spouses.

Both the union in being and the union of purpose manifest the Trinity. In the relationship of persons that constitutes the union in being, the bond is generated. In the relationship of persons which constitutes the unity of purpose, the generation of children is possible. Aquinas designated the procreative end primary and the union secondary. By primary he means that which is accomplished by man as an animal; by secondary that which is accomplished by man as man (Aquinas, *Summa Theologiae, Supplement*, q. 65,1). Conjugal intercourse is, as a matter of fact, always unitive and sometimes procreative. The understanding of conjugal intercourse as always unitive shifts the focus away from the organs of the spouses, away from the man and the woman each as individuals, to the marriage union itself.

This understanding is foundational to the differential designation of the ends of marriage as proposed by Saint Alphonsus Liguori. Liguori designates ends of marriage, the goods to be achieved in marriage, as intrinsic/extrinsic and necessary/contingent. The intrinsic and necessary good of marriage, according to Liguori, is the mutual giving of the right to one's body to each other. This giving and receiving constitutes the indissoluble bond of marriage. He designates the procreation of children and the satisfaction of the passions as intrinsic and contingent ends of marriage, that is, to be accomplished only within marriage and accomplished under the direction of practical reason whose role is to discern the existence of the appropriate conditions for bringing children into the world and the appropriate ordering of the satiation of the passions.

The characterization of the essential nature of marriage as a union found a central place in the work of the Pontifical Commission for the Study of Problems of the Family, Population, and Birth Rate and its widely publicized Majority Report which continues to exercise considerable influence within the Catholic community. The Majority Report affirmed the continuous teaching of the magisterium that (1) marriage is an intimate partnership of love and life; (2) the essential act of marriage is conjugal intercourse; (3) that the two intrinsic aspects of marriage are union and procreation; and as well, (4) the claim that reproduction is to be accomplished only within marriage. The Majority Report rejected the claim of the inseparable connection between the procreative signification and the unitive signification in every act of conjugal intercourse. The assessment of the Majority Commission was that the actualization of the procreative potentiality is to be understood as a requirement of the entire course of the marriage rather than a requirement of every single act of intercourse within marriage. The Report argued that the moral specification of marriage, considered as an act in itself, derives not from particular acts, that is, individual acts of conjugal intercourse, which constitute partial aspects of marriage but from the set of acts throughout the duration of the marriage.

In this understanding, the essential nature of marriage is a bond between a specific man and a specific woman. Conjugal intercourse, the act which signifies and contains the reality of marriage, is directed to the creation of the bond and is reserved to the spouses of the marriage. Reproduction, as the intrinsic and contingent end of marriage, is to be accomplished only within marriage and only in those circumstances conducive to the good of the child, the good of the family, and the good of the community. Hence, if it is appropriate to have children of this marriage, reproduction is to be accomplished within this marriage and over the course of the marriage. On the other hand, if it is inappropriate to have children of this marriage, reproduction is to be avoided, for that time during which reproduction is inappropriate even if this means for the entire course of the marriage. The objective criteria regulating the conjugal course and the reproductive finality in this conception of marriage would be derived from the understanding of marriage as a union of love and life. Sexual intercourse is limited to the partners of the marriage. Reproduction is limited to the marriage. Conjugal intercourse is always unitive and sometimes procreative. The objective criteria would prohibit those activities which are egotistical, hedonistic, violative of the dignity of the spouses, or directly abortive.

6 Human Cloning and Human Embryonic Stem Cell Use

This text of the Psalmist proclaims that the glory of God is manifest in the heavens and in the orderly transition of knowledge in time. The Psalmist wrote:

> See how the skies proclaim God's glory, how the vault of heaven betrays his craftsmanship! Each day echoes its secret to the next, each night passes on to the next its revelation of knowledge; no word, no accent of theirs that does not make itself heard, till their utterance fills every land, till their message reaches the ends of the world.
>
> (*Psalms*, 19: 2–5)

This manifestation of God's handiwork is evident not only in the visual spectacle of the majesty of universe but also in every word that constitutes the discourse that is knowledge.[1] The grandeur of God is no less evident in the human being, a creature who manifests the very image of God and who strives, in his life and work, to be like God.

The omnipresence of the majesty of God and the striving of humans to imitate that majesty can pose a challenge for humankind. This challenge lies between the poles of humble service and powerful temptation. While human control of the physical universe remains limited, the control of individual human life, while still somewhat limited, is quite possible in the presence of rapidly developing technology within the contemporary horizon. In this present context, technology often outpaces ethics and compassion often overwhelms reason. Technology figures out how to do things before it asks the question "ought this be done." Medicine suspects that a sick person might benefit from some available intervention and proceeds without asking the question "ought this therapeutic modality be undertaken for this person in this condition." Moreover, compassion, a rich human emotion in itself when untethered to reason, can blind reason's judgment. Science is propelled by the energy of the research imperative. Medicine is driven by compassion to the therapeutic imperative. But moral

DOI: 10.4324/9781003627197-6

questions intervene between knowledge and action. Among the questions which are needed to provide a bridge between knowledge and moral action are the following: (1) Is this a contribution to real human flourishing for this person or for this society? (2) Are the means to accomplish the desired end good? (3) Is the end itself a real human good? and (4) Is it a lesser good at the expense of a greater or is it a rightly ordered good? These moral imperatives do not enter consciousness at the same time and with the same exigency as the research imperative and the cure imperative, but the energy behind them must be cultivated if knowledge and compassion are to serve human flourishing.

Human cloning would be no exception to these observations, except for the fact that science so far has struggled at this point to achieve satisfactory results. The roadblock to the scientific and medical juggernaut to the industrialization of cloning in a manner that is relatively safe for the cloned human being lies in the refinement and perfection of the technique. This barrier is most likely a temporary delay caused by lack of understanding of the necessary elements required for epigenesis and the subsequent epigenetic reprogramming failures or abnormalities. Considering the history of science and technology, it is possible that these obstacles will be overcome in the near future. There will, most likely, be an insight into the art of human cloning, just as the insight into the spiraling double helix was the clue to the unraveling of the structure of the human genome. This pause in technological facility, however, provides the opportunity for careful consideration of the moral concerns surrounding human cloning before it becomes a routine practice.

This chapter will address the issue of human cloning in the following manner:

(A) A brief history of cloning;
(B) An introduction to significant reports on cloning;
(C) A description of the process and a clarification of terms;
(D) An examination of the scientific and ethical issues and the opposing views surrounding human cloning-to-produce-children;
(E) An examination of the issues and the opposing views surrounding human cloning-for-biomedical-research; and
(F) Afterword: some conclusions and some lingering questions for the culture and the Catholic tradition.

(A) Brief History of Cloning

Cloning of animals is a relatively new procedure in the biological sciences and its successes have been accompanied with much failure and wastage. In 1938, Hans Spemann was the first to envision cloning. Most of the early attempts at cloning were limited to frogs and, in 1952, Thomas King and Robert Briggs successfully cloned frogs. The first results, however, were dismal; no healthy frogs reached adulthood.

As scientists began to discover the reasons for their failure, they became more successful. In 1997, the first cloned mammal, Dolly the sheep, was born. Success with the production of Dolly was achieved only after the production and death of 277 sheep embryos. (Table 6.1 containing comparative data on live births from cloning animals is appended to this chapter.) Dolly was euthanized at age 6 because of illnesses associated with elderly sheep. Sheep of her breed generally live for 16 years.[2]

The work of cloning animals continues. Cattle including bulls, cows, and buffalo have been cloned since 1997. In 1998, the University of Hawai'i cloned healthy mice which have produced offspring. In 2001, Guar – a species of wild cattle – were cloned. In 2002, researchers at Texas A&M University cloned the first cat which was appropriately named CC or Calico Cat. In 2003, Banteng calves were cloned from frozen somatic cells of a calf that had died 20 years earlier. In the spring of 2003, a mule of particularly valuable traits was successfully cloned. Also in 2003, horses including Prometea who has since given birth to a foal were cloned. In 2009, a camel was cloned in Dubai and in that same year a Pyrenean ibex – a once-extinct species – was cloned. So, the science of animal husbandry marches forward as more complex animals are successfully cloned.

(B) Two Significant Reports on Human Cloning

The most recent significant reports on the issues of cloning, both cloning-to-produce-children and cloning-for-biomedical-research, are those presented by The Report of the National Academy of Science: *Scientific and Medical Aspects of Human Reproductive Cloning* (NAS) which was published in January of 2002 and The Report of the President's Council on Bioethics (PCBE): *Human Cloning and Human Dignity* (HCHD) which was published in July of 2002.

The National Academy of Science, from the outset, limited its work to the scientific and medical issues surrounding human cloning. In its report, The National Academy of Science made the following recommendation in regard to human reproductive cloning: "Human cloning should not now be practiced. It is dangerous and likely to fail. The panel therefore unanimously supports the proposal that there should be a legally enforceable ban on the practice of reproductive cloning" (NAS, 2). Significant in the report of the Academy were (1) the focus on the safety issues for the clone and the mother; (2) the call for attention to the need to follow already established rules of scientific research including success in animals; and (3) the recommendation that the Academy revisit the issue in five years.

Dr. Irving L. Weissman, chair of the NAS panel, summarized the position of the panel in the following:

> Data on the reproductive cloning of animals demonstrate that only a small percentage of attempts are successful, many of the clones die during all stages of gestation, newborn clones often are abnormal or die, and the procedures may carry serious risks for the mother. The proposed ban on human cloning should be reviewed within five years, but it should be reconsidered only if a new scientific review indicates that the procedures are likely to be safe and effective, and if a broad national dialogue on the social, religious, and ethical issues suggests that a reconsideration of the ban is warranted.
>
> (NAS, 3)

The NAS committee, however, approved cloning-for-biomedical-research. The Report had this to say:

> Finally, the scientific and medical considerations that justify a ban on human reproductive cloning at this time are not applicable to nuclear transplantation to produce stem cells. Because of its considerable potential for developing new medical therapies for life-threatening diseases and advancing fundamental knowledge, the panel supports the conclusion of a recent National Academies report that recommended that biomedical research using nuclear transplantation to produce stem cells be permitted. A broad national dialogue on the societal, religious, and ethical issues is encouraged in this matter.
>
> (NAS, 2)

Note the following from the recommendations. The NAS panel calls for broad national dialogue on both issues. In the recommendation on cloning-for-biomedical-research, there is a shift in the language from object to process and its product. The process is nuclear transplantation to produce stem cells. The object that is the end of the process is the embryo, which is the source of the stem cells.[3]

The President's Council on Bioethics, whose membership was broader in its expertise than was the membership of the National Academy of Science included scientists, philosophers, theologians, as well as those with expertise in law and public policy. The President's Council on Bioethics addressed the two issues of cloning-to-produce-children and cloning-for-biomedical-research.[4] The Council unanimously held that cloning-to-produce-children is unethical and recommended that this type of cloning ought not to be attempted. Moreover, it held that cloning-to-produce-children should be indefinitely banned by federal law no matter whether the project was supported by the use of private funds or the use of public funds.

The potential for physical harm to children in the process of cloning is so grave that all of the reputable scientific-ethical bodies to have studied the issue are at this time of one mind on the issue, namely, the possible risks to the new human being are greater than the benefits that might accrue from its existence. This consensus is found in the text of the Report of the President's Council is the following:

> These questions of the ethics of research – particularly the issue of physical safety – point clearly to the conclusion that cloning-to-produce-children is unacceptable. In reaching this conclusion, we join the National Bioethics Advisory Commission and the National Academy of Sciences. But we go beyond the findings of those distinguished bodies in also pointing to the dangers that will *always* be inherent in the very process of trying to make cloning-to-produce-children safer. On this ground, we conclude that the problem of safety is not a temporary ethical concern. It is rather an enduring moral concern that might not be surmountable and should thus preclude work toward the development of cloning techniques to produce children. In light of the risks and other ethical concerns raised by this form of human experimentation, *we therefore conclude that cloning-to-produce-children should not be attempted.*
>
> (HCHD, 96)

The Report of the President's Council on Bioethics did not enjoy the same unanimity on the issue of cloning-for-biomedical-research. Seven members of the Council voted to ban cloning-for-biomedical-research; three voted to place a moratorium for four years on cloning-for-biomedical-research; seven voted to go forward with cloning-for-biomedical-research. The compromise position reached by the majority vote (10–7) of the Council was to recommend a four-year moratorium on cloning-for-biomedical-researc h. In voting for this compromise recommendation, the Council, as did the NAS panel, called for broad dialogue on the issues and, in addition, the Council called for a comprehensive national review of all "current and projected practices of human embryo research, preimplantation genetic diagnosis, genetic modification of human embryos and gametes, and related matters, with a view to recommending and shaping ethically sound policies for the entire field."

(HCHD, X)

(C) Description of the Process and Clarification of the Terms

Cloning is a kind of asexual reproduction. It is distinguished from sexual reproduction in which the new human being arises from the union of the germ cells, the egg of the female and the sperm of the male, from two biological parents. Cloning is a procedure in which a somatic cell from an adult is reduced to a primitive stage and fused, either by electronic or chemical stimulation into an enucleated oocyte, an egg cell from which the nuclear DNA has been removed, of the same species kind as the somatic cell. A somatic cell is a body cell which contains the full complement or the diploid number of chromosomes rather than a germ cell which contains the haploid or half complement. Figures 6.1 and 6.2 describing the process and its goals are appended to this chapter. (Diagrams of this process and its goals as found in the NAS Report pages 7 and 8 are appended to this chapter.) Once placed within the egg cell, the reconstituted egg is activated, cell division commences, and the new organism begins its development.

The technical name for this procedure is somatic cell nuclear transfer and it is referred to in the literature as SCNT.[5] The embryo that was established in the SCNT process is sustained *in vitro*, in a laboratory dish, until its development is appropriate for its use. If pregnancy is the desired end, the resulting cloned embryo would be transferred to a female host whose body has been suitably prepared for implantation. And if all went well, a clone that is virtually identical, except for the mitochondrial DNA of the oocyte, to the human who donated the somatic cell nucleus would be born. If, on the other hand, research into the process of early human development is the goal or if the gathering and use of the pluripotent stem cells from the blastocyst for use in regenerative medicine is the goal, then the organization of the established embryo is interrupted, that is the embryo is destroyed, and its blastomeres become material for purposes of research.

Before taking up the ethical issues inherent in human cloning, a significant language issue needs to be addressed. Because there is considerable confusion about different kinds of cloning, it is important to use terminology that is precise and fair. To use a term such as "therapeutic" cloning in regard to the use of stem cells derived from human embryos, which were destroyed to harvest the stem cells, is to focus on the intention of the cloning without considering the source of the stem cells. It obscures the starting point in the process and the action – the destruction of the embryo – as it focuses on the goal of the action. To continue the use of the term "therapeutic" by itself tends to make compassion the sole value in decision-making. Recall that the integral goodness of an act requires more than a good intention. The object, the circumstances, and the intention must be good also.

The terms that will be used in this chapter are those adopted by the President's Council on Bioethics. That report used the following descriptive terms: "cloning-to-produce-children" and "cloning-for-biomedical-research." These descriptive terms embody a clear definition of the process which produces an embryo and, as well, the goals of the process. The summary of the Council's report contains the terms and their descriptions. They are

> *Cloning-to-produce-children*: Production of a cloned human embryo, formed for the (proximate) purpose of initiating a pregnancy, with the

(ultimate) goal of producing a child who will be genetically virtually identical to a currently existing or previously existing individual.

Cloning-for-biomedical-research: Production of a cloned human embryo, formed for the (proximate) purpose of using it in research or for extracting its stem cells, with the (ultimate) goals of gaining scientific knowledge of normal and abnormal development and of developing cures for human diseases.

(HCHD, XXIV)

Note that each process requires as a starting point the production of a human embryo, that is, a living developing human being in the early stages of its life. The scientific description of the process of cloning and the chosen ends of the process attest to the accuracy of the terms used by the President's Council on Bioethics.

(D) Ethical Views on Cloning-to-Produce-Children

With the understanding of the scientific process of cloning in place, the next step is the complex set of moral issues. The first set of moral issues centers on the question of cloning-to-produce-children. The second set of moral issues centers on the question of cloning-for-biomedical-research. However, there is a fundamental issue underlying the process of cloning despite the ultimate goal of the process, that is, the status of the embryo. Until there is a careful and satisfying resolution, that is, one that comports with experience and scientific data, of the ontological status of the embryo, there will be no consensus on the permissibility of its use. The question of the ontological status of the embryo was examined in Chapter 4 and concluded that individual human life commences with the union of the gametes. Hence, the embryo is a human being at a particular early and vulnerable stage in its human development.

The context of the question of cloning-to-produce-children will, of necessity, be set within the very human framework of human desires and human compassion. This is a good place to begin; it is not a sufficient place to end. There is a natural human desire to have children and there is a natural human emotion to love children and family members. Various reasons are offered as to why cloning might be desired. (1) If one cannot have a child sexually, that is, by union of the sperm of the father and egg of the mother or if having children sexually is undesirable because of the possibility of the transmission of inherited disease from either the mother or the father, cloning might appear as an acceptable alternative inasmuch as the biological tie to at least one parent might be maintained. (2) If a child or another family member is dying, the desire to duplicate that family member by the process of cloning might appear as an acceptable and merciful possibility. (3) Further, cloning might make it possible to produce genetically matched organs from new offspring for transplantation that would not be susceptible to rejection. (4) Finally, cloning might offer the possibility of duplicating the talent or the beauty or the intelligence or the athletic prowess of especially gifted human beings.

Cloning to produce a child under most of these circumstances presents a powerful case for compassion. But, to say that something is desirable is not to say that it is ethical. Cloning human beings of superior genetic endowment carries with it the worry of past eugenics programs gone awry. There are limits even to the alleviation of this suffering and there are limits to the attempts to fashion human beings with superior or culturally desirable traits. Recall that for an act to be morally good, the intention, object, and circumstances must also be good. The intention of compassion is both good and strong in itself, if it is directed to a good object under appropriate circumstances. However, if the object, here cloning-to-produce-children, is wrong then the act is wrong and must be resisted despite the strength or power of the passion or compassion. Reason must inform the heart. Similarly, cloning to produce human beings with desirable characteristics for the human good as a whole is an intention that has a tainted past. That tainted history is examined in Chapter 7.

Moreover, the worth of any intention must be measured along with the object and the circumstances of the act. Cloning to produce a child with characteristics desired by the parent or the parents, the right to have a particular *kind* of child, may be an attempt to exercise inappropriate control over progeny. Children have destinies of their own. Parents need to give their children the power – roots and wings – to discern and follow their own paths. To have a child to satisfy the particular desires of parents is to use the child from the very beginning of its existence. This may prove to be a terrible psychological burden for a child to carry.

In addition to the possibility that cloning might satisfy particular human desires or might be a compassionate human response to particular human needs, there are other more general goods that have been set forth to defend the right to clone to produce children. Among these goods are the goods of freedom, of autonomy, of existence, and of human well-being. There is no denying that these are human goods. However, the absolutization of any one of these goods as an individual right is dangerous for both the individual who makes the claim and for the society which permits such a claim. Human beings have a limited right to exercise freedom and the right to free exercise is accompanied by the obligation to exercise freedom rightly. The claimed autonomous right of one human being to exercise a procreative right to clone must be viewed within a context which includes the rights of the possible new human being generated in the process (the legal status of abortion and the current public ambiguity in regard to abortion tend to conceal these third-party interests), the rights of the family within which the cloned individual will be nurtured, and the rights of society to good order.

One of the most ardent defenders of human cloning-for-producing-children presents his position in the following:

> A society that bans acts of human creation that reflect unconventional sex roles or parenting models (surrogate motherhood, in vitro fertilization, artificial insemination, and the like) for no better reason than that such acts dare to defy "nature" and tradition (and to risk adding to life's complexity) is a society that risks cutting itself off from vital experimentation and risks sterilizing a significant part of its capacity to grow.
> (Tribe, 321)

Here is a very clear statement grounded in the prevailing philosophy of the contemporary culture. It promises human progress if human freedom is unhampered by claims of tradition and nature. To make this categorical claim is to forget the dismal history of human performance and to buy into the myth of inevitable human progress. Both tradition and understanding nature can serve as guides to human wisdom. Human decline is just as real a possibility as human advancement. It is important to note that "To ignore the fact of decline was the error of the old liberal views of automatic progress" (Lonergan, I, 260).

Existence is a basic human good and well-being is good for both individuals and for society. However, to choose to bring a human being into existence without regard for the significant probability of causing grave danger to that human being is to act irresponsibly regardless of whether the human life is brought forth by sexual or asexual reproduction. Responsible human beings ought not to knowingly and willfully behave in such a way as to risk grave danger for other human beings. To bring a human being into existence merely to satisfy one's own desires is selfish. Human reproduction requires careful attendance to duties to the newly generated human being. Hence, well-being as well as existence is a legitimate ethical concern.

There is an additional worry here. Concern for well-being of individual human beings ought not to be equated with the elitist notion that only the planned, perfect, and privileged have a rightful place in the human community. Those who are born with disabilities and those who become disabled later on in life do not lose human significance and worth on account of their limitations. Moreover, new dimensions of the meaning of human life are gifts to be received in them and with them.[6]

In regard to ethics of cloning-to-produce-children, the myriad questions are the following: (1) the safety of the procedure; (2) the concordance of the procedure with norms governing experimentation on human subjects; (3) potential harms and injustices to prospective human offspring; (4) potential harms and injustices to women; (5) potential harms and injustices to families and to society; and (6) violation of religious principles.

(1) *Safety Issues in Cloning-to-Produce-Children*

The National Academy of Science Report and the Report of the President's Council on Bioethics both concur that, at present, there is not sufficient technological expertise to successfully clone a human being. Both the law and ethics require prior experimentation of a procedure or a treatment modality on animals before it can be permitted on human beings. The Report of the National Academy of Science contains a rather complete collection of data on live births from the cloning of animals (NAS, Table 6.1, pp. 114–119). The Report of the President's Council on Bioethics contains a summary – taken from the NAS Report – of live births from the cloning of animals (HCHD, Table 6.1, p. 72).[7] The extensive data in the NAS Report summarize the cloning results for a wide variety of animals – sheep, cattle, mice, pigs, goats, and monkeys – and from a wide variety of cell types. The data in both reports show such low level of success and such high level of mortality and morbidity that, if these were transferred to human experimentation, would be ethically and scientifically unacceptable. The high rate of failure as fetal loss in the cloning of animals and the high rate of damaged and impaired offspring in animals preclude reputable scientists from moving beyond animal experiments to human experimentation at this time. Furthermore, those scientists, who experimented with the cloning procedure before the issue of the ethics of human cloning became a central ethical concern, were unable to move beyond the six-cell stage before the organism began to deteriorate. The scientific suspicion is that the lack of success results from failure in the epigenetic programming and/or in the imprinting mechanisms that have not been successfully activated or only incompletely activated in the cloning process. Epigenetic programming coordinates the processes required for the proper and orderly early development. Imprinting mechanisms direct the timely expression of appropriate genes. Mis-expression and/or perturbations in expression result in developmental failure.

For the present, the empirical evidence in regard to safety issues evident in cloning to produce offspring in animal experimentation precludes moving forward with cloning to produce children. Nonetheless, there are significant questions which require attention. They include: the concordance of the procedure with norms governing experimentation on human subjects; the potential harms and injustices to prospective human offspring; potential harms and injustices to women; potential harms and injustices to families; potential harms and injustices to society; violation of religious principles.

(2) *Norms and Codes on Experimentation on Human Subjects*

The issue of the concordance of the procedure with ethical codes for governing human experimentation is not unproblematic. Two international codes, the Nuremberg Code (1946) and the Helsinki Declaration (1964), as well as U.S. codes – the Belmont Report (1978), published by the National Commission for the Protection of Human Subjects of Biomedical and Behavioral Research, and the Code of Federal Regulations (HHS, 45 CFR 46) – are pertinent to the issue of cloning-to-produce-children. Each of these codes centers on the value of human dignity, the obligations that arise from particular human relations, and the limits of research. All prohibit experimentation that is dangerous to human beings.

The Nuremberg Code requires the following: in Article 1, the informed consent of the research subject; in Article 2 that the experiment provide a concrete good for society unavailable by any other means; in Article 3 that animal research precede research on human subjects; and in Articles 4, 5, 6, and 7 that the subject be protected from harm. The Declaration of Helsinki, by making a distinction between research directed to the medical care of patients and medical research directed to the advancement of knowledge, advances on the Nuremberg Code and retains many of the essential requirements of the Nuremberg Code, that is, that the subject be informed and that the benefits clearly outweigh the risks. The Declaration of Helsinki retains many of the essential requirements of the Nuremberg Code. It maintains that the subject be informed and that the benefits clearly outweigh the risks. It advances beyond the Nuremberg Code in that it makes a distinction between research directed to the medical care of patients and research directed to the advancement of knowledge. Other important advances enumerated in the Helsinki Declaration in medical research on human subjects are the following: (a) considerations related to the well-being of the human subject should take precedence over the interests of science and society; (b) special provisions are to be made for those who cannot give consent; and (c) in the case where consent cannot be directly attained that the research benefit be specific to the research-subject population.

The Belmont Report continues many of the same protections and distinguishes between ethical principles that guide research into medical care and ethical principles that guide experimental research. The Report lists as guiding the principles of respect for persons, beneficence, and justice.[8] The constellation of these principles requires: (a) respect for the autonomy and rights of persons and special protection for persons with diminished capacity; (b) that the scientific research be beneficial, in a concrete and meaningful way, either to the individuals involved in the research or to others; (c) that the harms and benefits be distributed justly; and (d) that the research subjects be selected fairly. The most recent regulations governing research in the United States are to be found in the Code of Federal Regulations at 45CFR46. These regulations hold that research involving those who are incompetent requires assent of the participant as well as consent of the person who has legal authority over the participant.

In summary, all four Codes have consent provisions, and protection from harm requirements. All four require some benefit calculation. All four have directions for the selection of subjects. The Belmont Report appears to have the broadest requirement for subject selectivity and for benefit, that is, benefit is not limited to the individual subject or to any particularity about the subject research group, but is directed to society as a whole.

In the application of the central requirements of these Codes to the issue of cloning-to-produce-children, there is concern for the informed consent of the adult participants in the process. But the assent provision, which would be impossible to get, is simply ignored. This means there is little concern expressed for the new human being to be generated. This disregard has its source in the myopia resulting from the lack of legal status for the unborn but conceived human being.[9] At a minimum, a best interest standard would need to be invoked. What is clear is that the strict application of the restrictions of these codes along with the recognition of – and respect for – the ontological status of the human being at the earliest stages of its development would prohibit both cloning-to-produce-children and cloning-for-biomedical-research.

(3) The Potential Harm to the Offspring

The potential harms to prospective human-cloned offspring are physical as well as psychological and social. The potential physical harms to cloned children, extrapolating from the real harms experienced by cloned animals, include a greater than normal risk of dying before birth, fatal abnormalities that cause death shortly after birth or after a relatively short life span, and nonfatal abnormalities such as "increased birth size, liver and brain defects, and lung, kidney, and cardiovascular problems" (NAS Report, Chapter 3). Some short-term consequences observed in cloned animals include failure of the immune system, premature aging, and sudden death.

Long-term consequences in cloned animals are simply unavailable, so no hypotheses about the long-term effects of cloning-to-produce-children are possible.

Among the possible psychological and social concerns for a cloned child are the following. The cloned individual would inherit a genetic identity already lived (in the case that the source of the somatic cell is someone who died) or would inherit a genetic identity that is being lived simultaneously by another (in the case that the source of the somatic cell is a contemporaneously living human being) or would inherit a particular genetic identity chosen by someone else (in the case that designer genes were selected or genes were manipulated). The first might cause a problem of expectations. For example, if the intention of the cloning were to produce a virtuoso violinist or an exceptionally gifted athlete or a brilliant scientist or a raving beauty, the offspring might experience unbearable pressure to live up to those expectations or suffer overwhelming guilt if other interests, self-chosen interests, became more directing of one's life.[10] The second might cause a problem of familial relationship. If one parent is the source of the somatic cell, then the offspring has genetic linkage to only one parent. The third possibility, if the somatic cell is taken from someone outside the biological family, then the cloned child would not have biological ties to the rearing family. While this might be considered similar to adoption, there are two concerns. Concern one is that adoption is, in a sense, a rescue act while the clone in this instance represents the deliberate choice to bring a human being into existence in a particular set of circumstances. Concern two is that adoption itself presents some obstacles to be overcome by the lack of biological relationship. A fourth possibility suffers the risk of cloned human being's being treated like any other consumer good or object of a parent's aspirations. Leon Kass cautions that "[p]arental control is a double-edged sword" which may be the source of psychological and physical harms for "the child whose genetic identity is selected in advance" (HCHD, p. 94). Children have an identity independent of their parent's desires and children ought to be understood as entitled to lives that are independent of their parents.

(4) The Potential Harm to Women

There are potential harms and injustices to women latent in the press for cloning-to-produce-children. The DNA of the somatic cell must be fused into an oocyte, a human egg cell, and there must be a womb to carry the newly conceived human being to term. All present cloning techniques require large numbers of oocytes. Recall that the production of one sheep, Dolly, required 277 sheep eggs. If a woman, on average, produces 12 to 13 mature eggs each year in her fertile years, it would take at least 20 years to produce eggs sufficient to produce one live birth, if extrapolation from the Dolly scenario were possible and if cloning-to-produce-children were no more complicated than cloning Dolly.

Of course, science does not have the time to wait 20 years and, of course, science has the technology to speed things up. Hormonal treatments are available to induce superovulation in women and surgical procedures are available to retrieve the eggs produced by superovulation. Hormonal treatments to induce superovulation have both physical and emotional risks – swings of emotional highs and lows – for women and no surgical procedure is without anxiety. Since only women have wombs, there must be some woman who is willing and able to carry the newly generated human being to term. This then requires an extension of the practice of surrogacy (treated in Chapter 5).

Furthermore, because animal cloning results in dangers to the clone-bearing mother that are not insignificant, human cloning-to-produce-children cannot be permitted to go forward at this time and at this level of experimental competence. Animal cloning is accompanied by increased morbidity and mortality for the host mother. The NAS Report lists the following:

> Increased maternal and mortality can result from late gestational fetal loss, increased size of the fetus, abnormal placentation, pregnancy toxemia, and most notably, hydroallantois and/or hydranminos (excessive fluid accumulation in the uterus often associated with fetal abnormality and maternal distress).
>
> (NAS, p. 42)

There is considerable debate among some feminists as to whether these new procedures present new economic opportunities for women and, hence a unique good for women, or if the new procedures present a whole new set of burdens rooted in biological structures unique to women. If financial incentives were offered for egg production or for womb use, it might be the case that only women in difficult economic circumstances might offer their bodily capacities for such projects. There are at least two risks here.

The first risk is that the acceptance of this role has the potential to reduce poor women to objects of production. The second risk is that if women are choosing from the position of economic necessity rather than personal flourishing or gift giving, then the consent to the procedure, whether egg donation or womb use, loses its voluntary character. The real possibility of both of these risks represents potential assault on the dignity of women. The issue of the commodification of women's bodies is a matter for all women. It is not restricted to women of limited means.

(5) The Potential Harm to Families and Society

The potential harms and injustices to families and to society at large are, for the most part, not physical harms but possible structural harms and injustices that might arise from a change in the order of relations in the family and in society. The potential harms to family include those of relationship and those of inheritance both genetic as well as economic. Those of relationship have to do with human dignity and human equality. The Report of the President's Council on Bioethics has this to say:

> a begotten child comes into the world just as its parents once did, and is therefore their equal in dignity and humanity . . . [and]. . . our emergence from the union of two individuals, themselves conceived and generated as we were, locates us immediately in a network of relation and natural affection.
>
> (HCHD, p. 112)

Among the potential and significant harms to society is the traversing of a major natural boundary in the transition from sexual to asexual reproduction and the probable industrialization of human production with the likely attendant practices of the destruction of those determined unfit or imperfect. It is a bold experiment to undertake to change that natural network and a bold assumption to presume that nothing will change as a result.

(6) Religious Principles

The Catholic tradition, which is central to the treatment of medical issues in these chapters, holds as normative that children are a good. Children are gifts of God. They should be conceived in the love of their parents and born in faith and into faith in the goodness of human life and in the hope of everlasting life. It holds the following: (1) children are to be born in marriage; (2) children are to be born of the marriage act, conjugal intercourse which unites husband and wife in an act that has both unitive and reproductive significance; and (3) that while all human beings have intrinsic dignity that commands respect, vulnerable human beings – "the least of these" – are to be the recipients of special care. Most instances of cloning-to-produce-children would be violative of (1) and all the instances of cloning-to-produce-children would be violative of (2). And cloning-to-produce-children, which accepts as ordinary practice, the direct destruction of those deemed less than perfect, violates (3). So, the Catholic tradition has principles in places that exercise a limit on the practice of cloning-to-produce-children. To these principles are to be added the potential physical, psychological, and sociological harms to children, to women, to families, and to society.

(E) Ethical Issues on Cloning-for-Biomedical-Research

The second set of moral issues centers on the question of cloning-for-biomedical-research. Here, the issue is the production of the human embryo for purposes other than the well-being of the human embryo itself. The embryo is produced for the harvesting and use of its stem cells or for observation of its development. Before proceeding, a basic clarification is necessary. Stem cells occur naturally both in the embryo and throughout the human body. The former are embryonic stem cells; the latter are adult stem cells. Stem cells can also be produced in the laboratory as induced pluripotent stem cells (IPSCs).

The production and use of embryonic stem cells has captured the imagination of scientists and the sympathies of the general public. The reason for this lies in the possible use of stem cells for increase in scientific knowledge and the possible therapeutic use of stem cells in regenerative medicine. Included in this possible use is the regeneration of nerve cells for spinal cord repair and the regeneration of brain tissue last to Alzheimer's or Parkinson's disease. It is important to note that, at the present stage of scientific and medical knowledge, such possible use of stem cells is largely promising. While the ends of knowledge and therapy are good ends, there remains controversy. What lies at the heart of the issue is the use of stem cells that have their source in the embryo and that, in their harvesting, bring about the destruction of the embryo.

An examination of stem cells follows in this order: (1) the power of stem cells; (2) the many possible goods that stem cells offer; (3) the sources of stem cells; (4) the ethical issues in stem cell use; and (5) the major positions in the stem cell controversy.

Stem cells are marvelously versatile cells. They are pluripotent in character, that is, they are unspecialized cells that have the capacity to give rise to many different kinds of cells including all 200 of the different types of cells – nerve cells, muscle cells, cardiac cells, etc. – in the human body. Stem cells are present in the bloodstream, in bone marrow, in the umbilical cord, in fetal tissue, in certain types of tumors, and in the inner cell mass of the embryo. Stem cells are considered potentially immortal; they have indefinitely continuous divisional ability without the loss of genetic structure. The potential limitless diversity and the potential immortality of stem cells make them very valuable.

Embryonic stem cells are the first cells of the human being. They are totipotent, that is they have the capacity to become every kind of cell in the body and to develop into a completely new organism of its kind. This is what makes them so remarkable. Adult stem cells have a more limited capacity. They have the capacity to become many different kinds of cells within a particular system within the body, but they cannot generate a new organism. In the early twenty-first century, scientists discovered how to create induced pluripotent stem cells (IPSCs). These are adult stem cells that are derived from the deprogramming of fully differentiated adult somatic cells into a more primitive or immature state. The primitive cells are then reprogrammed and inserted into the cytoplasm of an egg that has had its nucleus removed. As new growth commences, the expectation is that the proliferation of the appropriate IPSCs will occur and this will produce new tissue to be used in the regeneration and repair of lost or damaged tissue in the human body.

It has been suggested that stem cells might be able to generate new nerve cells and, hence, might be the source of a cure for spinal cord injuries, or that stem cells might replace impaired or disrupted or damaged brain cells and, hence, are a potential cure for Parkinson's Disease or for Alzheimer's Disease. It has been suggested that stem cells as a source of heart tissue or other solid organ tissue might make it possible to bypass the problem of organ rejection common in transplantation procedures. And it has been suggested that the study of early human development by using embryos generated in somatic cell nuclear transfer might be the key to preventing development damage for future desired children.

Use of adult stem cells, which are found in various parts of the human body, is unproblematic. A straightforward application of the principle of totality suffices – the part may be used for the good of the whole. Ethically, this is no different from a blood donation or a skin graft. And, as a therapeutic measure, there has been some success accomplished with the use of adult stem cells in the production of cardiac tissue. The problem with the use of stem cells taken from the inner cell mass of the embryo prior to implantation is that the embryo is destroyed in the harvesting of the stem cells. If the embryo is a living developing human being, then its life may not be destroyed to heal illnesses of other presently living, always developing human beings and its life may not be destroyed to serve the good of developmental correction for future living developing human beings. This would be an instance of experimenting on and using our children to improve our lives. The rules governing the principle of totality in an organism that is a moral community apply here. The most significant point here is that the principle of solidarity as refined by the distinctions of the principle of totality permits only the activities and not the life of the part (of the embryo) may be used for the good of the whole (the person or persons who would receive the stem cells or the society that would benefit from the research).

In its initial stages, the embryonic stem cell controversy was framed by two sides. The proponents focused on its goals, laudatory in themselves.

The opponents focused on the means which is accomplished through embryo destruction. The proponents claimed that embryonic stem cell research is imperative because of its promise. To deny the research is to prevent a whole host of cures from being developed. Preventing that research, and those cures, is immoral. On the other side, the opponents claim that embryonic stem cell research is immoral because it destroys a human being. While the promise of cures is great, it strikes the devil's bargain. There are some things that must not be done in order to improve our lives.[11]

The status of the embryo, that is, the embryo produced by the procedure of somatic cell nuclear transfer, is the first critical issue. A second critical issue is the need for embryonic stem cells. In contemporary medical ethics, there are different claims about the status of the early embryo. The status of the embryo was covered in depth in Chapter 4 where the conclusion was presented that every human life begins its existence as a zygote and becomes what it is by developing its potentialities. The becoming which is described in various stages is a time-conditioned unfolding of the possibilities given at fertilization. It is then a member of the moral community. Its life may not be directly taken to satisfy some human good other than life. Nonetheless, a brief summary of the specific set of claims and a response to each will be presented here.

Significant among the claims about the embryo are the following: (1) the embryo prior to implantation is simply a set of cells organized now in a particular manner; it is permissible to organize them in another manner so long as the reorganization serves a human good; (2) the embryo prior to implantation is the earliest stage of development in human life; it deserves profound respect, but not the respect owed to more developed forms of human life; and (3) the embryo prior to implantation is the earliest stage of development of every human being and deserves the same respect accorded to all other living developing human beings.

Those who defend (1) sometimes make the claim that the embryo produced by somatic cell nuclear transfer is an artifact. It is just a piece of tissue and it is different from the embryo produced by sexual reproduction. Now while it is true that the method of its coming into existence is different, it is still an embryo and as an embryo it is different from other types of tissue which remain, throughout the life of the tissue, simply that type of tissue, for example, cardiac tissue and bone tissue. The embryo is a living developing human being who, by its active natural potentiality, is destined to become a more fully developed human being. Those who defend (2) seem on face value to have the least defensible position. They recognize the embryo as an early stage in the life of an individual and require *profound respect* for that life, but allow the direct destruction of that life to serve the health or well-being of some other human being. There is something incompatible with the claim to proffer profound respect to something or someone in an act which countenances the killing of the object of the profound respect. (3) is left standing.

The second critical issue about embryonic stem cell research, however, is scientific. With the advent of Induced Pluripotent Stem Cells, are the embryonic stem cells even scientifically necessary? If the IPSCs have the pluripotent character embryonic stem cells without their being individual human beings, then they offer all the scientific benefits and none of the ethical drawbacks of embryonic stem cells. Of course, the scientific picture is not so neat and clean as that. Still, the advent of IPSCs has had an important effect – scientifically and ethically – on the debate.

(F) Afterword

In summary, both cloning-to-produce-children and cloning-for-biomedical-research, even if technically possible, are morally impermissible. The former is impermissible because of the complex set of issues described earlier. The latter for the simple reason that, at present, the proposed procedure causes embryo destruction. Concern for well-being as a societal good, that is, that the members of society be healthy and have effective treatment for illness and injury, is a limited good that should be sought within a context that accepts human finitude and that understands the limitation of the principle of totality as it applies to a physical organism and as it applies to a moral organism. This topic of the application of the principle of totality and the distinction between a moral organism and a physical organism will continue to be of considerable concern in the issue of cloning-for-biomedical-research.

An important question: if the physical risks to the mother and the child are shown to be statistically acceptable, that is, the mortality rate of each approximates the mortality rate of normal conception and childbearing and if the morbidity rate approximates that associated with normal conception and childbearing, would cloning then become morally acceptable? Could the objections to potential psychological and structural harms to the cloned human being, the family, and society be overcome, if the physical harms were overcome? Will those holding a particular religious tradition, such as committed Catholics, which proscribes cloning-to-produce-children, become an alien community in a culture which reduces progress to scientific progress, which values only human beings designed to meet certain standards of acceptability and which might permit, or even require, the early destruction of cloned human beings who do not meet such standards? If the tradition is the repository of truth, its alien status is to be endured – as sign of commitment and in the hope of transformation. It would not be the first time and it would not likely be the last time that the Catholic community was called upon to exercise endurance. The tradition, however, must be mindful of its obligation to continue to study its own tradition so that its understanding of the truth is a truthful understanding. In this, the tradition accepts the duty set forth by Pope Leo XIII in the encyclical *Aeterni patris* "*vetera novis augere et perficere*" – "to add to and perfect the old by the new" (*Aeterni patris*, §24).

Table 6.1 Comparative Data on Live Births From Cloning Animals, Adapted From Report of the President's Council on Bioethics, Human Cloning and Human Dignity, Washington, DC, 2002

SOME COMPARATIVE DATA ON LIVE BIRTHS FROM CLONING OF ANIMALS (HCHD, TABLE 6.1, P. 72)
[For a more complete collection of data, see the NAS Report Scientific and Medical Aspects of Human Cloning 114–119]

Animal species	*Donor cell*	*Number of cloned embryos transferred*	*Number of live births*	*Live births per embryo transfer*	*Reference*
Sheep	udder cells (frozen)	29	1	3.4%	1
Cattle	fetal fibroblasts	496	24–30#	4.8–6%	2a
	cumulus & oviduct cells	10	4–8*	40–80%	2b
Mice	cumulus cells	2468	31**	1.3%	3
Goats	transgenic fetal fibroblasts fetal fibroblasts transgenic fetal fibroblasts	97	5	5.2%	4a
		85	3	3.5%	4b
		184	5	2.7%	4c
Pigs	fetal fibroblasts	110	1	0.9%	5a
		335	5	1.5%	5b
Cats	cumulus cells	87	1	1.1%	6
Rabbits	cumulus cells	371	6	1.6%	7

Source: References:

1. Wilmut, I., et al., Nature, 385: 264–267 (1997)
2a. Cibelli, J.B., et al., Science, 280: 1256–1258 (1998)
2b. Kato, Y., et al., Science, 282: 2095–2098 (1998)
3. Wakayama, T., et al., Nature, 394: 369–374 (1998)
4a. Baguisi, A., et al., Nature Biotechnology, 17: 456–461 (1999)
4b. Keefer, C.L., et al., Biol Reprod, 64: 849–856 (2001)
4c. Reggio, B.C., et al., Biol Reprod, 65: 1528–33 (2001)
5a. Onishi, A., et al., Science, 289: 1188–90 (2000)
5b. Polejaeva, I.A., et al., Nature, 407: 86–90 (2000)
6. Shin, T., et al., Nature, 415: 859 (2002)
7. Chesne, P., et al., Nature Biotechnology, 20: 366–369 (2002)

Notes: # Six animals died shortly after birth; * four animals died shortly after birth; ** 20 animals died at a young age [Ogonuki, N.K., et al., Nature Genetics, 30: 253–4 (2002)].

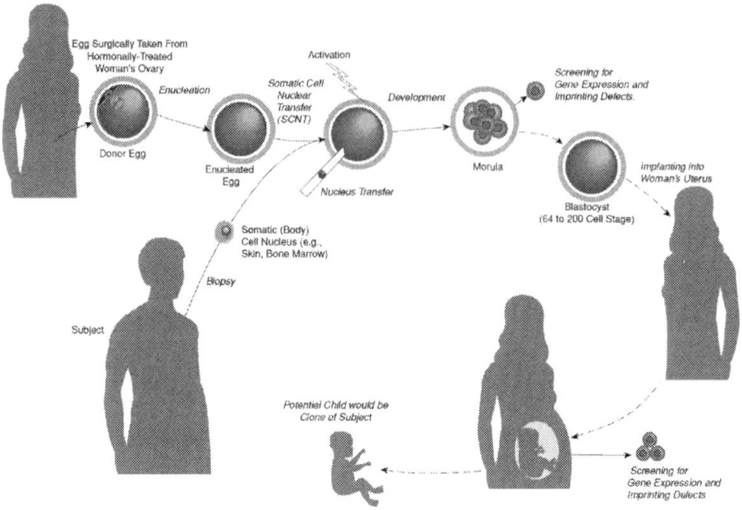

Figure 6.1 Cloning to Produce Children (NAS Report p. 7)

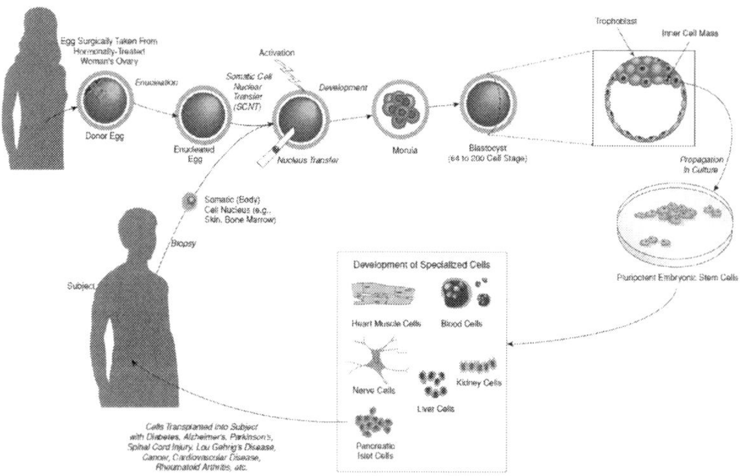

Figure 6.2 Cloning for Biomedical Research (NAS Report p. 8)

Questions for Reflection

1. In order to better understand the ethical issue of cloning-to-produce-children, describe the act in the ethical language of object, circumstances, and intention.
2. In order to better understand the ethical issue of cloning-for-biomedical-research, describe the act in the ethical language of object, circumstances, and intention.
3. How is the question of cloning shaped by the likelihood of success?
4. How is the issue of cloning shaped by the issue of whether the conceptus is a human being?
5. If cloning could be done safely, would it be ethical to do it? What are the most important ethical issues to be considered?
6. Examine the excerpt from the statement of Professor Lawrence Tribe. What values are embedded in that statement?
7. If cloning-to-produce-children is violative of your religious principles, why is this so?
8. The experiment of cloning-to-produce-children must be carried out in accordance with the legal norms governing experimentation on human subjects. What provisions of those codes apply here?
9. What are some of the potential harms and injustices to prospective offspring who might be cloned? What are the potential benefits?
10. What are some of the potential harms and injustices to women who might take part in the cloning process? What are the potential benefits?

Notes

1 The relationship between the Logos (eternal Word) and logos (spoken word) is not an accident in Christian thought.

2 Among the theories offered for the early demise of Dolly is the possibility that the shortened telomeres signifying already-aged cells contributed to her death. Telomeres are repetitive nucleotide sequences at the end of each chromosome. The telomeres protect the ends of each chromosome from deterioration or from the possibility of fusion with another chromosome. In the process of aging, the telomeres shorten.

3 If the position articulate in Chapter 4 on the status of the embryo as a living, developing human being is correct, then the recommendations of the NAS panel can be understood as the following: It is unethical to bring the cloned embryo to birth but it is reasonable to permit them to live for a time in order to experiment on them for the benefit of society.

4 Note the precise terminology here. The process is the same; the product is the same, that is, the creation of the embryo; the intentions are different.

5 Somatic Cell Nuclear Transfer (SCNT) is cloning. SCNT names the mechanism of cloning.

6 There is rich literature to serve (1) as an appropriate paradigm for the care of the vulnerable and (2) as an inspiration for the relatively autonomous. The

work of Stanley Hauerwas in his writing, his lectures, and his life provides a rich and profound source of reflection. *Living gently in a violent world: The prophetic witness of weakness.* InterVarsity Press, 2008) written with Jean Vanier allows readers to enter that world and be changed. *Critical reflection on Stanley Hauerwas' theology of disability.* Routledge, 2004 by John Swinton examines the 30-year work of Hauerwas on the theological significance of those with developmental disabilities.

7 This summary can be found in the appendix to this chapter.

8 Non-maleficence – do no harm – is a subset of beneficence.

9 This lack of legal status for the developing human being was adjudicated by the Supreme Court in *Roe v. Wade.* The effect of the *Dobbs* decision on the legal status of the preborn human being was not specifically addressed by *Dobbs*. It awaits resolution.

10 Note that these points also stand as critiques of the expectations that some parents place on children conceived in the natural way.

11 See Hans Jonas, H. (1980). Philosophical reflections on experimenting with human subjects. In *Philosophical essays: From current creed to technological man* (pp. 105–133). University of Chicago Press on the limits of the use of human subjects in experimentation. Jonas presents a counter-utility argument. The more vulnerable the subject, the less likely the permissibility of the experiment.

7 The New Eugenics

Therapy – Enhancement – Screening – Testing – Engineering

The Scriptures abound with messages of the Lord's power and providence. This Scriptural passage from Isaiah cautions humanity to take heed of that authority and to exercise providence over God's creation:

> Thus says the Lord, the Holy One of Israel, and Israel's maker, Of me you must learn, what times they be that are coming; trust me to do what I will with my sons, with my own creatures. It was I who framed the earth, and created man to dwell in it; it was my hands that spread out the heavens, my voice that marshalled the starry host; I, too, have summoned this man to perform my designs faithfully; go he where he will, my guidance will be his.
>
> (*Isaiah*, 45: 11–13)

It reminds us that all of the creation, the heavens, the earth, and humankind, are the work of God. In His creation of men and women, God endowed them with reason so that they might know His creation, marvel at its beauty, and know its power. In His creation of men and women, God endowed them with specific natures that they can come to know in order to protect, to heal, and to actualize those natures in a manner that is faithful to their end (telos). At the same time, the passage warns humanity of the limits of human authority. Men and women do not command God. Nonetheless, God calls humanity, as created in the image and likeness of God, to exercise dominion as responsible stewardship in the created order "to perform my designs faithfully." That exercise of stewardship includes healing what is broken in the world.

The focus of this chapter is genetics, the science of human heredity. In the contemporary period, this science has advanced from (a) observation of the phenotype and the attempt to discern the causes of the particular appearance evidenced in the phenotype to (b) the mapping of the human genome, with the consequent knowledge of and the possibility of manipulation of

DOI: 10.4324/9781003627197-7

the genotype, and the subsequent possibility of control of the course of its expression. The chapter will proceed in the following order:

(A) A bit of history about eugenics as a reminder of the perennial hope of improving the quality of the human race, and as well, the past history tainted by eugenics programs which were egregious violations of human dignity;
(B) An account of the development and progress in genetic testing and screening;
(C) A description of modern efforts at eugenics under the topics of genetic therapy and genetic enhancement in somatic cells and germ cells;
(D) A sketch of the remarkable recent advancements in genetic engineering;
(E) And finally, a reflection on the promise, power, and peril of the new genetics.

(A) A Bit of History – Eugenics

The desire to improve the quality of the human race and/or the quality of individual offspring is a perennial theme in human history. Plato's *Republic,* one of the earliest utopian works in Western philosophy, proposed selective breeding among the guardian class by arranging for the mating of the best men and the best women at the prime of their lives and in the most propitious seasons of the year for the good of the *Politeia*. There was to be no marriage and no nuclear family for these superior citizens, just coupling for the purpose of producing the best offspring for the city-state. Children born from this coupling were to be raised not by their parents but in the nursery of the city-state. Hence, the reciprocal loyalty and affection of parents and children for each other were to be replaced by loyalty and fidelity to the *Politeia.* Recall that in the *Republic* the activities of the individual are to be directed toward the flourishing of a well-ordered *polis* as the greater good.

The term "eugenics" was coined by Francis Galton in *Hereditary Genius*, his first major work, which appeared in 1869. The term from the Greek, simply means "well born" and it connotes a sense of contributing to or improving the stock of the race or the nation. In *Hereditary Genius*, Galton, concerned about the possibility that the human species was in the process of degenerating and informed by his own research on inheritance, advocated a system of arranged marriages between carefully selected men and women for the purpose of breeding to improve the British race. Inferior human beings were to be prevented from or discouraged from reproducing. The term "eugenics" may have been well-intentioned, but it would become one of suspicion when the goal of genetics was embraced by various political regimes and enforced through the coercive power of the state as an effective instrument for social engineering.

In modern times, the first extended programs in state-sponsored eugenics were developed in the United States in the late nineteenth and early twentieth century.[1] These eugenics programs grew from a constellation of ideas derived from (1) the establishment of the modern science of heredity transmission genetics; (2) organic evolutionary theory and the embrace of Social Darwinism; (3) contemporaneous criminology encouraged by a scientific hypothesis supported by postmortem studies of brains of criminals and from the findings of the famous studies such as the *Jukes Report* (1875) and *The Nam Family: A Study in Cacogenics* (1912) on inheritance and criminal behavior; (4) demographic concerns about dysgenics, that is, the growth of criminal population and the growth of the feeble-minded population because of their unrestrained breeding patterns; and (5) technical surgical advances in the practice of medicine such as vasectomy and salpingectomy.

The newly discovered scientific laws of heredity provided the impetus to purge the population of bad genes and to produce a more improved human stock. Social planners considered four possible means to curb what was considered the decline of the race. They were (1) the elimination of defective offspring; (2) restrictive immigration; (3) institutional segregation during the reproductive years of those deemed unfit to procreate; and (4) state-enforced sterilization. The first, the direct elimination of offspring, was considered morally unacceptable. The second was accomplished by exclusionary immigration laws which were fashioned to insure a decline in the number of Eastern and Southern Europeans and Jews permitted entry into the United States. The third, segregation by gender, was based on real practice. There were some actual segregated-by-sex colonies. However, this was found to be too expensive and too restrictive of the freedom of institutionalized persons. The fourth, compulsory sterilization, was considered more acceptable. The acceptability of compulsory sterilization, it was argued, would serve the goods of the elimination of the possibility of the reproduction of defective offspring, an increase in the liberty of those determined defective, and a cost-saving for the state.

Surgical sterilization became a major instrument of this modern attempt at eugenics. The idea of genetic sterilization, the pursuit of this end as a national goal, and the procurement of means to attain their desired result were pressed by some of the most influential families, by some of the most prestigious societies and foundations, by some powerful lawyers, judges, scientists, and physicians, and by some of the most elite universities in the United States. Various state legislatures defined categories of those deemed defective and crafted laws to effect their sterilization. Some of these laws were overturned by the courts as unconstitutional violations of due process and as cruel and unusual punishment or by veto of the governor. Pennsylvania was the first state legislature to approve a sterilization law in 1905. It was immediately vetoed by Governor Samuel W. Pennypacker who, in his veto, accused scientists of being afflicted with limited vision which in support of their narrow goals had lost sight of broader principles. In his veto message, Pennypacker wrote:

> The subject of the act is not the prevention of idiocy, but it is to provide that in every institution in the state, entrusted with the care of idiots and imbecile children, a neurologist, a surgeon and a physician shall be authorized to perform an operation upon the inmates 'for the purpose of procreation.' What is the nature of the operation is not described but it is such an operation as they shall decide to be 'safest and most effective.' It is plain that the safest and most effective method of preventing procreation would be to cut off the heads of the inmates, and such authority is given by the bill to this staff of scientific experts. It is not probable that they would resort to this means for the prevention of procreation, but it is probable that they would endeavor to destroy some part of the human organism. Scientists like all other men whose experiences have been limited to one pursuit, and whose minds have been developed in a particular direction, sometimes need to be restrained. Men of high scientific attainments are prone, in their love for technique, to lose sight of broad principles outside of their domain of thought . . . This bill whatever good might possibly result from it if its provisions should become law, violates the principles of ethics . . . To permit such an operation would be to inflict cruelty upon a helpless class in the community which the state has undertaken to protect.
>
> (Aronoff, pp. 148–49)

In 1907, Indiana was the first state to achieve legislative success in securing sterilization of those considered unfit. In 1914, Harry Laughlin at the center for the national eugenic movement, the Eugenics Record Office in Cold Spring Harbor, proposed a model sterilization law to serve the goal of eugenics. It authorized sterilization of the "feeble-minded, insane, epileptic, inebriate, criminalistic and other degenerate persons" (Cohen, p. 121). By the time the Model Law was published in 1914, 12 states had enacted sterilization laws. Notwithstanding legal challenges, the eugenic movement pressed forward and by 1927 achieved its most notable success. The central notion and the clearest articulation of the goals of this movement are best recorded in the words of Mr. Justice Oliver Wendell Holmes who, writing for the majority in a United States Supreme

Court decision, *Buck v Bell,* found involuntary sterilization to be a service to the common good and to be compatible with the guarantees found in the U. S. Constitution. Holmes concluded:

> We have seen more than once that the public welfare may call upon the best citizens for their lives. It would be strange if it could not call upon those who already sap the strength of the state for lesser sacrifices, often not felt to be such by those concerned, in order to prevent our being swamped with incompetence. It is better for all the world, if instead of waiting to execute degenerative offspring for crime, or to let them starve for their imbecility, society can prevent those who are manifestly unfit from continuing their kind. The principle that sustains compulsory vaccination is broad enough to cover cutting the Fallopian tubes (*Jacobson v. Massachusetts,* 197 U.S. 11, 1905). Three generations of imbeciles are enough.
>
> (*Buck v. Bell,* 274 U.S. 200, 1927)

By 1931, 28 states had laws authorizing eugenic sterilization. By the close of the twentieth century, it is estimated that some sixty to seventy thousand people were sterilized in the United States in the name of eugenics (Cohen, p. 319).

These eugenics programs in the United States exercised considerable influence on programs in other nations. A particularly noxious combination of scientism, utopianism, and millenarianism, along with German Nordic mythology, supported by the legitimating influence of practices and ideology imported from the United States, and empowered by a dictatorship, spawned the eugenics excesses of the Third Reich and contributed significantly to the flourishing of the work of the German Society for Racial Hygiene. Nazi eugenics programs are described often as eugenics run amok. The Nazis began with programs which encouraged healthy families and which restructured tax laws that favored childbearing. Both are benign in themselves. However, these programs were soon followed by what were considered complementary laws, that is, laws enacted to prevent the reproduction of defective human beings. Then the notion of defect was broadened from those with physical defects and illnesses refractive of treatment to debility associated with old age to the defect of being non-German. It is estimated that between the years of 1933 and 1945, through the agency of Nazi heredity health courts, three million five hundred thousand people were sterilized – most for no legitimate medical reason (Cohen, pp. 302ff.).

Eugenic sterilization, including nonvoluntary genetic sterilization, in the United States reached in apogee in the 1930s and continued until 1973. It is interesting to note that eugenic sterilization programs in the United States continued even after the Nuremberg Trial of physicians and the publication of the Nuremberg Code. It was not until 1973 that the debate over eugenic nonvoluntary sterilization became a public debate in the United States. What forced the debate was the public disclosure of the sterilization of young poor African American women and even some little girls in a family planning clinic located in Alabama and funded by the Department of Health, Education, and Welfare, and the public disclosure of programs of routine sterilization of retarded men institutionalized as wards of the state. In 1978, the Department of Health, Education, and Welfare (HEW) put into place a set of rigorous guidelines to protect minors and mentally incompetent persons from sterilization and to protect, with an elaborate consent mechanism, those competent persons who are dependent on public funds, from coercive sterilization.

(B) Genetic Testing and Screening

Developments in genetic testing and screening, coupled with the possible new genetic therapies to cure defects or illness, hold out great promise for human beings. But, as with all human progress, there is the possibility for abuse. First, there is a distinction to be made. Genetic *testing* refers to the determination of the genetic status of a particular individual thought to be at risk either because of clinical symptoms or family history for inherited disease. Genetic *screening* is the evaluation of populations or groups of people independent of known risk for inherited disease. If genetic testing and genetic screening are to be done, they must be accomplished without traversing fundamental human goods.

(B.1) Genetic Testing

There are several significant foci for genetic testing. They include (a) genetic testing to guide reproductive decisions, (b) genetic testing of children, and (c) genetic testing of adults.

Genetic testing wedded to reproduction is now becoming routine for those who are considering reproduction and whose medical history or genetic background indicates an increased risk for fetal genetic disorder. Several types of prenatal testing are now available: carrier testing, testing of the preimplantation embryo, and *in utero* testing of the fetus. Carrier testing is the evaluation of the prospective parents before conception to evaluate the likelihood of conceiving a child with a particular disease. Some population groups and communities, who are susceptible for serious inherited diseases, such as Jews of Eastern European ancestry who have a higher incidence of Tay-Sachs, encourage testing before marriage to alert men and women who would be parents of the potential risks for their children. Evaluation of the preimplantation embryo is part of the process of *in vitro* fertilization and is done prior to transfer of the embryo to the uterus of the woman. *In utero* testing of the fetus, including ultrasonography, amniocentesis, fetoscopy, and chorionic villus sampling, has been in place for some time now to evaluate the genetic condition of the fetus. As technology advances in DNA determination so too will testing modalities advance.

Genetic evaluation combined with counseling affords couples the opportunity to know and understand the risks for the child they might conceive. It allows the couple to make a prudential judgment as to whether or not the possible harms for the child are greater than the benefit of existence for that child. Evaluation of the preimplantation embryo or the fetus, by any means available, allows for the possibility of treatment prior to birth, if treatment is available, or allows the parents to make plans for appropriate care for their child, if their child has a problem for which there is no medical remedy at this time, or allows the medical team that will care for the mother and child to prepare for problems that might attend the birth of the child or allows the parents to rejoice in the knowledge that their child is well as they wait in joyful anticipation and the expectation of a safe birth. Evaluation of the preimplantation embryo and evaluation of the fetus that permits the destruction of the embryo or the fetus is an act of directly killing a vulnerable developing human being. The fact that the killing is done in a hospital by those whose profession commits them to protect human life and done with the consent of the mother, or the mother and father, does not change the nature of the act.

Genetic testing of children for the possibility of genetic disease represents a particularly difficult decision. The ethical principles that have been operative in the testing of newborns provide some guidance here. A particular set of difficulties present here when the child is asymptomatic and there is no cure for the disease and/or no amelioration of its course. In general, genetic testing should not be done on children unless there are serious reasons for the testing. Symptoms of illness or a familial history of a treatable disease are cogent reasons for limited testing. Pre-symptomatic testing of children for diseases such as Huntington's whose clinical manifestations occur later in life and for which, at this time, there is no cure ought not to be pursued. The calculation of risk in the risk/benefits ratio is too great. Despite pleas of parents for the information as a way of preparing for their child's future, clinical observations suggest that the social and psychological risks to the child and to the family structure are too grave. The future of any human being is not guaranteed. The child upon achieving adulthood may choose, for serious reasons, to have that information as a way of life planning including the possibility of marriage and children.

Genetic testing of adults has a set of potential benefits and burdens that must be weighed carefully. Among the potential benefits are: knowledge of diagnosis or risk; intervention for prevention or treatment; assessment of risk for members of family; guidance for reproductive decisions; and facilitation of economic planning decisions. Among the potential harms are: psychological and emotional harm; economic harm including exclusion from insurance and employment; stigmatization; and serious physical harm.

(B.2) Genetic Screening

The evaluation of populations or groups of people independent of known risk for inherited disease is not new. Its first application was the development of a simple screening test of newborn children for phenylketonuria (PKU) in 1961 by microbiologist Robert Guthrie. PKU is an error in the metabolism of phenylalanine that, unless treated by diet restriction, results in mental retardation. PKU testing is essentially testing for the presence of a disease or disability in a situation where there is a relatively simple way of ameliorating the effects of the condition. With the success of the PKU screening, all the states adopted mandatory newborn screening programs and expanded these programs as more tests became available. Requirements in the states were varied. Some states mandated testing for as few as 3 conditions while other states mandated testing for 30 or more conditions. Some states mandated a limited panel of tests and offer an additional supplementary panel that parents may request. Most states have informed consent requirements which, for the most part, are casually administered. Some states, but not all, have opt-out opportunities, for religious or other serious grounds, for parents.

Nonetheless, it was the case that a standard set of ethical requirements were in place to guide newborn screening. They were (a) there is a clear indication of benefit for the child; (b) a system is in place to confirm the diagnosis; and (c) treatment for the disease is available. These simple guidelines were developed out of the set of principles presented by James Wilson and Gunnar Jungner in a World Health Organization monograph in 1968. The ten Wilson-Jungner criteria for including a condition in a screening program are the following:

1. The condition sought should be an important health problem.
2. There should be an accepted treatment for patients with recognized disease.
3. Facilities for diagnosis and treatment should be available.
4. There should be a recognizable latent or early symptomatic stage.

5. There should be a suitable test or examination.
6. The test should be acceptable to the population.
7. The natural history of the condition, including development from latent to declared disease, should be adequately understood.
8. There should be an agreed policy on whom to treat as patients.
9. The cost of case-finding (including diagnosis and treatment of patients diagnosed) should be economically balanced in relation to possible expenditure on medical care as a whole.
10. Case-finding should be a continuing process and not a "once and for all" project.

(The President's Council on Bioethics: *Newborn Screening*, p. 22)

In the specific application of the Wilson-Jungner principles to newborn screening, William K. Frankenberg in 1974 offered the following: (a) the disease should be important; (b) the disease should be relatively prevalent; and (c) the disease should be amenable to early treatment. Of particular importance here is Frankenberg's emphasis on the benefit of treatment to the child. He also suggested that screening without consideration of these criteria might be detrimental in the utilization of limited medical resources and in the possible consequential increase in harm (The President's Council on Bioethics: *Newborn Screening*, pp. 24–25).

A similar set of recommendations for newborn screening was presented by the Institute of Medicine in 1994. That report recommended the following:

> newborn screening [should] take place 1) for conditions for which there are indications of clear benefit to the newborn, 2) when a system is in place for confirmatory diagnosis, and 3) when treatment and follow-up are available for affected newborns.
>
> (Institute of Medicine, 1994)

This was followed in 1995 by the joint report of the American College of Medical Genetics and the American Society of Human Genetics which maintained that the focus of genetic testing should remain the medical benefit to the particular child. The report stated: "timely medical benefit to the child should be the primary justification for genetic testing in children and adolescents" (American Society of Human Genetics and American College of Medical Genetics, p. 1233). Similar recommendations were made by the American Academy of Pediatrics in 2000. The Academy recommended that newborn screening be done if there is an effective, accepted, and available treatment for the condition. In observing this "enduring consensus," the President's Council on Bioethics noted the following in 2008:

> In all these statements of principle, *direct benefit to the newborn child* was identified as the paramount and indispensable criterion for inclusion of a disease in a uniform screening panel. To justify such inclusion, the natural history of the disease must be well understood, the diagnostic test for its presence must be clear and precise, and an effective treatment must be available.
>
> (The President's Council on Bioethics: *Newborn Screening*, pp. 25–26)

The presence of an apparent consensus notwithstanding, the rapid advances in testing and screening techniques have resulted in the expansion of the list of diseases targeted and tested and have resulted in a tension and a difference in assessment in the principles guiding newborn screening. As early as 1975, the National Research Council, one of the four National Academies, in its consideration of newborn screening expanded the notion of the benefit of screening beyond the direct benefit as treatment to the child. This expansion encourages screening even when treatment for the child is not presently available and if there might be a benefit to the family and/or to society. These benefits other than treatment of the child are the following:

> 1) to the infant (to provide management and support even when direct treatment is unavailable), 2) to the family (to inform subsequent reproductive decisions), and 3) to society (to provide knowledge of the true range and incidence of the condition.
>
> (National Research Council Committee for the Study of Inborn Errors of Metabolism, p. 1)

With the advance of research, new screening techniques provided the opportunity to test for more targets. The new screening techniques, which include tandem mass spectroscopy (MS/MS) along with the anticipated development of affordable DNA-based multiplex platforms, indicate a horizon within which both phenotype and genotype testing will become readily available. These changes are evident in the 2005 recommendations of the American College of Medical Genetics. The College studied 84 heritable disorders in order to provide and propose a uniform screening panel from these for all the states. At the conclusion of its work, the College proposed that a mandated, two-tier, uniform screening program be available in all the states which included screening for the 29 core conditions as well as the 25 secondary conditions. The criteria for the core condition designation were (1) that the condition be well understood, (2) that beneficial treatment be available for the child, and (3) that the test be specific and sensitive. The secondary conditions, determined by the ability of identification by the screening technique, were included, even though they did not meet the traditional criteria. They were included because either they could be used in differential diagnosis or simply provide a set of samples or a database for further studies that might benefit families or society. It is no longer the case that the list is limited to diseases that are well understood and for which there are effective treatments. The Center for Disease Control and Prevention, an agency of the federal government, maintains a site (cdc.gov) which lists the complete set of conditions that are screened in each state.

By 2008, most of the states had adopted screening for the 29 core conditions and many had adopted screening of the secondary panel. The research imperative continued to press the expansion of the list and the expansion of the concept of benefit. In addition, various governmental agencies, including the federal government in the Newborn Screening Saves Lives Act of 2007, lent support by way of increased financial aid to that expansion. This Act also directed the establishment of regional centers as storage banks for the newborn blood samples and for the data gathered from the samples. The pharmaceutical industry and the gentech industry, aware of new markets for their products, lobbied in support of the expanded program. Parent advocacy groups whose voices provided poignant testimony from the needs of their children joined them in this enterprise.

In the presence of these competing pressures, the President's Council on Bioethics, concerned by the rapid expansion from screening for treatment to screening for research, placed the issue of newborn screening on its agenda. The President's Council presented its report: *The Changing Moral Focus of Newborn Screening* in 2008. From the beginning, the Council noted that the newborn screening program continues to move forward with little public discussion and little real understanding of its reach on the part of parents and the public. The Council noted that an effective newborn screening program must include the following: "education, screening, follow-up and diagnosis, treatment and evaluation" (The President's Council on Bioethics: *Newborn Screening*, p. 7). The Council recognized both the good of screening to find those at risk in order to treat and the good of research for the advancement of knowledge, but acknowledged, at the same time, the risks involved. The testing for treatment, on the model of the phenylketonuria (PKU) program and the congenital hypothyroidism (CH) detection, offers early identification of a disorder and the possibility of a successful treatment. The latter, screening for research, while supplying a large set of samples and a large database for research, includes several risks. Among the risks are: the significant numbers of false positives; the medicalization, sometimes unnecessarily, of the life of a child; the identification of conditions that are not presently treatable; the identification of conditions that are poorly understood; the possible disturbance of the bond between child and parent; the continuing concerns over privacy and ownership of the samples being stored; valid informed consent; and the measure of cost of the program vis à vis other public health initiatives. After weighing the risks and benefits, the President's Council offered a compromise position. That position is the following:

1. Reaffirm the essential validity and continuing relevance of the classical Wilson-Jungner screening criteria.
2. **Insist that mandatory newborn screening be recommended to the states only for those disorders that clearly meet the classical criteria.** Such a disorder must pose a serious threat to the health of the child, its natural history must be well understood, and timely and effective treatment must be available, so that the intervention as a whole is likely to provide a substantial benefit to the affected child.
3. **Endorse the view that screening for other conditions that fail to meet the classical criteria may be offered by the states to parents on a voluntary basis under a research paradigm.** Such screening programs should be presented forthrightly as pilot studies, whose benefits and risks to the infant are not certain, and for which IRB approval should be obtained in each state. A condition included in a pilot screening study should be moved to the mandatory screening panel only if the evidence clearly establishes that it now meets the classical criteria.
4. **Affirm that, when differential diagnosis of some targeted disorders entails detection of other poorly understood conditions that would not otherwise be suitable candidates for newborn screening, such results need not be transmitted to the child's physician and parents.** It should be left to the states to formulate rules governing whether and when to disclose those results.
5. **Encourage the states to reach a consensus on a uniform panel of conditions clearly meriting mandatory screening.** In contrast, diversity among the states in regard to the pilot conditions for which they offer optional screening is to be welcomed, as it permits the states to learn from each other's different experiences.
6. **Urge a thorough and continuing re-evaluation of the disorders now recommended for inclusion in the mandatory screening panel, to ascertain whether they genuinely meet the classical criteria that would justify mandatory screening of all newborns, or whether they instead are suitable candidates for pilot screening studies.** In support of such continuing reevaluation, states should be encouraged to collect and share data on the short- and long-term outcomes for children who test positive for a genetic disorder, both those on the mandatory screening panel and those targeted by pilot programs.

7. **Reject any simple application of the "technological imperative," that is, the view that screening for a disorder is justified by the mere fact that it is detectable via multiplex assay, even if the disorder is poorly understood and has no established treatment.** There should be no presumption that multiplex screening platforms are to be used in "full profile mode"

(The President's Council on Bioethics: *Newborn Screening*, pp. 105–106. Bold in the original).

Notice how these points (a) clearly embrace the benefits of limited genetic screening, while (b) neither simply rule out nor simply embrace broader programs of screening.

By 2012, all states adopted newborn screening for the 29 conditions in the core panel, many included screening for the conditions in the secondary panel of 25 conditions, and a few states expanded beyond the 54 to include screening for additional conditions such as Krabbe disease, a late onset, little understood genetic disorder of the nervous system. The list continues to expand. The list of the core conditions and secondary conditions is available at:

(http://www.hrsa.gov/advisorycommittee/mchbadvisory/heritabledisorders/recommended panel/uniformscreeningpanel.pdf)

Concerns about genetic testing and population-wide genetic screening along with attempts to fashion responsible national policies continue. The issue of informed parental consent remains even while insufficiently attended. The federal government has a well-developed albeit elastic set of consent requirements in place to guide research whether on children or on competent adults. These can be accessed at the Health and Human Services site (HHS.gov) at 45CFR46 and at the Federal Drug Administration site (FDA.gov) at 21CFR50. Ownership of the blood samples, especially the samples taken from newborns in the mandatory screening programs, and the existence of the databases without sufficient privacy protections have been and will continue to be challenged. The sufficiency of treatment and effective follow-up programs continue, as does the expansion of the medicalization of life.

(C) Genetic Engineering – Therapy and Enhancement

Forced sterilization is no longer a respectable means to accomplish a eugenic vision in developed and developing, free nations. But, the vision of a better human life, whether as relief from disease or enhancement, continues. Advances in science, including the unraveling of the DNA structure of the human gene, the mapping of the human genome, and the development of technologies that allow the alteration of human genes, present amazing challenges, opportunities, and risks for humanity. As with all new knowledge and technology, there are also possibilities for misuse in the violation of human dignity, of human rights, and of the ordered good of society. Eugenics now has at its disposal the sophisticated tools of genetic engineering whose possibilities seem endless now that the human genome map has been completed and along with it advances in the understanding of the function and interaction of the genes. The anatomy of the human genome is likely to provide both a new basis for biological study such as evolution and comparative anatomy and, as well, a new model for application in medical treatment tailored to the individual. This last has been designated genomic medicine and is heralded as being able to fashion individualized treatment for a particular patient based on that person's genetic information.

There are four types of genetic engineering. They are classified by type and are designated as types I, II, III, and IV in order of location and intention from which follow potential medical and scientific implications and ethical seriousness. Type I is somatic cell gene therapy; Type II is germ cell gene therapy; Type III is somatic cell gene enhancement; and Type IV is germ cell gene enhancement.

	Therapy	**Therapy**	
Somatic Cell	Type I *Somatic Therapy*	Type II *Germ Cell Therapy*	Germ Cell
Somatic Cell	Type III *Somatic Enhancement*	Type IV *Germ Cell Enhancement*	Germ Cell
	Enhancement	**Enhancement**	

Type I is therapeutic genetic engineering. It is directed to the cure and prevention of diseases which has their source in somatic cells such as blood, bone, nerve, and cells specific to solid organs. Type I therapy is limited in scope to the disease of the specific individual receiving the therapy.

Type II is also therapeutic. It is genetic engineering that is directed to the cure and prevention of disease that has as the locus of its intervention the germ cells – the gametes essential for reproduction. This type of therapy has the potential to affect future human beings – offspring born of the person whose germ cells were modified.

Type III and Type IV are not, strictly speaking, therapy. They are attempts to manipulate genes in order to enhance some desired capabilities or some desired traits. Type III is somatic gene enhancement; the effect of the manipulation is limited to the individual. Type IV is germ-line gene enhancement; it has the potential to affect future generations and perhaps, at its farthest reach, to alter the human species.

While much of the promise of genetic engineering remains just that – a promise – there has been some success in Type I somatic cell gene therapy. In 1990, a 4-year-old girl, who suffered from a rare genetic disease – a severe combined immune deficiency (SCID) – became the first patient to undergo gene therapy. SCID is caused by the absence of an enzyme required for the proper function of the immune system. People suffering from this disease are required to live a restricted life in a sterile environment.[2] Physicians from the National Institutes of Health used a vector[3] to insert autologous lymphocyte cells, cells taken from the patient, with the desired gene that produces the enzyme adenosine deaminase to compensate for the defective gene. The corrected lymphocytes were returned to the child by intravenous infusion. The child was being treated with PEG-ADA, a version of the ADA enzyme, but this treatment had not been sufficient to restore immune function to desired levels. The new treatment was successful and it, in combination with PEG-ADA, continued for the child. With her immune system strengthened, she was able to attend school. Four years after the inception of this new protocol, the child weathered chicken pox with no more difficulty than that experienced by any other child with chicken pox.

This success was followed by the development of gene marker and therapy protocols. Within five years of the first treatment of a patient with gene therapy, there were more than a hundred protocols. Some are up and running; others in the process of review.

The use of recombinant DNA techniques to treat diseases involving missing or impaired genes seems unproblematic. Its use to treat such diseases as SCIDs, cystic fibrosis, types of anemia, and some types of cancers seems an appropriate human good and an intervention that allows human beings to exercise a providential role for the created world. It appears to be little different from any other curative measure practiced in the realm of medicine. Furthermore, it may offer better options for patients who suffer from severe illness.

Cystic fibrosis provides a clear example of the potential benefit of somatic cell gene therapy. As the disease progresses, lung transplantation becomes the treatment of last resort. If lungs become available – a very big if – the patient is required to undergo an invasive surgical procedure and is required to ingest immunosuppressant drugs for a lifetime. A further, and not inconsequential, aspect of the lung transplantation is the considerable cost. As somatic cell gene therapy develops, it may prove to be less invasive than transplant surgery; it may be immune to rejection; it may be cost-effective; and finally, it might be able to cure or regulate the disease so as to permit normal or close to normal human function.

While the development of somatic cell gene therapy presents great hope for those suffering from serious disease, there is always the possibility of unanticipated consequences. A graver physical danger might be the eventual outcome rather than the hoped for good, so careful risk/benefit analysis must be considered. With this possibility in mind, great care must be taken that the approved steps for developing therapeutic medical treatments be carefully adhered to and there be no rush to embrace "miracle" cures.

Another possible danger lies in the current reductionism that is a consequence of a narrow focus on a single gene. The risk here is the potential failure to understand how the gene operates in relation to other genes and in the whole person. A final concern relates to the distribution of the therapy. Because it is therapy, not research or enhancement, its end is to serve sick people. Procedures for distribution must aspire to be just and must be public. With these caveats in mind, it seems appropriate to go forward with the additional caution in regard to possible harms which lie in the potential to misallocate the energy of science and the resources that society and medical science have available for medical relief. The excitement of the new-fangled technology in the developed world can become the occasion of forgetfulness of the need to supply basic medicine such as vaccination to all the children of the world.

Of course, with the development of any new protocol, there exists the possibility of unimagined complications and subsequent harm. The tragic death of Jesse Gelsinger[4] in a clinical trial of gene therapy at the University of Pennsylvania in 1999 provides a reminder of experimentation gone awry and a reminder that progress is neither guaranteed nor without costs. Gelsinger suffered from ornithine transcarbamylase deficiency (OTC) which is the inability to metabolize ammonia. He was enrolled in a Phase I trial to test the toxicity of a potential genetic therapy. He was injected with a corrected gene carried by an adenoviral vector. Gelsinger died within a few days following the injection. His death was attributed to a massive immune response triggered by a reaction to the viral vector. The immune reaction led to multiple organ failure and brain death. His death is the first to be acknowledged publicly in a gene therapy clinical trial.

Type II therapy, germ line therapy, has not yet been performed in the United States because of its complexity and because of the serious ethical issues involved. The risk of Type II germ-line genetic therapy lies in its potential unknown effects on future generations. The unlocking of the anatomy, both mapping and function, of the human genome combined with sophisticated assisted reproductive techniques would allow for new levels of genetic testing and screening, genetic diagnosis, and treatment.

These effects could be good or they could be bad. A possible good effect is cure of the disease or defect in the individual and in subsequent offspring. The possible deleterious effects, both material and social, include the same ones listed for somatic cell therapy, that is, unanticipated consequences, the danger of reductionism, and the potential for injustice in distribution. Moreover, an additional potential bad effect may be the destruction of nascent human life, if, after the treatment is attempted, the subsequent testing reveals a problem with the new human being. The direct destruction of defective genes is not problematic; the direct destruction of defective human beings is problematic.

If medical interventions are understood strictly as healing, then Type III and Type IV are not medical interventions. They represent a new set of issues that touch on the very definition and proper use of medicine because here the use of a medical technology is to satisfy human desires for enhancements of some characteristic or trait. Now enhancement of itself is not problematic. Think of all the ways human life is enhanced by some aspect of science and medicine and by human choices in the contemporary world. Better nutrition makes humans stronger and when combined with disease control, increases the life spans. Vitamins delivered before birth through the mother across the placenta give babies a healthier start in life. Laser surgery is used to improve vision and to eliminate glasses. On the other hand, athletic performances enhanced by chemicals are disdained; these are judged as unfair. So lines are drawn and ought to be drawn. The placement of the line must be capable of being defended, that is, it must be drawn for such important reasons as grave harm or uncertainty for the future or misuse of resources.

In a developed and affluent society in which choice and power to effect that choice control the direction of science and technology, some of the concerns are: the reason for the enhancement, the degree of enhancement, and the means of enhancement. In developed and developing nations, there appears a normal progression of enhancement of human life and human living. This normal progression might even be designated natural. One example is the Flynn Effect, the progression of IQ over time. The studies by James Flynn, taken from a variety of sources from 20 countries over 60 years and supported by significant and reliable data, show steadily increasing IQs. If there is a natural progression of improvement, might it be possible to use that as a model to guide enhancement that is an incremental progression of enhancement? The important concerns in regard to genetic enhancement in addition to why, what degree, and by what means, are concerns about (1) the distribution of the good of enhancement, (2) the direction of financial resources toward enhancement and away from cure (think of the millions of dollars spent in developed nations on cosmetic surgery), and (3) the possible change of perception of normal versus disabled human being with a consequence of increased discrimination against those who are not enhanced and decreasing sensitivity toward those who are perceived as less than perfect.

Type IV germ cell genetic enhancement has all the potential problems as somatic cell enhancement and two additional risks. The first is the risk of "made to order" children, a topic treated in Chapter 6 on human cloning. Here, the genetic identity is chosen as an object of someone else's aspirations. Failure to live up to these aspirations adds an additional pressure to one's life. The second is the possible destruction of those embryos or fetuses who, when examined before birth, do not live up to the specifications of the genetic enhancement.

Each of these types of genetic engineering presents complicated scientific, medical, and ethical questions that touch on the very definition of medicine, the use of medicine within culture, and the distribution of medical resources around the globe. These questions will continue to arise. They will continue to arise at points where all the disciplines intersect with each other. Therefore, it is important that people being trained in any one discipline receive some training in the others, and that institutions develop the means to bring individuals trained in the different disciplines into meaningful conversation with each other. We cannot afford to "silo" these areas of expertise.

(D) Advancements in Genetic Engineering

With the completion of the mapping of the human genome, the identification of specific genetic markers including those of genetic diseases, and the increased understanding of the possibility of its manipulation, genetic engineering of the human genome has become the new reality. A number of tools have been developed including TALENs – transcription activator-like effector nucleases, ZFNs – zinc finger nucleases, and, more recently, the CRISPR-Cas9 mechanism. All of these utilize prescription enzymes that are engineered to cut specific sequences of DNA. Once cut, the DNA is susceptible to repair or editing. The constructed repair DNA can be conveyed by a bacterial or viral vector or inserted into a plasmid to be delivered by way of messenger and guide RNA to the nucleus of the cell where its genome is accessed and repaired. The last, the CRISPR-Cas9 mechanism, was observed as an adaptive immune system generated in some pro and eukaryotic organisms as a response to viral infection.

The mechanism of CRISPR-Cas9 emerged from the work of American biochemist Jennifer Doudna and French microbiologist Emmanuelle Charpentier in their independent and then cooperative studies to yield a more efficient genetic engineering tool. The system operates by means of the CRISPR-associated protein Cas9 which cuts the DNA of the infecting virus, constructs a specific sequence of the genome, and delivers it to produce in the host genome a set of Clustered Regularly Interspaced Short Palindromic Repeats (CRISPR) which include DNA fragments from the infection and which now were capable of detecting and destroying the DNA of subsequent infections. This adaptive immune system of CRISPR-Cas9 is simpler, less expensive, and more effective as a genome editing tool than its predecessor mechanisms. Therein lies its promise as well as its peril and its excitement as well as its unease.

The application of this new technology requires that it be performed safely and ethically. To ensure safe and ethical delivery of the new technology requires the protective action of legal regulation and ethical consideration. Manipulation of the genome, while offering great hope for the alleviation of illness and disability caused by hereditary disease, is not unproblematic. The potential biological problems include off-target alterations, on-target alterations with unintended consequences, unknown immunogenic factors, lack of efficient delivery, and uncertainty in binding.

To address the issues presented by the amazing possibilities suggested by the application of this new technology, a group of experts in the fields of science and medicine along with an interest in law and ethics gathered in Napa California in 2015 to initiate a discussion on its governance as it might apply to the human genome. They issued a statement *A prudent path forward for genomic engineering and germline gene modification*. The statement contained four recommendations:

1) Strongly discourage, even in those countries with lax jurisdictions where it might be permitted, any attempts at germline genome modification for clinical application in humans, while societal, environmental, and ethical implications of such activity are discussed among scientific and governmental organizations. (In countries with a highly developed bioscience capacity, germline genome modification in humans is currently illegal or tightly regulated.) This will enable pathways to responsible uses of this technology, if any, to be identified.
2) Create forums in which experts from the scientific and bioethics communities can provide information and education about this new era of human biology, the issues accompanying the risks and rewards of using such powerful technology for a wide variety of applications including the potential to treat or cure human genetic disease, and the attendant ethical, social, and legal implications of genome modification.
3) Encourage and support transparent research to evaluate the efficacy and specificity of CRISPR-Cas9 genome engineering technology in human and nonhuman model systems relevant to its potential applications for germline gene therapy. Such research is essential to inform deliberations about what clinical applications, if any, might in the future be deemed permissible.

4) Convene a globally representative group of developers and users of genome engineering technology and experts in genetics, law, and bioethics, as well as members of the scientific community, the public, and relevant government agencies and interest groups, to further consider these important issues, and where appropriate, recommend policies.

(Baltimore, pp. 37–38)

These recommendations remain a set of guidelines to initiate conversation and, as well, to understand and manage risks arising from the new promising technology. The responsible use of the technology requires that issues of safety and efficacy be addressed in a manner that is not overwhelmed by compassion. The press for exemption from normal regulatory oversight, except in the case of a national emergency, should be initially greeted with suspicion.

In the United States, all research projects utilizing federal funds are governed by international and federal guidelines for the protection of human subjects. The federal guidelines are both legislative and agency-driven. These guidelines are subject to modification in the presence of the rapid expansion of the science. As is often the case, science advances more rapidly than reflection on its appropriate use and limits. Genetic engineering provides a case in point. Lawmakers have supported legislation to fund this emerging field and, at the same time, they have limited procedures deemed unethical. For example, in 2020, the Appropriations Committee of the U.S. House of Representatives banned the FDA from considering any request to approve clinical trials in which a human embryo is intentionally created or modified to include a heritable gene modification. (Recall that the production of human embryos in the infertility industry for possible implantation and gestation is for the most part an unregulated industry in the United States.) The presidents and the courts have and will continue to weigh in as the field develops.

The governing regulatory agencies in the United States have been the Department of Health and Human Services (HHS), the U.S. Food and Drug Administration (FDA), and the Recombinant DNA Advisory Committee of the National Institutes of Health (NIH). The FDA applies the same standards to genome research and application that it applies to any drug application. These standards include a phased process that begins with preclinical studies on nonhuman subjects to determine efficacy, toxicity, and action on the body. Phase 1 tests a *nontherapeutic* dosage on healthy volunteers to determine safety. Phase 2 tests a therapeutic dosage on a small group of patients (100–300) to determine therapeutic *efficacy*, *safety*, and *side* effects. These three effects – efficacy, safety, and side effects – do not require perfect performance. They require high probability of success and low probability of harm. Efficacy is the determination of the effectiveness of the medication, that is, does it have the effect that is intended. Measures of efficacy guard against wasteful spending and fraud in health care. Safety and side effects are measured in degrees of risk as compared to the benefit of treatment. Phase 3 studies continue to monitor the drug while it offers a therapeutic dosage to a larger group of patients. Phase 4 is the study of long-range effects.

HHS applies the standards contained in the Common Rule – Code of Federal Regulations Title 45, Part 46 (45CFR§46). The Common Rule was updated in 2018. Its focus is the protection of human subjects who participate in medical research. In this role, regulations are in place to guide research and to require informed consent on the part of participating subjects. Because informed consent requires a subject capable of knowing the issues at hand and situated as to be free, the Rule considers special populations and the limitations of informed consent in those populations. These special populations include pregnant women, fetuses, neonates, prisoners, children, and wards of the state.

While on its face the Rule appears stringent, there is considerable elasticity in the operational policies. Examples of this elasticity can be found at 45CFR§46.207 which sets in place a process to approve "[r]esearch not otherwise approvable which presents an opportunity to understand, prevent, or alleviate a serious problem affecting the health or welfare of pregnant women, fetuses, or neonates" and 45CFR§46.407 which similarly sets in place a process to approve of "[r]esearch not otherwise approvable which presents an opportunity to understand, prevent, or alleviate a serious problem affecting the health or welfare of children." It is instructive to view the movement from 45CFR§46.404 to 45CFR§46.408 as the possible experimentation on children traverses a gradation of risks and a parallel gradation of assent and permission. Here assent of the child and permission of the parent(s) take the place of informed consent. The assent of the child is ascertained by the appropriate Institutional Review Board (IRB) when in its judgment that a child is capable of providing assent. In making its determination, the IRB must take into account the ages, maturity, and psychological state of the children involved. However, this assent can be waived. If the IRB determines that

> the capability of some or all of the children is so limited that they cannot reasonably be consulted or that the intervention or procedure involved in the research holds out a prospect of direct benefit that is important to the health or well-being of the children and is available only in the context of the research, the assent of the children is not a necessary condition for proceeding with the research.
>
> (45CFR§46.408 (a))

At 45CFR§46.404, the research must involve *no greater than minimal risk* to children. Here, the assent of the child and the permission of the parents or guardians must be solicited. At 45CFR§46.405, the research is described as "involving *greater than minimal risk* but presenting the prospect of *direct benefit* to the individual subjects." Here, the greater risk is justified by the potential benefit to the child. The assent of the child and the permission of the guardians must be sought. At 45CFR§46.406, the research involves "*greater than minimal risk* and *no prospect of direct benefit* to individual subjects, but likely to yield *generalizable knowledge about the subject's disorder* or condition." Here, the research has no direct benefit for the child subject but can go forward as a *social contribution*, that is, generalizable knowledge to gain understanding about the child's condition or disorder.

At 45CFR§46.407, a process is in place that approves "[r]esearch not otherwise approvable which presents an opportunity to understand, prevent, or alleviate a serious problem affecting the health or welfare of children." Here, the research has *no relation* to the child or the child's condition or advancing knowledge related to the child's condition. The research under consideration is permitted to move forward as a contribution to advancing knowledge about children in general. It is again a social contribution within which the child is rendered experimental material. To this last move toward approval of the research project, there is added a requirement of consultation with experts in science, medicine, law, and ethics along with public review to determine the reasonableness of the opportunity presented by this experiment and to assure that sound ethical principles are applied. As in the previous levels of experimentation on children, the assent of the child and the permission of the parent(s) or guardians are to be solicited. Here, the research imperative appears to obliterate informed consent.

NIH established its Recombinant DNA Advisory Committee (RAC) in 1974 to provide recommendations to the NIH Director and to provide a public forum for discussion of the scientific, safety, and ethical issues related to basic and clinical research involving recombinant or synthetic nucleic acid molecules. In its early work, RAC set guidelines and reviewed for approval all DNA research. Its original mandate was to follow and provide advice on safety and ethical issues associated with emerging biotechnologies. These emerging areas of research include technologies involved in human gene transfer. In 2019, NIH refocused RAC and the committee was renamed the Novel and Exceptional Technology and Research Advisory Committee (NExTRAC). In order to streamline oversight of human gene therapy (HGT) research by eliminating duplicative review and reporting requirements, RAC would no longer require individual HGT protocol submissions and no longer require reporting to NIH. That review and oversight is now the task of the FDA and local institutions. Local oversight is to be provided by institutional review boards and institutional biosafety committees. Insofar as HGT protocols include research on human subjects, these protocols are to be governed by the Common Rule, FDA regulations, and local oversight.

At this point, research is moving forward in genetic engineering in somatic cells for therapeutic reasons. This is Type I and if safe, it is ethical. No experiments are going forward that effect germline therapeutic, somatic enhancement, or germline enhancement genetic engineering in the United States. The world scientific community met a report of germline therapeutic genetic engineering in China with widespread disapproval. Several trials in genetic engineering of somatic cells for therapeutic reasons are in process. Clinical trials as Phase II – a therapeutic treatment in a small sample – are going forward to treat retinal blindness and as preclinical studies in sickle cell anemia.[5] Oversight of these trials lies in the domain of regulatory agencies – FDA, HHS, and local IRBs – in the United States. This strict oversight remains an important protection of vulnerable human subjects and ought not to be ignored or bypassed.

(E) Afterword

Genetic testing and genetic screening are powerful tools in the detection of genetic anomalies. Genetic engineering – as therapeutic – suggests the possibility of the elimination and/or control of genetic disease in a manner similar to the control of other diseases. Identification of those that can be successfully treated with the tools at hand serves the human good as individual and as common.

Attempts to arrive at appropriate sets of guidelines are fraught with difficulty. In regard to testing and screening, the following must be considered: (1) there should be compelling reasons for the testing or screening; (2) the burdens-to-benefit ratio should be favorable, that is, there should be an available treatment that ameliorates the condition; (3) there should be a careful assessment of the vulnerability of the person in the case of serious negative outcomes; and (4) there is a caring and compassionate well-informed family or network in place.[6]

At this point in time, a set of guidelines for genetic engineering is a moving target. Nonetheless, some guidelines from the past are helpful. Safety to the patient and distribution of health care resources are the central concerns. In regard to the safety of patients, careful attendance to the FDA guidelines – outside of an emergency – requiring phased trails is necessary. Informed consent is necessary where possible and where not possible, limits to the elasticity of assent and permission must be tightened.

Genetic engineering raises fundamental questions about the human condition that cannot be answered by science and medicine alone. That fact has implications for how scientists and physicians are trained. They will have to answer some of those questions in their own work, but they will need help from other disciplines. However, the sciences and medicine have a specific role in helping society engage in evidence-based conversation about those questions. That contribution cannot be ignored.

Questions for Reflection

1. The desire to improve the quality of the human race and the quality of individual members is as old as the history of mankind. Cite some significant historical and personal instances of the press of this desire.
2. The goal of genetic engineering is to contribute to the improvement of human life. This goal becomes suspicious when it becomes the tool of the state as part of a eugenics program. In the late nineteenth century and in the early twentieth century, the United States was a leader in a eugenics program that was advanced by way of nonvoluntary sterilization. Read the excerpt by Mr. Justice Oliver Wendell Holmes in the *Buck v. Bell* decision. What values are presented in that excerpt?
3. How should the line be drawn between the promise and the peril of genetic engineering in humans? How does the "law of unintended consequences" factor into your analysis?
4. Because of its past history with nonvoluntary sterilization, the United States now has in place a formidable set of protections surrounding the important right to procreate. These protections can be found in Court decisions and in the guidelines of the Department of Human Services which proscribe sterilization of the mentally incompetent. Do these guidelines provide the proper balance of protection for procreative rights and for children?
5. Early criteria for genetic screening included the point that an effective treatment had to be available. More recently developed criteria have expanded, on the grounds that (a) it can simply be good to know if a genetic disorder is present, even if it cannot currently be treated, and (b) knowing that a disorder is present allows further research to be done. If you were a legislator, or a hospital administrator, with limited resources, and considering the issue of false positives, where would you draw the line and why?
6. What are the limits of the research imperative? How should the competing goods of research, consent, privacy, and the potential for abuse be balanced?
7. Do Type III (somatic enhancement) and Type IV (germ cell enhancement) genetic engineering count as *medical* interventions? Why or why not? What definition of "medicine" underlies this answer?

8. What qualifies certain forms of *therapy* or *enhancement* as legitimate or illegitimate uses of medicine?
9. The genetic testing of children presents a particularly difficult decision. What guidelines should be in place to protect the child and the family?
10. What effects might easy access to genetic enhancement modalities have on society?

Notes

1 In addition to the Cohen (*Imbeciles: The Supreme Court, American Eugenics, and the Sterilization of Carrie Buck*) and the Aronoff, "The Constitutionality of Asexualization Legislation in the United States," texts, the collection of papers in *A century of eugenics in America*. Indiana University Press, 2011 provides an interesting set of readings that moves from the history of the eugenics movement in the USA from the passage of the Indiana eugenic sterilization law to the present moment of eugenics operative in the era of the mapping of the human genome. The set of readings, edited by Paul Lombardo, was part of the Indiana Legacy project launched in 2007 to mark the centennial of the Indiana Eugenic Sterilization Law. Embedded within the readings is the perennial nature/environment debate as individuals, families, particular groups, society, and governmental policies press for the betterment of offspring and the human race.

2 Recall David the Bubble Boy.

3 A vector is a vehicle that delivers the genetic material to the proper site.

4 Jesse Gelsinger died on September 17, 1999 while participating in a phase 1 clinical trial for gene therapy at the Institute for Human Gene Therapy at the University of Pennsylvania. Phase 1 trials are *generally* understood to be testing the toxicity of the experimental therapy at various dose levels. In "Are Phase 1 trials therapeutic? Risk, ethics, and division of labor," *Bioethics*, March 2014, *28* (3), 138–146, James A. Anderson and Jonathan Kimmelman examine the differing perspectives of the various stakeholders – drug regulatory agencies, institutional review boards, clinical investigators, referring physicians, and patients – in their understanding of the purpose of Phase 1 trails. The different understanding is seen in Anderson's account of the trajectory of the ratio of safety/effectiveness. For the regulatory agencies, the focus is the toxicity profile. At the distant end, the patient holds a hope for therapeutic effectiveness. The 18-year-old had a mild or partial type of ornithine transcarbamylase deficiency (OTCD) which was identified when he was 2 years old. In his case, the deficiency was managed by a low-protein diet and medication in the form of 50 pills a day. Jesse volunteered for the project because he thought it might help him and children with the more deadly form of the disease. Jesse received an infusion of the OTC gene attached to an adenovirus to integrate the added gene into his chromosomal DNA. Four days later, apparently having suffered a massive immune response triggered by the use of the viral vector to transport the gene into his cells leading to multiple organ failure and brain death, Jesse was declared dead and removed from life support. His death halted all gene therapy for a time and his death continues to raise questions about the ethics of human experimentation.

5 One site of this Phase II trial is at the Casey Eye Institute at Oregon Health and Science University. It uses the CRISPR tool to attempt to repair mutations in the *CEP290* gene that cause a rare form of inherited blindness called Leber congenital amaurosis type 10; also known as LCA10 and *CEP290*-related retinal

dystrophy. The preclinical studies in sickle cell are centered on red blood cell genotyping.

6 Every year, when I (MMH) teach the issues of gene therapy, gene enhancement, and genetic engineering, the students raise an important question. Their question is: "What human emotion might be lost, if there were no persons with disabilities to draw forth sympathy, compassion, and finally love. What kind of society might we have then?" No doubt, this is an important question to ponder. In response, I always ask them if they had a child with a disability and they had the opportunity to correct that disability, would they? The subsequent questions are: Who is to choose? By what criteria would they choose the qualities and characteristics that best serve human flourishing whether for the individual or for society? How should the goods at hand be distributed? And here the issue is joined.

8 Special Relationships/Special Responsibilities

This scriptural passage from Saint Paul's *Letter to the Romans* notes distinct part-to-whole relationships. Saint Paul wrote:

> Each of us has one body, with many different parts, and not all those parts have the same function; just so we, though many in number, form one body in Christ, and each acts as the counterpart of the other. The spiritual gifts we have differ, according to the special grace which has been assigned to each. If a man is a prophet, let him prophesy as far as the measure of faith will let him. The administrator must be content with his administration, the teacher, with his work of teaching, the preacher, with his preaching. Each must perform his own task well; giving alms with generosity, exercising authority with anxious care, or doing works of mercy smilingly.
>
> (*Romans* 12: 4–8)

The first relation is the relationship of the parts of the body each of which has a distinct function to serve the good of the person. The human being and these parts constitute a physical whole that is a union in being. Human beings are given a particular kind of body with particular parts whose integration and accomplishment serve human flourishing. The second part-to-whole relationship is that wherein each person, with particular assigned gifts, is part of the body of Christ. This relationship constitutes a spiritual whole that is captured in the theology of the mystical body. A third relationship is that of the reciprocal relationship of the human person and the human community. This set of relationships constitutes a moral whole, that is, a union of purpose, which by its reciprocal activities fashions a community in which human flourishing as individual and societal is possible. Properly understood human flourishing, as individual, as societal, and as spiritual, accomplishes its final end in union with God. This final end orders the other ends of the maintenance of life, the sustaining of the good life, and the receptivity of the insertion of

DOI: 10.4324/9781003627197-8

grace. As a member of the Body of Christ, each human being is called to order one's life and to serve God's people. Each person is called to exercise a particular set of gifts in service to that body. The scriptural text also acknowledges a difference in the distribution of gifts, exemplified here as prophecy, service, and teaching. It continues with a reminder that all gifts received are to be used, and used well, in the service of others. Moreover, the reception of the gift places its possessor in a relationship rooted in the need of others of that particular gift. Note too that the passage draws attention to the fact that the gifts flow primarily from the grace of God with human agency adding its cooperation to the gifts of grace. Hence, there can be no proprietary claim to these gifts; they are not the exclusive private property of the recipient. While it is true that they are given to the individual, the deeper truth is that they are meant to be a gift to the world through the individual.[1]

Finally, because the human person is created in the image and likeness of the Trinity, it ought to be expected that every aspect of human existence would be experienced as a call into relationship and communion. Saint Catherine of Siena, in her *Dialogue*, says that God explained to her that this is part of the reason for the unequal distribution of gifts among human beings:

> I distribute the virtues quite diversely; I do not give all of them to each person, but some to one, some to others . . . And so I have given many gifts and graces, both spiritual and temporal, with such diversity that I have not given everything to one single person, so that you may be constrained to practice charity towards one another . . . I have willed that one should need another and that all should be my ministers in distributing the graces and gifts they have received from me.
>
> (*Dialogue*, I.7 in *Catechism of the Catholic Church*, 1937)

The simple fact of diversity in abilities points toward relationships.

This chapter focuses on the special part to whole relations of the human condition as found in the individual as composed of many related parts and as found in the human condition as social, that is as related to and needing others. This chapter will proceed in the following fashion:

(A) Framing the Issue: Human Life in Relationships;
(B) Maternal–Fetal Relationship;
(C) Physician–Patient Relationship;
(D) Mentally Ill and Their Families and Society;
(E) Human Person and the Gift of the Body;
(F) Afterword: the Limits of Responsibility.

(A) Framing the Issue

As individual, the human being subsists as a whole whose integrated parts serve its flourishing. Human life is embodied in a particular way. The social situation of human living derives from the fact that individual human flourishing requires the existence of a society capable of nurturing that flourishing. There is a reciprocal relationship between the good of the individual and the good of society. This places human beings in a variety of relationships. The distribution of gifts required to serve human flourishing is unequal. This distribution results in sets of relationships that are simultaneously asymmetrical and symmetrical. The relations are symmetrical inasmuch as they are relationships between human beings as human beings. This requires appropriate mutual respect. The relationships are asymmetrical because the more powerful have been given particular gifts to serve the less powerful. This requires appropriate care. Hence, specific obligations fall upon the recipients of special gifts to serve others if individual human life and human society are to flourish.

The reality is that human life is lived in relationships – a fact that is charged with philosophical and theological meaning. This truth, recognized from the writings of antiquity to the persistent and consistent contemporary claims of solidarity, puts to rest the enlightenment myth of human beings as autonomous rights-bearing individuals. Recall Aristotle's claim of need of man *qua* man for social structure from both the family and the political structure, if man is to flourish. In the *Politics,* he described the human who might live outside of social structures in the following: "so that he must be either a lower animal or a god" (Aristotle, 1253a). These relations function across and sustain society. Human beings begin their lives in a relationship. Human flourishing is dependent upon a content-thick matrix of specific goods to be accomplished within particular relationships. Among these relationships are the mother and child, husband and wife, parent(s) and the family, teacher and student, physician and patient, researcher and subject, lawyer and client, and citizens and the commonweal. This chapter will treat three real social relationships. They are the maternal–fetal relationship, the physician–patient relationship, and the relationship between the mentally ill and those whose obligation is their care. It will then turn to the individual human being as an integrated whole whose body, understood as gift of God, empowers and limits the individual in its use. The gift of the body requires its acceptance and its care throughout a lifetime that will witness its development, its flourishing, and its diminishment unto death.

The three social relations can be described, isomorphically, as the relation between the powerful and the vulnerable. Each relationship can guide and serve as an exemplar for the direction of other relationships encountered in society. The asymmetry of these essential relationships is obvious.

Power has its source in position, competency, and knowledge. Vulnerability derives from a variety of limitations such as inadequate knowledge, immaturity, dependence, incapacity, and the deficit caused by illness. Each position of power is marked by special gifts that, as the Scriptures remind, are to be used in service to the vulnerable. The model for this service is God who created each human being in His image and likeness. As God is a communion of persons, humanity is called into community; as God is creative, humankind is called to be creative; as God is providential, humankind is called upon to be providential; as God is sacrificial, humankind is called upon to be sacrificial; as God is love, humankind is called upon to love and to be loved. The exercise and duty of creativity, of stewardship, of sacrifice, and of love flow from the particular gifts that have been given to those who have been chosen to care for God's creatures in a particular way.

(B) Maternal–Fetal Relationship

In the not-too-distant past, the topic of maternal–fetal relations would be covered in a sentence or two. Pregnant women ought to care for the children they carry. Society, including medicine and law and business as parts of society, ought to have in place protections for pregnant women and the children they are carrying. However, that was the past; the present is different. This section will proceed in the following fashion: (1) examination of elements in the contemporary culture that are problematic for this relationship; (2) examination of the elements in the reality of the relationship itself that might serve human flourishing; and (3) an examination of practical problems that arise in this relationship.

(1) The Present Context

Among the reasons for the cultural difference of the present are three that together have exercised a catalytic effect in the transformation of the underlying culture. The first is the power in the public sphere of a particular form of feminism. The second was the removal of legal protection for the developing but conceived preborn human being, the *conceptus*, by U.S. Supreme Court decisions and state laws.[2] The third is the remarkable advance of medicine and medical technology. These advances allow medicine to be not only effective in the cure of illness, in the care of those whose illness cannot be cured, in the amelioration of the effects of disabilities, and in service to human flourishing but also to use its skills beyond medical indication or medical necessity to serve human choices. Two examples of the last are the increasing incidence, without medical necessity, of cosmetic surgery and elective abortion.

The characterization of women that operates from within this contemporary matrix is that of women as isolated, autonomous, rights bearers, who, within a zone of privacy, claim among their important rights the liberty to abortion if pregnancy interferes with their interests or is a burden in any way to their definition of their lives. A woman may, if she chooses, isolate herself from the father of the child even in those instances where he is her husband and where he wants the child and is committed to the support of the woman and the child. A pregnant minor girl, now an emancipated minor, may isolate herself from her parents in making this important decision in her life. In some cases, the relation of women and girls to spouses and parents is now supplanted by a relationship to the State.

Decisions of the Courts, including the 1973 decisions *Roe v. Wade* and *Doe v. Bolton* and the 1992 decision *Casey v. Planned Parenthood*, and as well the decisions which presented challenges to these Court rulings, constructed the values that from 1973 forward ordered and continue to order the present cultural matrix. While the Court rulings speak of the possible protection accorded to the fetus as a function of its development, there is, as a matter of fact, little real protection. These judicial rulings, by designating the fetus as a nonperson and by refusing to address the issue of its humanity, rendered invisible the human being developing within the body of the pregnant woman. Considered simply as the product of conception or considered simply by reference to the condition of the woman, her pregnancy, it could be removed from her body or her pregnancy could be terminated at her request. Subsequently, the remains of this nascent human life became accessible and manipulable as embryonic tissue and fetal tissue to provide possible material for harvest and use of its stem cells.

Women in developing nations were accorded similar protections in the name of women's liberation to destroy the human beings developing within their bodies. Nations and businesses, which do not fall into line and grant this liberty to women, are considered oppressive and reactionary. Access to abortion as part of total reproductive services is required to be included in many aid programs, both nationally and internationally, that focus on the health of women.

The most significant result of the change in the culture has been the number of abortions performed in the United States in the wake of these judicial interventions. The narrative of a national need to legalize abortion for those rare instances in which the pregnancy was a threat to the life or health of the mother, the pregnancy was the result of rape or incest, or the problem of serious irremediable fetal deformity has been shown to be false. The supposed rarity of abortion has been displaced by the reality that, by and large, abortion was to be sought and granted now as a choice for an unplanned pregnancy. That this is the case illustrated by the fact that from

1973 to the present, the culture of the United States has witnessed the transition in the understanding of the practice of elective abortion from that of a heinous act, spoken of in whispers, if spoken of at all, to that of the most common surgical procedure performed on young women.

The data regarding the frequency of elective abortion and the data regarding the procurers of abortion are striking (Jones, Finer, and Singh, pp. 5ff.). From 1973 until the present, the number of abortions in just the United States has averaged approximately 1.3 million per year, that is, 60 million conceived unborn children killed at the request of their mothers. The year 1990 marks a high point in the procurement of abortion with approximately 1.5 million human lives aborted. From 2001 forward, the average has leveled to approximately 1.2 million per year. Of the women procuring abortions, 65% self-identify as Christian; 85% are either not married or not in a significant relationship; and 54% used, albeit some inconsistently, some form of contraceptive (Jones, Finer, and Singh). Some of the reasons that have been offered by women for the choice of elective abortion are (a) responsibility to other individuals; (b) inability to afford a child; (c) the perceived interference of a child with work or school or other dependents; (d) the unwillingness to be a single parent; (e) or the experience of a difficult relationship with the putative father of the child (Jones, Finer, and Singh). Some women choose abortion because of fetal defect that can range from the devastation of anencephaly to tetralogy of Follot to Down syndrome to deficiencies caused by maternal drug and alcohol abuse. The abortion rate for children diagnosed with Down syndrome (Trisomy 21) in the U.S.A. has been estimated, according to statistics drawn from theory-based demographic models, to be 30% (Graaf, p. 765).

As the technology for identifying fetal anomalies grows more sophisticated, the list of indications for elective abortion grows longer. Note well the absence of abortion because the life or health of the mother is at risk. Various surveys from the Alan Guttmacher Institute to the state and federal registries to the data of the National Right to Life Committee are fairly consistent in reporting relatively low percentages of abortions in the category of the "hard" cases even while it is the case that the numbers from the Alan Guttmacher Institute triple the numbers from the National Right to life Committee.

Three things are undeniable. The first is that there are problem pregnancies. The second is that the vast majority of abortions now performed in the United States are not performed for medical reasons; they are elective procedures. The third is the fact that so many women and girls are choosing abortion. In regard to the first, the life of the pregnant woman must continue to be protected in the law and by medicine. So too must the life of the child that is developing within her. Moreover, men and women, members of a society that is committed to human flourishing, must address this issue of problem pregnancy and fashion the essential solutions that are conducive to a culture that does not choose killing as a solution to its problems. This must include the care of the mother and child when it is the case that the child, *en ventra sa mère* (within its mother's womb), has a condition incompatible with life. It must include the care of the child and the family when it is the case that the child will be born with disabilities. It must include care for the mother and the child, if it is the case that the familial structure does not exist or is broken. This last must be accomplished in a way that does not facilitate the destruction of the family, that hinge unit of society that is essential for the flourishing of individuals and society.

In regard to the second, that is elective abortion, if most abortions are not performed for medical reasons, then the role of physician as physician is transformed in the practice of medicine in this procedure. That is, physicians abandon the commitment to their professional life and become technicians, albeit skilled technicians, to what is simply the facilitation of the choices of some women. In regard to the third point, the magnitude of the number of abortions in the U.S.A. calls into question, on one hand, the quality of the women's and girls' consent as both informed and free in regard to the object of abortion, and, on the other hand, the possibility of willed ignorance or scotosis[3] in regard to the life developing within the body of the woman.

(2) A Context of Real Relations

Pregnancy provides a concrete and paradigmatic example of human lives embedded in a relationship.[4] In the normal course of events, all human beings begin their lives in this relationship. Two human beings, both the woman and the conceived yet unborn human being, exist as really related to each other. An adequate morality requires attention be directed both to the relationship and to the beings who constitute the relationship. Directing attention to the relationship reveals the union to be asymmetrical. Directing attention to the beings in the relationship reveals an isomorphic symmetry, that is, each related being is a human being but at a particular point on the human development trajectory.

Examination of pregnancy as a relationship reveals several things. Pregnancy is a temporary physical and moral union of two whole human beings. There is a physical union which is a union in being. There is a moral union also and this is a union of purpose. As a physical union, it is more complex than most physical unions. In most physical unions, the relationship is of whole to part where the part is not necessary for the continuation of the whole and where it may be the case that if the part threatens the life of the whole, the part may be destroyed. The amputation of a cancerous organ provides a sufficient example. Pregnancy is temporary physical relationship between two physically whole human beings, one immature and one mature. In most instances, the continuation of the temporary relationship does not endanger the life of either.

The temporary physical relationship is also a moral union, a unity of purpose. Neither of the human beings who constitute the relationship is determined to accomplish the totality of its existence within this relationship. Each of the two entities has meaning outside the relationship. The woman is a relatively autonomous being. Her life is characterized by a set of ends that extend beyond the pregnancy. For the duration of the pregnancy, the fetus is a radically dependent human being. While its growth and development are intrinsically directed, its continued existence is possible only within the nurturing environment supplied by the woman. Accomplishment of the ends of the fetus which lie outside the pregnancy requires the cooperation of the woman. When the union is chosen, either implicitly or explicitly, its status and the obligations of the more powerful member are less problematic from an ethical perspective. The more powerful accepts the disadvantages which occur for the sake of the more dependent. When the union occurs without consent, a more problematic relationship is constituted. The obligations that arise from a non-voluntary or involuntary relationship are a function of the need fulfilled by that relationship and the status of the beings who constitute that relationship. In attending the pregnancy relationship as a physical union, the appropriate question is: What obligations might be claimed to arise where the life of one human being is so radically dependent on the other for such a limited period of time? In attending the relationship as a moral union, the appropriate question is: What limitations may be placed on the activities of the more powerful when they find themselves in relationships that are not of their own choosing?

Two things are worthy of note here. First, while there are many relationships in society that follow the pattern of the weaker and the stronger relationship (physical, political, educational, and financial), what might be the assessment if, in every case, the stronger were permitted to eliminate the weaker because the weaker got in the way. Second, the fact is that in every day life every human being is radically dependent on others. If only the independent have dignity, then most are at risk.

The most powerful agents in the possible transformation of culture are women. Women must reclaim the responsibility of bearing witness to the proper ordering of love and marriage and procreation, and of sharing that understanding of that responsibility with those – other women, men, boys, and girls – in their lives. The advances that women have made are important advances and feminism has been an important catalyst in the opening of wonderful opportunities for women. Women rightly affirm these as good. However, these advances must not be purchased by the failure to recognize the real differences between men and women and the real differences in obligations for men and women. Both men and women live their lives embedded in sets of relationships and from these relationships advantages and obligations arise. These relationships exercise a limiting function on the exercise of autonomy and an enabling function on the exercise of limited autonomy. If, when she is pregnant, she accepts the child that is growing within her and refuses to deliver that child to death, her witness may serve as the catalyst that initiates the transformation of the culture. But, she cannot do it alone. She and her child need the father of their child and the society within which they live so that they might flourish.

(3) *Practical Problems*

With the understanding of our lives embedded in relationships in place, the examination of problematic issues follows. They are (a) the justification for abortion in pregnancies considered a maternal and fetal conflict and (b) the protection of pregnant women in the workplace.

(a) *Maternal–Fetal Conflict*

In the contemporary culture, this potential conflict can be addressed from within the differing feminist perspectives, namely, the gender equality feminist and the gender equity feminist. Each examines and resolves the conflict from within the elements that define her understanding of her place in the world. The gender equality feminist holds a position that she is an autonomous, rights-bearing human being. Because she claims equality to men, which includes a right to be free from pregnancy, she asserts her rights to elective abortion in her rights of privacy, of liberty, and of freedom from burden as fundamental. Furthermore, because the conceived but not yet born human being is not an autonomous, rights-bearer, hence not a person who has standing in the law, she is free to end her pregnancy and the life developing within her whenever the pregnancy interferes with her life, physical health, mental health, economic circumstances, familial or social circumstances, or if the conceived but not yet born human being is deformed or if the conception of the new life is the consequence of rape or incest. Arguments to the contrary notwithstanding, there are no external limitations on elective abortion except physician restraint.

The gender equity feminist recognizes that women and men, while they share a common humanity, have different gifts as male and female. She recognizes that these special gifts provide for human life to be lived and to flourish as embedded in relationships. Her rights to autonomy and to freedom are limited by the legitimate claims of others. She understands that our being in the world as related human beings is the source of our traditions of community and hospitality and solidarity, of mutual respect, and of liberty as ordered, of beneficence, and of intersubjectivity. These relationships constitute the links in the web of society. From these specific relationships to one another, concrete duties arise and are defined. At the same time, the human beings who anchor these relationships possess individual identity. They have significance in themselves apart from these relationships. An adequate moral theory considers both the beings who constitute the relationships and the link which defines the relationship.

The equity feminist ought then to recognize the fact every pregnancy involves at least two human beings, both herself and the child she carries. So, the question becomes under what circumstances the immature and dependent human being may be killed at the request of the more mature and more independent human being. She should present a set of answers different from her sister, the equality feminist, to the question of the permissibility of abortion. Her starting point ought to be that is inasmuch as abortion takes the life of a living developing human being (a position developed in Chapter 4), the moral rules that apply to the taking of human life apply here. This understanding is affirmed in the *Ethical and Religious Directives for Catholic Health Care Services* which in Directive 45 recognizes that abortion is the direct taking of the life of the preborn human being regardless of its stage of development and which forbids abortion at any time in the pregnancy. The directive states:

> Abortion (that is, the directly intended termination of pregnancy before viability or the directly intended destruction of a viable fetus) is never permitted. Every procedure whose sole immediate effect is the termination of pregnancy before viability is an abortion, which, in its moral context, includes the interval between conception and implantation of the embryo. Catholic health care institutions are not to provide abortion services, even based upon the principle of material cooperation. In this context, Catholic health care institutions need to be concerned about the danger of scandal in any association with abortion providers.
>
> (ERDs, 45)

So unless the life of the woman is threatened by the continuation of the pregnancy, abortion is not an option for her.

However, a special case arises for consideration if the life of the pregnant woman is directly threatened by the continued existence of the preborn human being. With the advances of medical science in monitoring pregnancy and caring for the mother and her child, the direct threat to the life of the mother is seldom the case. However, when it is the case that her life is threatened, abortion is permissible under the guiding rubric of the principle of double effect. The act has two effects: (1) saving the life of the woman and (2) the destruction of the child. The fact that the choice here is a choice of one life over another is acknowledged and the principle is applied. The intention of the act is the saving of her life; the death of the preborn human being is foreseen but not intended and if its death can be averted, it must be averted. The most common medical instance of this dilemma in contemporary medicine is ectopic pregnancy. An ectopic pregnancy is the result of the implantation of the embryo in the fallopian tube rather than in the uterus. Its position in the fallopian tube is inappropriate for two reasons: the fallopian tube does not provide a suitable environment for its development and the growth of the embryo in the fallopian tube poses a risk of rupture of the tube and serious medical consequences, including the possibility of death, for the mother. The preborn human being, in cases where the life of the mother is at risk, cannot, however, be viewed as an unjust aggressor in the formal sense. Unjust aggression requires the intention to commit an act of aggression. The preborn human being is not capable of forming an intention. Its position, in the situation of permissible abortion, is to be viewed as material aggression, that is, as a matter of fact, its continued existence poses a threat to the existence of the mother.[5]

The same application of the principle of double effect allows the pregnant woman to go forth with the medical treatment necessary for the continuation of her life and health in the presence of disease or illness. Sometimes the treatment has a second effect of causing the death of the preborn human being. The health of the mother is the intended effect; the death of the child is the unintended and undesired effect. This understanding is affirmed in Directive 47 which states,

> Operations, treatments, and medications that have as their direct purpose the cure of a proportionately serious pathological condition of a pregnant woman are permitted when they cannot be safely postponed until the unborn child is viable, even if they will result in the death of the unborn child.
>
> (ERDs, 47)

It may be the case, however, that the mother, who is faced with a serious illness that requires treatment which poses a threat to the life of her developing child, may choose to forego the treatment for the sake of her child. Her choice, usually made out of religious commitment, such as in imitation of the Christ, is an instance of supererogation, that is going beyond what can be asked. That choice may not be made an obligation for other women. There can be no fetus first rule in ethics or in the law. Both the woman and the preborn human being have equal value as human beings and an equal right to have their life protected.

The case of fetal deformity, no matter what its etiology and no matter what its degree and no matter what its consequent disability, presents a particular problem to be faced by pregnant women and their families. These problems, some quite significant, have been put forth as reasons adequate to justify abortion. Of course, no one wants a child to suffer. But, whether the preborn human being is perceived as a child with intrinsic rights depends on the perspective of the culture. In the world as defined by the gender equality feminist, the preborn human being does not have the rights of a person, hence it is not viewed as a child. Furthermore, its continued existence, especially if it is disabled, may impede the activities or interfere with the lifestyle of the woman. So, whether it is allowed to continue its existence or not is her choice. Its death, as a beneficent or compassionate killing, is to be preferred to its suffering and her freedom is to be preferred to its care. If, on the other hand, the preborn human being is recognized as a dependent member of the human community, a member to whom some other human beings are already related, a different set of responses should arise. The disability of the human being should be compensated for by the ability of the community into which it is born to care for it. Those who suffer disability, and whatever suffering is attendant upon the disability, more frequently than not attest to the fact that they prefer their existence, albeit limited, to their not being born. In the case of a preborn human being with disabilities so grave that it may never be able to attest to the goodness of its existence, its goodness may be affirmed by the impact that its life has on others and those who commit themselves to its care. Here, the first voice that should speak on its behalf is the voice of the woman who is related most intimately to the child. Her choice can initiate societal change, first in her own small society and then as witness to the wider society. The choices that human beings make affect the quality of the society whose progress or decline is fashioned by human choices.

In addition to those pregnancies in which the fetus is known to have a disability, there are some pregnancies in which the fetus has a condition incompatible with life. Once the diagnosis of a condition incompatible with life has been confirmed, the significant question is to determine the appropriate care for the human beings, both mother and child, in this sad, perhaps devastating, and temporary situation. The two possible courses of action are to continue the pregnancy until birth or to seek a termination of pregnancy by early induction. The former response directs attention primarily to the child and the sanctity of the child's life. The latter response directs attention primarily to the woman, her grief, and the desire to move on with her life. In response to this difficult and poignant situation, Catholic

Health Care Institutions have provided different responses. In some institutions, intervention, understood as a kind of direct abortion, is forbidden. In other institutions, very close attention to Directives 45 and 49 in the *Ethical and Religious Directives for Catholic Health Care Services* allows the early induction of labor, the delivery of the child, and care for the child until it dies. Directive 49 states: "For a proportionate reason, labor may be induced after the fetus is viable." It is argued that there is no direct intention to destroy a viable fetus, there is a proportionate reason for the induction, and the resources of the hospital will be made available to sustain the life of the child at delivery.

Neither response is unproblematic. The first response which forbids intervention and which may, if the woman is seeking help in a Catholic institution, force her to seek help elsewhere is claimed to be dismissive of the woman and of her concerns and of the concerns of her family. Some women report feeling abandoned by the institutional church when they needed its comfort most. The child that they so desperately longed for will not be and they wish to bring closure to the tragedy by early induction. Some women, on the other hand, find comfort in carrying their child to term. They experience consolation in the fact that they cared for their child in the only way still possible, that is, in the patient accompanying of the child in its brief life until the child returns to the God who gave it life. Here there needs to be a sustained conversation. In the conversation, the voices of women must be heard. Rather than being dismissed as having vested interests, women must be accorded respect as the voice of experience. The recording of the conversation is important. We shall have listened and we may learn.

The second response, induction and delivery at the point of potential viability, is also problematic, even while it intends to stay within the letter of the law. There is a very real sense in which the child with such a condition is never viable. These children have conditions incompatible with human life; they are not disabled as is the child with Down syndrome. So, an early induction with all the equipment on hand for resuscitation may have the appearance of performance without purpose. A better response might be to have all the appropriate comfort care measures in place for this child who is born dying.

When a woman is pregnant as the result of rape or incest, the woman is rightly the subject of compassion. She has been injured by a violent act and the consequences do not end with the violence of the act. The injury violated her body and her person, and the individual who perpetrated the act should be punished. What she is capable of doing – not just physically capable of doing but also emotionally and spiritually capable of doing – will depend on the society, both large and small, within which she lives and the perspective from which she understands her condition. If she views herself solely as an autonomous, rights-bearing individual and if she views the human life as it develops within her to be possessed of no rights and if she lives in a community that offers her no support in her sad and stressful situation, then abortion appears to be her solution. If, on the other hand, she views herself as related to this new life, despite its origin, and if she views the human life as it develops within her to be a human being possessed of the same rights as every other human being and if she lives in a community that offers her support in her sad and stressful situation, then she may have the capacity to choose life. Women have the strength of character to bear adversity, even great adversity such as presented in pregnancy as a consequence of rape or incest. But it is difficult to bear that weight alone and she is not meant to be alone.

In addressing this difficult question of pregnancy by violation at least two important questions arise. The first question is: what obligations might be claimed to arise where the life of one human being is so radically dependent on another human being for such a limited amount of time? The second question is: what limitations ought to be placed on or expected of the activities of the more powerful members of society when they find themselves in relationships that are not of their own choosing? Note that both questions are not limited to the question of pregnancy. The answers establish principles that apply to many other situations. We shall often find ourselves in situations not of our own choosing. We shall sometimes find ourselves as the stronger party; we shall sometimes find ourselves as the weaker party. The choices that we make under both those circumstances create the kind of person we become and the kind of society we constitute by our membership.

(b) Women in the Workplace

The issue of pregnant women in the workplace has become particularly convoluted within the contemporary horizon marked by gender equality feminism and the legal status of abortion. In the not-too-distant past, there were protections for pregnant women in the workplace. It used to be considered enlightened policy, beneficent even, for businesses to put into place protections for women who are pregnant. The protections were mindful of the fact that she was in a changed condition, not disabled, but carrying a developing new life within her. Now these policies have come to be considered paternalistic and in violation of the right of women to be considered equal to men. As a consequence, the protections for pregnant women and their unborn children have gradually diminished. An example can be found in the case of the *United Automobile Workers v. Johnson Controls (1991)*.

The company, Johnson Controls, produces automobile batteries and during the production of the batteries lead and lead oxide particles are released into the air. This lead can enter into the bloodstream and remain there for a considerable time period. The levels of lead in the air and the levels of lead absorbed into the bloodstream were low enough to be considered safe for adults. However, because the level of lead in the factory was considered high enough to lead to brain and central nervous system damage to the preborn human being, Johnson Controls in an attempt to protect the developing human being and in an attempt to save itself from possible future liability, put into place restrictions on women in the workplace. The company tried a variety of remedies including the exclusion of pregnant women and women at risk for pregnancy from employment by the company to the exclusion of all women from work sites where the risk of contamination was considered significant. The case wound its way through the courts and finally reached the U.S. Supreme Court. The Supreme Court ruled against the protective policy of Johnson Controls. Justice Blackmun who delivered the opinion for the Court wrote:

> Johnson Controls's fear of prenatal injury, no matter how sincere, does not begin to show that substantially all of its fertile women are incapable of doing their jobs . . . [i]t is no more appropriate for the courts than it is for individual employers to decide whether a woman's reproductive role is more important to herself and her family than her economic role.
> (*UAW v. Johnson Controls, Inc.* 111 S. Ct. 1196 EPD 40, 605,1991)

The decision of the Court was framed in the presence of the following elements: (1) the claim of equality of men and women in the workplace; (2) the choice of the women in the exercise of her reproductive role and in the exercise of her economic role; and (3) the lack of standing in the law for the fetus. A better choice might have been had in a company policy that made it possible for pregnant women to have the opportunity to have a position of comparable worth and to continue to work within the company for the duration of their pregnancy.

The appropriate balance in maternal–fetal relationships will be recovered only by the reversal of the cultural bias that has been created by the failure to recognize the preborn human being as a bearer of rights and by the assertion of women of both radical equality and the fundamental right to abortion. With this reversal in place, it may be possible for companies to put into place policies which respect the equal dignity and real differences of men and women and their right to work, the economic needs of women as well as men, and the health needs of developing human beings.

(C) Physician–Patient Relationship

The physician–patient relationship is a temporary relationship between two persons that occurs at the point of clinical practice. While both the physician and the patient live their lives embedded in other relationships including familial, professional, social, and civic, the focus of this section is the complex relationship between the physician *qua* physician and the patient *qua* patient and the physician as human being and the patient as human being. This complex relationship is simultaneously asymmetrical and symmetrical. It is asymmetrical because, on the occasion of the clinical encounter, it is a relationship between unequals. It is, at the same time, symmetrical because it is a relationship between two human beings. Both relationships are directed by what in 1919 William Osler, often called the father of modern medicine, designated *philotechnia* – love of the art – and *philanthropia* – love of humanity (Pellegrino, 1988, p. 22).

The relationship begins most acutely on the occasion of illness when the patient turns to the physician to access the art and practice that the physician professes to hold. The patient, because of the fact of illness, is in an altered existential state. The patient is vulnerable. The condition of illness has been aptly described in the following:

> In the state of illness the body is no longer our ready instrument; it becomes, instead, the center of our concern. It begins to tyrannize, to make demands . . . there is a split between self and body: one steps back, as it were, and begins to look at one's body; the unity of the body and self that had previously existed is fractured . . .
>
> . . . [T]he person who is ill has lost some of his freedom. He does not have the knowledge to discern the answer to three fundamental questions . . . *What's wrong? What can be done?* and *what ought to be done?* . . . [H]e puts himself into the hands of another person. He becomes dependent upon that person and therefore vulnerable.
>
> . . . The underlying thought in illness for most persons, even with trivial and certainly with important symptoms is: *Is this the beginning of the end of my existence?*
>
> (Pellegrino, 2008, p. 67)

The physician, on the other hand, operates from a position of power that has its source in knowledge, training, and experience. The physician presents as competent in the practice of medicine and as willing to employ that competence in the care of the person who presents as patient. Sometimes this care is curative, sometimes it is preventative, sometimes it is palliative, and sometimes it can be only presence. It must always be guided, first, by doing good, that is, practicing the art of medicine in the interest of the patient. The relationship requires trust; it is a fiduciary relationship. It lasts as long as the patient needs the care that comes from the competencies of the physician. Furthermore, it lasts as long as the patient is willing to acquiesce to that care.

In the contemporary era, the question of a structure, the nature, and the appropriate ends of this relationship seem uncertain. In the not-so-distant past, there was a common set of medical/moral principles that directed medical practice. These principles and practices were set out in Antiquity in the Hippocratic Oath, which even while it was violated occasionally, served for centuries as a standard for medical practice in the West. The swearing of the Hippocratic Oath marked entry into the practice of medicine for many. The principles of the Oath were reaffirmed and amplified by the Greek physicians/philosophers of the Roman Empire. Among these were Galen of Pergamon, Aretaeus of Cappadocia, and Scribonius Largus. These principles appear later at the core of *The Prayer of Maimonides.* Despite the longevity of this tradition, few medical schools in the United States swear some form of Oath of Hippocrates. Some schools report swearing the Oath of Geneva; some the Prayer of Maimonides; some an oath written by the faculty and the graduating class; and some report that there is no oath taken by those entering the profession.

An examination of the Hippocratic Oath might, despite its limitations, make concrete some of the obligations of the physician in this relationship to the patient. The Oath states:

> I swear by Apollo the Healer, by Asclepius, by Hygieia, by Panacea, and by all the gods and goddesses, making them my witnesses, that I will carry out, according to my ability and judgment, this oath and this indenture.
>
> To hold my teacher in this art equal to my own parents; to make him partner in my livelihood; when he is in need of money to share mine with him; to consider his family as my own brothers, and to teach them this art, if they want to learn it, without fee or indenture; to impart precept, oral instruction, and all other instruction to my own sons, the sons of my teacher, and to indentured pupils who have taken the physician's oath, but to nobody else.
>
> I will use treatment to help the sick according to my ability and judgment, but never with a view to injury and wrong-doing. Neither will I administer a poison to anybody when asked to do so, nor will I suggest such a course. Similarly I will not give to a woman a pessary to cause abortion. But I will keep pure and holy both my life and my art. I will not use the knife, not even, verily, on sufferers from stone, but I will give place to such as are craftsmen therein.

> Into whatsoever houses I enter, I will enter to help the sick, and I will abstain from all intentional wrong-doing and harm, especially from abusing the bodies of man or woman, bond or free. And whatsoever I shall see or hear in the course of my profession, as well as outside my profession in my intercourse with men, if it be what should not be published abroad, I will never divulge, holding such things to be holy secrets.
>
> Now if I carry out this oath, and break it not, may I gain for ever reputation among all men for my life and for my art; but if I break it and forswear myself, may the opposite befall me.
>
> (*Hippocrates*, pp. 299–301)

It is important to note here that the physician *swears* the oath, "I swear by Apollo the Physician, by Asclepius, by Hygieia, by Panacea, and by all the gods and goddesses." It is a serious undertaking. The named gods and goddesses are invoked because of their connection with healing. The invocation of these gods in particular and all the others indicates the seriousness of the undertaking. The gravity of the oath is reinforced in its closing words with the two conditionals. The first is: "If I carry out this oath . . . may I gain forever reputation among all men for my life and my art." The second is: "[I]f I break it . . . may the opposite befall me." The physician here acknowledges accountability in real consequences that are attendant upon adherence to the oath. The physician's awareness of the double role as physician and as human being appears twice in the Oath as the physician swears to "keep holy both my life and my art" and in the closing words to have the physician's reputation measured by an account of both life and art.

There are ten specific commitments that give content to the oath. The first is the bond between the physician and the teacher. The physician swears to respect the teacher in a manner equal to the relationship between the physician and the parents. The swearing physician promises "to make him [his teacher] partner in my livelihood," to provide financial support when necessary and to teach his family members the art of medicine. The second is a commitment to students of the art of medicine, including his sons, the sons of his teachers, and indentured students, to instruct "without fee or indenture" only those "who have taken the physician's oath."

These obligations to the profession are followed by the commitment of the physician to treat the patient "to help the sick according to my ability and judgment, but never with a view to injury and wrong doing." Two limitations are important here; the first is the specification of the domain of the practice to the sick; the second is limitation of action to the competence of the physician with a positive end first to help and a negative proscription never to harm. What follows next is the list of prohibitions.

The prohibitions are: not to "administer poison to anybody when asked to do so;" not even to suggest poison as a course of action; not to "give to a woman a pessary to cause abortion;" not to have recourse to use of the knife even "on sufferers from stone" (that competence belongs to some other craft); "to abstain from all intentional wrong-doing and harm, especially from abusing the bodies of man or woman, bond or free;" and finally the affirmation of the obligation of confidentiality in the practice of medicine, that is, to keep everything seen or heard as "holy secrets."

Five centuries later, Greek physicians of the Roman Empire claim to be in the line of Hippocrates. Evidence for this can be found in the displeasure of Galen that the contemporaneous medical culture fails in regard to the virtue, the excellence to be accomplished both in life and in the practice of medicine. Galen wrote, as can be found in *The Best Doctor Is Also A Philosopher*, that (1) "doctors pay lip-service to Hippocrates," but are too lazy to actually reach his level of expertise, (2) because they don't follow Hippocrates properly, they lack training in logical theory, and (3) [their] "bad upbringing in our times" which encourages people to value wealth over virtue (Rosen, p. 18).

Scribonius Largus, a contemporary of Galen, in a similar fashion, reminds physicians that "Hippocrates, the founder of our calling, transmits the beginnings of this discipline in the form of our sworn oath." His list of prescriptions and proscriptions can be found in the Preface of his *Compositiones Medicamentorum* which presents a list of 271 medical remedies. Here, he admonishes physicians to be competent. The proper use of drugs is a vital area of their art of healing. This proper use is to be regulated by the appropriate character of the physician as compassionate and kind. This limitation precludes the physician "bound by the sacred oath of medicine" from giving a harmful drug even to an enemy. He wrote:

> Medicine, however, does not measure a man's worth according to his wealth or character, but freely offers its help to all who seek it, and never threatens to harm anyone.
>
> Hippocrates, the founder of our calling, transmitted the beginnings of this discipline in the form of our sworn oath, which ordains that no physician should give, or even show, an abortifacient drug to a pregnant woman. In this way, Hippocrates long ago prepared his students' hearts and minds to learn humane feeling. How much more evil would this man, who thought it wrong to destroy even the tenuous possibility of a man, judge the harming of a living human being! In truth, he believed it to be the utmost importance that each and every physician preserve the name and honor of medicine by working conscientiously, even reverently, in accordance with the maxim which he himself set

> down: "Medicine is the science of healing, not of harming." If, while aiding the suffering, the doctor does not concentrate his whole being on following this ideal in every way, then he does not truly practice the compassion he promises.
>
> (Pellegrino, 1988, p. 26)

The respect for the dignity of the physician requires the recognition of the expertise of the physician. This offering of the competencies of the physician to the patient is to be an exercise of benevolence, not paternalism, to care for the medical needs of the patient. This protects the professionalism and freedom of the physician who cannot be seen as a mere technician directing skills to satisfy the desires of the patient. The patient may not ask the physician to violate the physician's ethical principles and the physician, except under special circumstances, may not ask the patient to accept procedures not directed at the patient's care.

The American Medical Association, since its inception, has developed sets of ethical principles for practitioners. The most recent iteration of its code of ethics is the following:

AMA Principles of Medical Ethics

Preamble

The medical profession has long subscribed to a body of ethical statements developed primarily for the benefit of the patient. As a member of this profession, a physician must recognize responsibility to patients first and foremost, as well as to society, to other health professionals, and to self. The following Principles adopted by the American Medical Association are not laws, but standards of conduct that define the essentials of honorable behavior for the physician.

Principles of Medical Ethics

I. A physician shall be dedicated to providing competent medical care, with compassion and respect for human dignity and rights.

II. A physician shall uphold the standards of professionalism, be honest in all professional interactions, and strive to report physicians deficient in character or competence, or engaging in fraud or deception, to appropriate entities.

III. A physician shall respect the law and also recognize a responsibility to seek changes in those requirements which are contrary to the best interests of the patient.

IV. A physician shall respect the rights of patients, colleagues, and other health professionals, and shall safeguard patients' confidence and privacy within the constraints of the law.
V. A physician shall continue to study, apply, and advance scientific knowledge, maintain a commitment to medical education, make relevant information available to patients, colleagues, and the public, obtain consultation, and use the talents of other health professionals when indicated.
VI. A physician shall, in the provision of appropriate patient care, except in emergencies, be free to choose whom to serve, with whom to associate, and the environment in which to provide medical care.
VII. A physician shall recognize a responsibility to participate in activities contributing to the improvement of the community and the betterment of public health.
VIII. A physician shall, while caring for a patient, regard responsibility to the patient as paramount.
IX. A physician shall support access to medical care for all people.

In the contemporary era, the rights and duties of patients and physicians are often presented in "Bills of Rights" and/or "Bills of Rights and Responsibilities." Patients are advised of these at appropriate times and physicians are instructed in these throughout their careers. They appear in every medical setting. The core commitments to patient rights are similar and can be found in the Code of Medical Ethics of the American Medical Association in the following:

Code of Medical Ethics Opinion 1.1.3

The health and well-being of patients depends on a collaborative effort between patient and physician in a mutually respectful alliance. Patients contribute to this alliance when they fulfill responsibilities they have, to seek care and to be candid with their physicians, for example.

Physicians can best contribute to a mutually respectful alliance with patients by serving as their patients' advocates and by respecting patients' rights. These include the right:

(a) To courtesy, respect, dignity, and timely, responsive attention to his or her needs.
(b) To receive information from their physicians and to have opportunity to discuss the benefits, risks, and costs of appropriate treatment alternatives, including the risks, benefits, and costs of forgoing treatment. Patients should be able to expect that their physicians

will provide guidance about what they consider the optimal course of action for the patient based on the physician's objective professional judgment.

(c) To ask questions about their health status or recommended treatment when they do not fully understand what has been described and to have their questions answered.

(d) To make decisions about the care the physician recommends and to have those decisions respected. A patient who has decision-making capacity may accept or refuse any recommended medical intervention.

(e) To have the physician and other staff respect the patient's privacy and confidentiality.

(f) To obtain copies or summaries of their medical records.

(g) To obtain a second opinion.

(h) To be advised of any conflicts of interest their physician may have in respect to their care.

(i) To continuity of care. Patients should be able to expect that their physician will cooperate in coordinating medically indicated care with other health care professionals, and that the physician will not discontinue treating them when further treatment is medically indicated without giving them sufficient notice and reasonable assistance in making alternative arrangements for care.

(AMA Code of Medical Ethics Opinion 1.1.3)

Note that in these Codes the preponderance of responsibility falls upon the physician to deliver certain goods, namely, treatment, information, respect, privacy, continuity of care, and so forth, to the patient. The major obligation of the patient appears to be to accept or reject care. If the patient accepts care, then it becomes the responsibility of the patient to follow the directives of the physician. If the patient chooses to reject care that is ordinary care for the patient, then the patient–physician relationship no longer exists. The patient should seek treatment from another physician. The physician ought to facilitate that transfer provided that the sought-after treatment accords with the physician's medical and moral judgment. If the sought-after treatment contravenes the physician's medical expertise or moral judgment, the physician is not obliged to provide the care or to make a referral. This is not a case of medical abandonment but the termination of the patient–physician relationship by the patient. If the patient chooses to reject care that is extraordinary care in favor of a different modality or comfort care, then the patient–physician relationship may continue as both the patient and the physician seek the same end of the best medical care for this particular patient in these particular circumstances.

Occasionally, a conflict may arise between the physician and the patient, or more often between the medical team and the family, in regard to appropriate care for a patient. This sometimes occurs at the point of end-of-life decision-making where the medical team assesses the proposed treatment as futile. The resolution of this difficulty has required both institutional and legal attention. Most institutions have put into place policies to guide the resolution of the conflict. These policies follow the framework supplied by the American Medical Association. That framework offers the following:

(1) All health care institutions, whether large or small, should adopt a policy on medical futility; and
(2) Policies on medical futility should follow a due process approach. The following seven steps should be included in such a due process approach to declaring futility in specific cases.

   a. Earnest attempts should be made in advance to deliberate over and negotiate prior understandings between patient, proxy, and physician on what constitutes futile care for the patient, and what falls within acceptable limits for the physician, family, and possibly also the institution.
   b. Joint decision-making should occur between patient or proxy and physician to the maximum extent possible.
   c. Attempts should be made to negotiate disagreements if they arise, and to reach resolution within all parties' acceptable limits, with the assistance of consultants as appropriate.
   d. Involvement of an institutional committee such as the ethics committee should be requested if disagreements are irresolvable.
   e. If the institutional review supports the patient's position and the physician remains unpersuaded, transfer of care to another physician within the institution may be arranged.
   f. If the process supports the physician's position and the patient/proxy remains unpersuaded, transfer to another institution may be sought and, if done, should be supported by the transferring and receiving institutions.
   g. If transfer is not possible, the intervention need not be offered ("Medical-Futility in End-of Life Care," Chicago 1997).

Moreover, many states provide legal protection for physicians in the exercise of their professional judgment. The following is an example from the state of Pennsylvania.

From Pennsylvania Law

20 PA CSA 5431(a)(6):

(a) General rule – A health care provider or another person may not be subject to criminal or civil liability, discipline for unprofessional conduct or administrative sanctions and may not be found to have committed an act of unprofessional conduct as a result of any of the following:

. . .

(6) Refusing to comply with a direction or decision of an individual based on a good faith belief that compliance with the direction or decision would be unethical or, to a reasonable degree of medical certainty, would result in medical care having no medical basis in addressing any medical need or condition of the individual, provided that the health care provider complies in good faith with sections 5424 (relating to compliance) and 5462(c) (relating to duties of attending physician and health care provider).

The symmetry of the relationship of physician and patient has its sources in the relationship of equals, one human being to another human being. In antiquity, this relationship was characterized by the notion *humanitas*, the set of qualities that formed a traditional albeit unwritten code of conduct expected of properly cultivated human beings. This relationship requires respect for human dignity. Every human being has intrinsic value. While the grounding of that dignity may vary, in the religious tradition that is foundational here dignity has its source in the realization that every human being is created by God in the image and likeness of God. Every human being is an end in himself/herself; no human being is to be used solely as a means. The respect for the dignity of the patient requires informed consent, inasmuch as that is possible, regarding the treatment. Informed consent requires knowledge and freedom both of which may be compromised by the fact of the patient's illness and medical understanding of the situation. The respect for the physician requires that the patient inform the physician of all the pertinent information regarding the patient's health. Respect for the autonomy of the physician requires the recognition of the set of values that the physician holds. To request or to attempt to coerce a physician to violate those values is an attack on the integrity of the physician as a person. This relationship of equals is marked by a reciprocal set of operative, albeit limited, values including truth-telling, informed consent, confidentiality, and mutual respect.

This presentation of the social contract/covenant between the individual patient and the individual physician is clearly idealistic and aspirational.

Inasmuch as the physician facilitates the well-being of individual patients, this serves a social good in and of itself. However, the relationship between the physician and society as a whole is more problematic both in its grounding and in its delivery. Attention to the grounding serves to make physicians more aware of their obligations. The physician as professional assumes greater obligation for proper distribution of the goods of medicine. The issue of distribution is addressed in Chapter 9. Physicians are or have been the recipients of certain goods that allow them to practice medicine. A consideration of the nature of the profession provides the grounding of the obligations of the profession and sheds some light on how the profession can contribute to the amelioration of the distribution problem. Membership in any profession is a privileged position whose purpose is to serve the public good. This commitment to serve the public good is paramount, even while the practice of the profession provides the livelihood for the professional. The privilege of membership in a profession confers status to those so admitted and confers obligations upon the professional. The physician receives knowledge and power from institutions that the society has put into place to allow the physician entry into the profession. While physicians work very hard for their education and physicians pay a great deal of money, which represents only part of the cost, for that education and physicians have the right to expect a fine level of compensation, they ought not to consider their profession their private property. The institutions, the medical schools, the colleges, and universities of which they are sons and daughters, the scientists, both the famous and those who labored in relative obscurity, who came before them, the teachers who invested so much in them, the country that sustained peace and offered them the liberty that permitted their course of study and their practices, were not created by them. All of these were put into place by society so that some might have the privilege of becoming physicians in order to serve the needs of society. Physicians, by accepting these opportunities to become physicians, enter implicitly into a social contract between themselves and society for the purpose of caring for the sick and disabled members of society. At this difficult time in medicine, physicians ought to remember this social contract, reflect on its meaning, and explicitly affirm it by their actions. Having accepted these particular goods of this society, physicians now have certain obligations/certain duties toward it and its members to use the skills that they have learned and the competencies they have mastered for the good of their patients and for the good of their society. Moreover, physicians who adhere to the religious traditions informed by a creative, providential, merciful God in whose image they are created have grounding for their obligations as they live out the obligations inherent in that image.

While the great majority of physicians commit their lives to the ethical practices demanded by their codes, there remain some issues that require attention. Among them are the following related issues: the social contract between physicians and patients and physicians and society, real informed consent, trust in the profession, conflicts of interest, medical errors, and monitoring the profession. The social contract between physicians and patients requires real informed consent. Informed consent, as carried out in many clinical settings, is more often procedural than real. The procedure usually involves giving the patient a clipboard with several papers on the board or presenting the patient with multiple computer screens to read. The patient is told what each form says and is asked to sign each. The patient rarely has medical knowledge sufficient to make informed judgment about the medical issue at hand. This ignorance includes the progression of the illness, the potential remedies and resources, the economic impact, and the familial impact. Most patients, because they trust the physician and/or the institution simply sign the documents.

The image of medicine as the scientific authority altruistically healing the ills of the nation needs the rectification of reality supplied by the admission of medical error that results in disability or death and, as well, the economic connections of the physicians and medical institutions (a) with pharmaceutical firms, (b) with manufacturers of medical devices, and (c) with the frequency of the choice of more radical, that is, and more remunerative, procedures over more conservative ones. Physicians as members of a professional guild claim the right to govern their profession by setting up qualifying training programs and monitoring the practices of their members. They have put into place many review boards, both national and local, to accomplish these tasks.

(D) The Mentally Ill – Their Families and the Community

Caring for persons with mental illness presents a unique and difficult set of problems for them and the families that love them and a society that claims both *parens patriae* obligations to care for the sick and police power to protect society. For much of human history treatment of mental illness was limited to three options, namely, institutional confinement, homelessness, or remaining within the family while disrupting family life. While the contemporary period has witnessed a change in its assessment of mental illness with the gradual but incomplete removal of the stigma attached to mental illness and the recognition of it as a condition that calls for medical intervention and continuous appropriate care, treatment is difficult to accomplish. The reasons why treatment is difficult to attain are to be found (1) in the law, (2) in the very nature of the effect of mental illness on decisional capacity, and (3) in the advance of the pharmacological treatment of mental illness.

(1) The Law

In the U.S.A., a new era in the care of mentally ill persons was inaugurated by the *O'Connor v. Donaldson* (422 U.S. 563, 1975) decision of the Supreme Court. The case on behalf of Kenneth Donaldson moved through lower courts and rose to the U.S. Supreme Court. Donaldson had been committed by his parents to a mental health facility and remained there for 15 years. All attempts by him to gain his release were thwarted by the superintendent of the facility. Donaldson claimed that he was (a) not dangerous, (b) not mentally ill, and (c) that he had not been provided with treatment. The Court, in narrowly addressing the specific issue at hand, acknowledged a constitutional right to freedom for those mentally ill persons who are not dangerous and who are able to live safely on their own. They cannot be involuntarily civilly committed. For an involuntary commitment to occur for a mentally ill person who is not dangerous and who is able to live safely, the Court required "something more." This "something more," although not specified in the Court decision, has usually been translated as treatment.

The *O'Connor v. Donaldson* case is a landmark in mental health law. The confinement option for the mentally ill, who are not dangerous and therefore not subject to the police power of the state, was severely restricted. In the exercise of its *parens patriae* role, most States have put into place policies and procedures for involuntary commitment and for treatment guided by an ongoing treatment plan. Among these procedures are (a) the person requesting the commitment must have first-hand knowledge of the danger from or to the mentally ill person; (b) an emergency psychiatric examination must be provided; and (c) a time limitation, usually 120 hours, is imposed on holding the patient unless a mental health officer determines a longer, albeit specifically limited, commitment is necessary and presents a specific plan for treatment. Subsequent to that initial commitment, regular review of time-specific treatment plans is necessary to extend the commitment.

While the *Donaldson* case is generally viewed as a progressive step toward achieving better care of the mentally ill, the unforeseen consequences are increased incidence of homelessness and increased entanglement of loving and caring families who are subjected to dealing with complicated administrative court procedures as they navigate the rigorous due process limitations now in place. The continuing presence of the homeless mentally ill seems to be refractive of solution in the major cities in the U.S.A. The major reasons for this are the legal requirement of the "least amount of restrictions" and the inability of the polity to provide sufficient and safe housing for the homeless who are mentally ill. For families coping with family members who suffer with mental illness, the problem of finding appropriate care can be daunting. While there are practical standards in place, accessing this relief through administrative court procedures is difficult for families when the mentally ill person refuses medical intervention. An example from the state of Pennsylvania illustrates the process and its difficulty in caring for the mentally ill. The first step requires the judgment that the person poses a danger to themselves or others. The latter is easier to determine as a fact than the former. Once this judgment of potential danger is made, a 302 commitment petition must be submitted to a mental health hearing officer. The person who signs or calls for the 302 commitment must have direct first-hand knowledge of the person and the danger the person poses for themselves or others. In order for a person to be considered a danger to themselves or others, there must be several things that occur within 30 days prior to the submission of the 302. Among those items are the inability to feed or care for themselves without supervision of another person, attempted suicide or suicidal threats, and self-mutilation. Under a 302 commitment, the hospital can hold the admitted person for a maximum of 120 hours. To be held longer, a new petition – a 303 petition – must be filed by the same person who filed the 302. The 303 petition must be approved by a mental health hearing officer. A 303 commitment lasts for a maximum of 20 days. At that point, the reasons for the commitment are reviewed. If during the time of the commitment the patient has been restored to an appropriate functional level, the person is released. If the person has not been restored to an appropriate functional level, the reasons for the continuation of commitment and the treatment plan must be submitted and reviewed by the administrative agency.

(2) *The Impact of Mental Illness on Decisional Capacity*

Pre-Planning Mental Health Care: The onset of an acute episode of mental illness renders the patient cognitively impaired, even if only temporarily, and hence unable to exercise real informed consent. An effort to overcome the obstacle of temporary loss of cognitive ability to exercise informed consent can be found in a psychiatric advance directive and/or a mental health care declaration document with or without the designation of a power of attorney for mental health care. These documents can serve as legal instruments that record a competent person's specific instructions or preferences regarding future mental health treatment when the person, because of a mental health crisis, is determined by a mental health professional to be incapable to give informed consent to specific treatment. The directives can be used to plan for the possibility that someone may lose capacity to give or withhold informed consent to treatment during acute episodes of psychiatric illness.

The National Association for the Mentally Ill (NAMI) supports the use of psychiatric advance directive and/or a mental health care declaration document with or without the designation of a power of attorney for mental health care. All states have advance directives for medical care including mental health care in some form and many states have a separate and very detailed form for a psychiatric advance directive. Important items included in these forms are a time limitation on the declaration itself, treatment preferences and treatment rejections, choice of facility, participation in experimental studies and drug trials, appointment of a guardian of the person, the determination of the power of attorney for care, choice of care for minor children as well as the protection of parental rights. Most directives include a limitation of revocation which states that the patient may revoke the declaration or any part of it at any time either in writing or orally as long as the patient is no longer incapable of making mental health decisions. The inherent ambiguity of the notion of incapable appears to incline health care providers, when in doubt, to accede to the choice of the moment of the patient. These mental health care directives are relatively new legal documents that have had limited testing in the law. Furthermore, because the person in a mental health crisis may express choices different from those expressed in the advance directive, a preexisting relationship between the patient, the mental health care providers, and the family or health care proxy is essential to navigate this situation.

(3) The Treatment

Advances in pharmacotherapy have, in some instances, alleviated, diminished, or controlled, for a time, some of the debilitating effects of mental illness. The appropriate and consistent use of medications, along with appropriate counselling, has allowed some mentally ill persons to lead relatively normal lives. This represents a significant advance over institutionalization. The broad spectrum of mental illnesses described in the *Diagnostic and Statistical Manual of Mental Disorders V* (DSM-V) and in the *International Classification of Diseases 10* (ICD 10) presents a range from substance abuse, addiction, depression, schizophrenia, and paranoia, to a variety of personality disorders. These differences are so significant that treatment modalities cannot be generalized. Furthermore, the side effects associated with the medications appear so significant that the prescribed medications are sometimes refused by the patient. Monitoring by a health care provider or a family member is required to prevent a relapse which is followed sometimes by a diminished recovery and is followed occasionally by homelessness.

The care of a family member who suffers from mental illness is often a lifetime project that requires the support of the entire family, if the burden is not to be overwhelming for one or two members of the family. Some families have the financial and emotional resources to partner with the medical and social services community to care for their family members. Others do not. Here, the application of the principle of solidarity, tempered by subsidiarity, must be applied. The plight of the homeless mentally ill in the major cities is sad. Sheltering is a temporary and ineffective solution. Many of the homeless are shelter-resistant because of the perceived physical dangers to themselves and the possible loss of their possessions. Surely the citizens of major cities that can approve and build facilities ranging from massive athletic arenas to concert venues to dog parks can develop, if they will, adequate housing that recognizes the dignity and the struggle of the mentally ill.

(E) The Human Person and the Gift of the Body

This section treats first the reality of embodiment as male and female and then the reality of the tension of human living in the struggle to integrate the physical, psychological, affective, and spiritual aspects of every person in the trajectory toward possible unity of these powers in maturity. This integration provides the basis for the very possibility of human flourishing both for the individual and for society. It then treats departures from this path as found in disorders (a) of sexual development, (b) of same-sex attraction, and (c) of gender confusion.

(1) Embodiment as Male or Female

Human beings are embodied and, moreover, embodied in a particular way as male or female. Sexual differentiation is a significant feature of this embodiment. Sex as a noun is an objective biological trait of the person; this trait is carried in every cell in the body. Sex as a verb describes a particular capacity of the person. Sex is a way of being in the world and, as a way of being, it is the foundation of a way of relating in the world. As a way of being in the world, the differentiation of human beings as male or female has a material basis in the sex chromosomes as XX or XY with a consequent difference in anatomy, physiology, and function. A concise, albeit imperfect, summary of this differentiation can be found here:

> [Sex]is a bias and orientation in a large number of potencies, a typical and complementary differentiation within the species, with a material basis in a difference in the number (sic) of chromosomes, with a regulator in the secretions of endocrinal glands, with manifestations not only in anatomical structure and physiological function but also in the totality of vital, psychic, sensitive, emotional characters and consequently,

> though not formally, in the higher nonorganic activities of reason and rational appetite.
>
> (Lonergan, FLM, p. 42)

In regard to sex as a way of relating in the world, there exists an inherent complementarity, and hence attraction, between male and female, as one of these capacities as a principle of dimorphic union and a principle of bi-fecundity presses toward fulfillment in some human beings. The dimorphic nisus intends ontological completeness in the union of male and female in marriage wherein the partners are complementary principles constituting the marriage itself. The good of bi-fecundity is offspring. This principle of union as attraction begins as *eros* and, if properly ordered and sustained, provides the upward dispositive thrust through *philia* to reach fulfillment in *agape*. Sex as a way of relating is accomplished appropriately in marriage wherein the ends of this complementary dimorphism and bi-fecundity as real and rational are accomplished. The topic of sex as a complex human activity with a set of multiple ends and its regulation is treated in Chapter 5.

While this objective biological binary characterization of sex is the norm for human beings, its ordering is not without difficulty. The difficulties lie within the human nature itself as both complex and fallen. Each human being manifests a substantial unity within which there are specific potentialities – intellect, will, and passions – to be actualized on a variety of levels – nature, reason, and grace – and integrated appropriately in the direction of perfecting the human person. The variety and press of the different appetites, including the spontaneous drive of our sexual nature, give rise to inner tensions as reason and will strive, usually imperfectly, to direct this natural appetite toward human flourishing. Accomplishing this integration requires knowledge and virtue and grace whose gifts are attained, if at all, only over the course of a lifetime.

(2) Issues With Embodiment

Notwithstanding the fact that sex is an objective trait with a material basis in human beings that is ordinarily expressed as either male or female, there are occurrences of ways of being, and hence ways of relating, that lie outside this norm. This too is a fact. Some are disorders of sexual development (DSD) and these are readily medically recognized. Others, such as same-sex attraction, commonly designated homosexuality, present as a specific way of being in the world as physically either male or female but with a way of relating in the world that inclines one toward members of the same sex and, sometimes, a way of acting in sexual intercourse with a member or members of the same sex. Others still, such as gender dysphoria, present as a disjunction between the material observable sexual development in the body and the claimed experience of gender identity. This section will present a brief account of the disorders (a) of sexual development, (b) of same-sex attraction, and (c) of gender confusion. While recognizing the contentious nature in the contemporaneous culture regarding discussions of homosexuality and gender dysphoria and as well the unsettled science, it is important to examine these occurrences in order to serve the flourishing and well-being of those persons whose lives are marked by a particular orientation or a claimed identity. Difference in orientation or dissonance in biological and claimed identity cannot be the occasion for unjust discrimination. Moreover, while every human being possesses intrinsic dignity in his or her person, the acts of human beings are still to be judged in relation to their appropriate flourishing and their final end. Hence, these differences are appropriate subjects of study inasmuch as information gained might alleviate clinically significant social or biological distress or impairment and inasmuch as the study might facilitate spiritual and psychological flourishing.

(a) The disorders of sexual development are capable of clinical verification in specific biological indicators. These indicators include sex chromosomes, gonads, sex hormones, and ambiguous genitalia. Among these along with their estimated frequency/100 live births are: non-XX or non-YX (0.0639); Turner's Syndrome (0.0369); Klinefelter's Syndrome (0.0922); disorders of androgen insensitivity (0.00760); and congenital adrenal hyperplasia (0.00770) (Blackless, 159). In addition, there is the true intersex condition of gonadal dysgenesis where the genitalia are ambiguous and the gametes a complex combination of XY configurations. These results suggest that less than 0.2% of human beings depart materially/biologically from the norm of unambiguously male or female in bodily presentation. When the study is expanded to include later onset congenital adrenal hyperplasia (CAH), the total percentage increases to 1.7%. If these results are correct, then approximately 99.8% or 98.3% of human beings are clearly recognizable as biologically either male or female.

In addition to these materially determined sexual development anomalies, there are two categories of sexual claims isomorphic to the description of sex as a way of being and sex as a way of relating that require attention. They are homosexuality and gender dysphoria. In the contemporary culture, it is quite difficult to come to a clear understanding about these two presentations. It is difficult to find the science and separate it from the multiple voices and multiple agendas in the public domain. Claims run the gamut that includes the following notions: (1) sex is not an objective reality; it is a social construct used to generalize specific empirical observations; (2) sex is a choice and the choice of its expression must be respected by others; (3) sex has a variety of normal manifestations across a spectrum; (4) sex and gender identification are separable and when they conflict remedies including radical surgical transformation of the body are appropriate; and (5) sex and gender are normally inseparable; sex as femaleness and maleness are written into the person as a biological, psychological, and spiritual unity whose integration is accomplished over time.

This last is the understanding of the Catholic tradition and it provides the framework for the consideration of homosexuality and gender dysphoria. The difficulty and dis-ease of these topics cannot be an excuse from entering into the discussion. Entering the discussion requires caution and respect. The need for caution has its source in the lack of data because of the imperfections in the studies such as size of cohort, length of study, and appropriate control groups. The need for respect lies in the obligation to respect the dignity of every human being and to be mindful of the many manifestations of human suffering.

(b) Those persons who experience erotic inclinations toward members of the same sex present, biologically, as male or female. Homosexuality is experienced as a pattern of attraction – emotional, romantic, and/or sexual to persons of the same sex rooted in a particular way of being – as a person with same-sex inclinations. At this point, there is no single scientific theory on the cause of same-sex orientation in some persons. Attempts to determine its etiology suffer from the contemporaneous hypersensitivity of the issue because of the possible consequences resulting from prenatal testing and genetic profiling. It may be the case that some biological factors predispose to a same-sex attraction. Studies that reported a possible linkage between same-sex attraction and the X chromosome at the tip of its long arm have not been replicated. Other studies, including the examination of the posterior corpus callosum which appears larger in some men who experience same-sex attraction than in men who are attracted to women, the examination of the methylation pattern found in specific regions of the genome, and the presence of prenatal androgens continue at this point without clear conclusions. Some theorize that same-sex attraction occurs in some persons as a result of a complex interplay of genetic, hormonal, and environmental influences that occur prior to birth. Some claim that same-sex attraction has its origin in childhood sexual or psychological abuse. To this is added the claim that the occurrence of same-sex attraction is simply a normal occurrence on the human sexuality spectrum and persons with homosexual inclinations are capable of living satisfying lives precisely by acting on these inclinations. Some, on the other hand, claim that homosexual orientation is marked by unnatural and disordered inclinations which, if acted upon, have negative social, psychological, and spiritual effects over a lifetime.

One thing that is beyond dispute is that there are persons who experience same-sex inclinations. The claim that there is a material basis for deep-seated same-sex attraction, that is, some persons are by nature homosexual, is to be distinguished from homosexual behavior that is situational or psychologically rooted. If the cause is situational or psychological, that is, it is transitory, then the remedy is, respectively, change the place or pursue psychological therapy. But, even given the claim that a person having homosexual inclinations has a material basis and it is an enduring erotic attraction that does not in itself answer the question of acting on those inclinations. There are other characteristics found in human beings that have a material basis, but no one presses the argument that they ought to act on them or that social structures should be put in place to signal approval and to enable their actualization. For example, the double Y chromosomes found in some males dispose them to violence. Society does not fashion structures for these males to satisfy their violent drives. Instead, society attempts to protect both society and these individuals from their violent proclivities. Schizophrenia and manic depression appear to have material bases in the brain. Nonetheless, they are still recognized as disorders and those who suffer these disorders are recognized as in need of help. Cystic fibrosis disease results from a CFTR gene mutation; it is recognized as a departure from the norm; and it requires lifelong medical intervention. So, while some forms of same-sex attraction may naturally occur in some individuals, the question remains whether these are disordered inclinations as not natural to human beings as human beings. This distinction is made in the following:

> For it happens in an individual that some one of the natural principles of the species is corrupted, so that something which is contrary to the specific nature, becomes accidentally natural to this individual . . . Consequently it happens that something which is not natural to man, either in regard to reason, or in regard to the preservation of the body, becomes connatural to this individual man, on account of their being some corruption of nature in him. And this corruption may be either on the part of the body, – from some ailment; thus to a man suffering from a fever, sweet things seem bitter, and vice versa, – or from an evil temperament; thus some take pleasure in eating earth and coals and the like; or on the part of the soul; thus from the custom some take pleasure in cannibalism or in the unnatural intercourse of man and beast, or other such like things which are not in accord with human nature.
>
> (*Summa theologiae* I-II, q.31, a.7)

The contemporary teaching of the Catholic Church on sexual relations between members of the same sex centers on the assessment of the acts as disordered inasmuch as they cannot accomplish the ontological completion of the marriage union intended by dimorphism and they cannot accomplish the end of offspring intended by bi-fecundity. Because this is the case, the inclinations toward those acts are judged to be disordered. Inasmuch as the act itself, that is sexual intercourse between members of the same sex, is judged as objectively evil, then the inclination toward that act is assessed as objectively disordered. The teaching is summarized in the Catechism of the Catholic Church in statements 2357–2359.

> 2357 Homosexuality refers to relations between men or between women who experience an exclusive or predominant sexual attraction toward persons of the same sex. It has taken a great variety of forms through the centuries and in different cultures. Its psychological genesis remains largely unexplained. Basing itself on Sacred Scripture, which presents homosexual acts as acts of grave depravity, tradition has always declared that "homosexual acts are intrinsically disordered." They are contrary to the natural law. They close the sexual act to the gift of life. They do not proceed from a genuine affective and sexual complementarity. Under no circumstances can they be approved.
>
> 2358 The number of men and women who have deep-seated homosexual tendencies is not negligible. This inclination, which is objectively disordered, constitutes for most of them a trial. They must be accepted with respect, compassion, and sensitivity. Every sign of unjust discrimination in their regard should be avoided. These persons are called to fulfill God's will in their lives and, if they are Christians, to unite to the sacrifice of the Lord's Cross the difficulties they may encounter from their condition.
>
> 2359 Homosexual persons are called to chastity. By the virtues of self-mastery that teach them inner freedom, at times by the support of disinterested friendship, by prayer and sacramental grace, they can and should gradually and resolutely approach Christian perfection.
>
> (Catechism of the Catholic Church)

Note here the movement from the assessment of the acts to the assessment of the inclination to the call to chastity and the resultant effective freedom. These actions are forbidden because of their nature as contrary to the purposes of sexual intercourse. They are not consistent with the objective goods of sexual expression and they have negative consequences for the character of the persons involved. There is no condemnation of the person with same-sex tendencies; the teaching is directed only to acting on those inclinations in a particular way and to fostering them in a particular way.

Is it appropriate for two homosexual people to form a union of friendship? Yes, but remember true friendship is based not on pleasure or utility but on virtue. Should this particular kind of friendship include the satisfaction of sexual desires for reasons of enhancing the union of friendship? If, as a matter of fact, homosexual activity is not in accord with the objective goods of sexual expression, then No. The actualization of disordered desires or inclinations corrupts the character of the person. This corruption affects the human being in two ways: first, the satisfaction of the disordered passion reinforces or strengthens that particular passion which habituates the person in a particular direction, thus determining disordering of character, and, second, powerful passions can override and interfere with the development of other potentialities appropriate for integrated human life. Possible consequences for the individual are the interference with the attainment of the rational and transcendental ends of human life. Moreover, this corruption of character has social consequences, which cannot fail to have an impact on the individual person, on the friendship, and on the common good. This corruption of character has eternal consequences. The eternal consequence is that it places at risk our relationship to God. A true friend does not desire the destruction of a friend. True and deep friendship is possible without sexual intimacy. To require sexual activity as a necessary enhancement of friendship is to have a narrow vision of the person, an impoverished understanding of friendship, and to give sex primacy over the person.

Should the friendship between homosexual persons include the type of intimate sexual activity reserved for marriage? No, and for several reasons. First, while genital stimulation is possible within a homosexual relationship, conjugal intercourse is not possible. Second, self-gratification rather than self-donation appears to be the end of intimate sexual activity outside of marriage whether that activity be engaged in by heterosexual persons or homosexual persons. Third, to seek sensual pleasure for its own sake is to engage in a particular type of hedonism. Further, pleasures are differentiated as appropriate or inappropriate – a distinction as old as at least the *Nicomachean Ethics* of Aristotle. Appropriate pleasure accompanies an act of human flourishing; it is the delight that is attendant to activities which accomplish human goods. Pleasures are designated good or evil following the kinds of activities that pleasures complete. And finally, the intimate sexual activity of conjugal intercourse is reserved to those who are married. Its pleasures facilitate the accomplishment of the multiple goods of marriage. It is an activity inappropriate to those who, whether they are heterosexual or homosexual, are not married.

(c) Those with gender dysphoria describe and claim a particular way of being that is different from the range of normative appearances and normative behaviors expected from their XX and XY biological determination. The person with gender dysphoria presents physically as male or female but claims to experience the self as the opposite sex. The discrepancy is described as causing great distress and/or impairment in social functioning. It is sometimes present with a disorder of sexual development and sometimes without. Gender dysphoria is different from the clinically verifiable disorders of sexual development which are marked by specific biological indicators. Because of the distress and suffering caused by this difference in the way of being and acting, persons who claim gender dysphoria often seek medical treatment including lifelong cross-sex hormones and surgery to align natal gender with experienced gender.

The *Diagnostic and Statistical Manual of Mental Disorders-V* of the American Psychiatric Association describes gender dysphoria in adolescents and adults in the following:

A. A marked incongruence between one's experienced/expressed gender and assigned gender, of at least six months duration, as manifesting two of the following:

   1. A marked incongruence between one's experienced/expressed gender and primary and/or secondary sex characteristics (or in young adolescents, the anticipatory secondary sex characteristics).
   2. A strong desire to be rid of one's primary and/or secondary sex characteristics because of a marked incongruence with one's experienced/expressed gender (or in young adolescents, a desire to prevent the development of the anticipated secondary characteristics).
   3. A strong desire for the primary and/or secondary sex characteristics of the other gender.
   4. A strong desire to be of the other gender (or some alternative gender different from one's assigned gender).
   5. A strong desire to be treated as the other gender (or some alternative gender different from one's assigned gender).
   6. A strong conviction that one has the typical feelings and reactions of the other gender (or some alternative gender different from one's assigned gender).

B. The condition is associated with clinically significant distress or impairment in social, occupational, or other important areas of functioning (DSM-V, pp. 452–53).

The criteria for determination of gender dysphoria in children are similar but with appropriate modifications. These modifications include concrete behavioral actions such as the choice of clothing, friends, games, play, and toys not typical for children of the natal gender.

While the occurrence of gender dysphoria is quite small, 0.005%–0.014% in adult males, 0.002%–0.003% in adult females, and slightly higher in children and adolescents, it does cause significant distress in those who experience it. The psychological experience of disconnecting from the body is not to be minimized. There does seem to be an affective and cognitive disconnect in the person in regard to the body. Persons who experience this disconnect have been reported to be at greater risk than the general population for adverse health outcomes including depression, substance abuse, and suicide attempts (Mayer, pp. 59ff.). Recognition of the misalignment is important and appropriate care for the person is crucial. If it is the case that the attempt to remedy this condition by way of cross-sex hormones and sex reassignment surgery, which in the short term may appear satisfactory, fails in the long term to remedy the adverse psychological and social health issues, then such radical treatment is inappropriate. The logic intrinsic to the practice of medicine would dictate that priority be given to the least intrusive intervention. Given that, at this point, there is no physical evidence for the occurrence of gender dysphoria in persons without a disorder of sexual development, an account for this misalignment might be sought elsewhere. Cognitive therapy seems to be an appropriate first-step intervention. The brain is plastic; the body is not.

Despite a failure to identify a specific physical cause for gender dysphoria, it is important to recognize the profound suffering of persons and psychological stress of those who experience this disparity. It is evident that some who suffer from gender dysphoria do experience adverse health outcomes including depression, substance abuse, and suicide attempts that are significantly more frequent than the general population. Some adults with sufficient means and willing physicians will seek remedies found in the arsenal of medical possibilities. Bodily reassignment by way of cross-sex hormones and sex reassignment surgery in adults seems a mutilation without justification, that is, without the proportionate expectation of freeing the person from the adverse health outcomes. If the prior adverse clinically significant conditions, such as depression, substance abuse, and suicide attempts, continue, then the patient – despite expressed satisfaction with the new appearance – has been poorly served by the skills of medicine.

Bodily reassignment by way of social affirmation, prepubertal blockers, cross-sex hormones, and sex reassignment surgery in children seems particularly problematic for several reasons. The reasons are (1) children are not capable of informed consent; (2) the radical nature of the proposed remedy; and (3) the possibility of the reversal of the child's understanding of the integrity of the biological sex and the experienced sex and the difficulties attendant with that reversal. The American College of Pediatricians reported in their statement *Gender Dysphoria in Children* (2016) that in 80–95% of children who are diagnosed with prepubertal gender dysphoria, when provided with appropriate cognitive therapy throughout the normal maturation process, the dysphoria resolves at puberty. However, it is also reported that children who receive prepubertal blockers and cross-sex hormone therapy go forward to complete the process of transitioning.

The notions of the fluidity of gender and the fixity of biological sex present challenges in the contemporary culture. Ideas do have practical consequences. The idea of eugenics in the late nineteenth and early twentieth centuries propelled a powerful sterilization movement in the U.S.A. The idea that some human beings might be fit objects for experimentation to serve the well-being of other human beings or the advance of knowledge resulted in Tuskegee and Willowbrook – tragedies for the nation and scandals for medicine. The particular challenge to medicine is that of using its tools – surgery and drugs – in a way that provides good outcomes for patients. At this point in time, it is difficult to discuss or even to gather evidence on these contentious topics. Nonetheless, the uncertainty about diagnosis and outcomes as well as the radical nature of the surgery should serve to caution medicine. Moreover, children as children should be protected. Those responsible for children including their parents and their physicians should exercise patience on behalf of their children.

The claim that the objective biological binary characterization of sex is the norm for human beings has consequences. While it can serve as the basis for distinctions that define roles and obligations, it cannot be the cause of unjust discrimination. Moreover, those who claim the Catholic tradition must meet those who present as outside the norm with love and compassion in the manner that Jesus accepted those who came to Him. All human beings are possessors of intrinsic dignity; all human beings are possessors of rights. All are to be respected in their persons. But, rights claims are not trump cards to be played to silence discussion. Rights claims are claims that require articulation and defense if they are to have standing before the bar of reason.

(F) Afterword

This chapter on special relations is rooted in the anthropology that reveals that human beings live their lives in relationships as related to God, to each other, and to their bodies. The primary relationship is to God as the source of life for every human being and the end toward which all tend. The relationship of God to humanity serves as the model for the relationship of human beings to each other and, as well, for human beings toward the gift of their nature. Human beings, as created in the image of God as creative and providential, are called to care for each other and themselves according to the gifts they have been given. The right ordering of these relations is the source of first of our worship and then of our traditions of community, of hospitality, of solidarity, of mutual respect, and of liberty as ordered, of beneficence, of intersubjectivity, and also of medicine. Right ordering of our lives as accomplishing the integration of the press of the different appetites, including the spontaneous drive of our sexual nature, gives rise to inner tensions as reason and will strive to direct this natural appetite toward human flourishing. Accomplishing this integration requires knowledge and virtue and grace; it is the task of a lifetime.

Questions for Reflection

1. List the many relations in society that involve interactions between the more powerful and the less powerful. What are the effects on culture when habits of treating the less powerful as "disposable" develop? In what ways does the culture's choosing "care" or "dispose" as its paradigm for treating the vulnerable affect culture?
2. How have you experienced *individuals* using their gifts well or poorly to serve community life? How have you experienced *institutions* using their gifts well or poorly to serve community life?
3. Have you ever witnessed the conversion of an individual or institution from poor stewardship to good stewardship, or vice-versa? Describe the essential features of the transition.
4. Feminism has a set of significant values that have brought about many advances for women and society yet the contemporary feminist movement is fractured by ideology. Describe the successes of feminism and the features that distinguish equity feminism from equality feminism.
5. Examine and evaluate the justification for abortion from the perspective of a gender-equity feminist. Examine and evaluate the justification for abortion from the perspective of a gender-equality feminist.
6. In the contemporary culture, abortion is sometimes suggested as a remedy for risk to the mother, as a remedy for fetal deformity, and as a remedy for a pregnancy resulting from rape or incest. Identify the starting principle that grounds your argument, other principles that guide your resolution, and the role of the communities, large and small, that can contribute to the resolution. What changes are needed in cultural norms to protect and elevate maternal–fetal relations?
7. Should physicians take an oath to guide the practice of medicine? If so, what should be included in the oath? If not, why not? What is the source of violations of professional/ethical conduct in medicine?
8. Medicine and medical research have made wonderful contributions to the maintenance of health and care of the sick. What would medicine and medical research look like if the model were God's creative and providential care of creation?

9. What does, or should, informed consent mean in cases of mental illness? How does care for the mentally ill make questions about society's distribution of resources particularly acute?
10. How can (a) recognition of human dignity and (b) the need for moral evaluation in cases of homosexuality and gender dysphoria be combined? What does it look like, concretely, to respect persons and their decisions, while disagreeing with their moral claims? What role does medicine have under such circumstances? On what basis might medical noncooperation operate with a person's course of actions?

Notes

1 The treatment of talents is parallel to the treatment of private property in the Catholic tradition. Private property is a real right but it is a right that serves the universal destination of goods. See CCC 2402–2406, 2446, and 2459.

2 Chapter 4 at Section D-3-c describes the change in Federal Law as a consequence of the United States Supreme Court decision *Dobbs v. Jackson Women's Health Organization*, No. 19–1392, 597 U.S. ___ (2022). At this point in 2025, it is impossible to tell the effects of the overturning of *Roe, Doe, and Casey*. The almost 50 years of legal abortion on demand did change the contours of the culture. The legality of elective abortion now lies in the hands of the state legislatures and the citizens of the states.

3 Scotosis means choosing intellectual blindness. It is usually defined as "the hardness of the mind against unwanted knowledge."

4 It is no accident that the notion of the human being as simply an autonomous rights being individual is associated with the Deism of the Enlightenment. The emphasis on relations has resurfaced at a time when Trinitarian thought is being emphasized. The notion of God and the notion of human being are linked.

5 The Phoenix case: In 2009, a particular case captured the attention of Catholic ethicists, physicians, and the Catholic Health Care system. A 27-year-old woman who was ten weeks pregnant was admitted to a Catholic hospital with very severe pulmonary arterial hypertension with profoundly reduced cardiac output, right heart failure, and cardiogenic shock. The medical team recommended termination of the pregnancy – abortion. The case was referred to the hospital ethics committee for guidance. The controlling directives from the ERDs are Directives 45 and 47. Directive 45 forbids "the directly intended termination of pregnancy." Directive 47 permits

> Operations, treatments and medications that have as their direct purpose the cure of proportionately serious pathological conditions of a pregnant woman are permitted when they cannot be safely postponed until the child is viable even if they will result in the death of the unborn child.

The ethics committee at the hospital identified the placenta as the problem. The demands of the placenta for the additional volume of blood placed an overwhelming strain on the heart of the woman. Continuation of the pregnancy would most likely result in the death of the mother and the child. The committee decided that the application of Directive 47 was controlling and the pregnancy was terminated. Controversy as to whether this was a direct abortion or an indirect abortion followed. The Bishop of the diocese determined that the abortion was direct and subsequently informed the head of the ethics committee that she had incurred excommunication. For analysis of this case, see M. Therese Lysaught's, "Moral Analysis of a Procedure at Phoenix Hospital" (2011). Theology Faculty Research and Publications. 373. https://epublications.marquette.edu/theo_fac/373. Lysaught maintains that in this particular clinical situation the life of the child could not be sustained. The only life possible of medical rescue was that of the mother.

9 The Provision of Health Care

This scriptural passage from the Gospel of Saint Luke records the Lord's command of hospitality. While the passage refers to dinner, it serves as an apt analogy to health care.

Luke wrote:

> When thou givest a dinner or a supper, do not ask thy neighbors to come, or thy brethren, or thy kindred, or thy friends who are rich; it may be they will send thee invitations in return, and so thou wilt be recompensed for they pains. Rather when thou givest hospitality, invite poor men to come, the cripples, the lame, the blind: so thou shalt win a blessing, for these cannot make thee any return; thy reward will come when the just rise again.
>
> (*Luke*, 14:13–14)

For the rich and the relatively rich in developed nations, health care is not a problem. For the poor and developing nations, it may be a matter of life or death. This passage reminds us that to serve the underserved is a blessing.

The distribution of health care in a just manner is a vexing problem in the contemporary developed world. It seems so overwhelming as to be refractory of solution. Some of the best minds in the U.S.A. business world, including Amazon.com Inc., JPMorgan Chase & Co., and Berkshire Hathaway Inc., attempted a joint venture – the Haven Venture – in 2018 to understand and to transform health care. After three years and a cost of $100 million, the venture collapsed. Haven cited lack of data, lack of transparency in health care cost information, and lack of scale to provide negotiating power with insurers and providers as the major reasons for failure (*WSJ*, January 8, 2021). This failure indicates the complexity of health care in the U.S.A. and the intransigent problems of lack of transparency and lack of power to untangle its operations.

DOI: 10.4324/9781003627197-9

In the contemporary developing world, the virtual nonexistence of health care, which dooms all but the powerful to debilitating disease and early death, is tragic. Challenges in the developed world in the distribution of health care are economic, political, ethical, and just plain human. The just plain human challenge starts with the simple acknowledgment of the matter of fact that the goods that can be delivered by the medical profession are finite while the human need and demand for the goods of health care seem infinite. The political is marked by claims at both extremes which toggle between the notions of health care as either a right or a privilege. The economic data make clear that expenditures on health care as a percentage of gross domestic product (GDP) are rapidly rising. In addition, expenditures in the final six months of life seem often disproportionate to the good accomplished. This rapid increase in health care expenditures translates into fewer funds for other needs that serve the common good such as education, social welfare, and defense. The ethical challenge lies in determining the meaning of justice in the distribution of health care.

When to these challenges is added the commitment to Christian practice, it seems that the complexity is compounded. In describing the aspiration of health care informed by the values of the Catholic tradition, the document *Ethical and Religious Directives for Catholic Health Care Services* (ERDs) has recourse to the understanding of the banquet in the parable of Jesus found in the Gospel of Luke at 14:13. The theme is extending hospitality not as a medium of exchange – you invite your friends and your family and important people to the banquet and they are understood to have a duty to reciprocate – but rather of extending hospitality as a way of rendering care for the vulnerable. Jesus instructed the disciples with these words: *When thou givest hospitality, invite poor men to come, the cripples, the lame, the blind.* The *Directives*, in quoting the words of Jesus, stop there in mid-sentence. It is instructive to complete the sentence. The text continues, *so thou shalt win a blessing, for these cannot make thee any return.* Caring for those who cannot reciprocate is a blessing. The text concludes with the promise that compensation will come from God, *on the day the just rise again.*

The claim that Catholic health care is a response to the challenge of Jesus means that Catholic Health Care Institutions are not primarily economic entities, although a sound economic base is required for their continuous operation. Furthermore, a robust commitment to mission inspires financial support that must be wisely stewarded. They are institutions that are called, first and foremost, to extend hospitality, as medical care, to the vulnerable. The vulnerable are *all* those who are sick. Hence, Catholic health care has a particular identity and an additional set of challenges that derive from its special mission and identity.

This chapter will proceed in the following fashion:

(A) An examination of the current challenges in the provision and distribution of medical care in the United States;
(B) A consideration of the role and limits of Catholic Health Care Institutions;
(C) A consideration of scarce resources in ordinary and extraordinary times;
(D) Afterword.

(A) Challenges to Medical Care in the United States

(1) The Background

This country has witnessed and has been the beneficiary of marvelous advances in medicine and in medical technology. These benefits are the result of many forces including (a) the expertise and dedication of those who practice medicine; (b) the refinement of the instruments, procedures, and anesthetics that make possible the success of surgery; (c) the discovery, creation, and availability of antibiotics and vaccines from the research of both the private and public sectors that brought a safety and security to childhood never before known in human history[1]; (d) the advances in pharmacology including immunosuppressant drugs that facilitate the success of the transplantation of human organs; and (e) now on the horizon the possibility of genomic medicine. The very success of medicine spawned the problem that now confronts us, namely, the goods, now efficient and safe, that medicine can provide are desirable. As demand increases, the limits of the goods become increasingly evident. So, the distribution of medical care and medical resources is, and will continue to be, a refractory problem for medicine and for society. This is true whether the resource be the more general resource of health care itself or a specific resource such as promising new drugs or organs for transplantation. The supply is finite; the need appears infinite; and human nature remains human nature.

The problem is further convoluted by the operative language of the contemporary discussion and the ideas that fill and overrun the cultural matrix within which the discussion goes forward. Among the most egregious examples in the health care debate are the "right" to health care, "free" health care, and "government" money. Add to these the ever-competing and largely misunderstood notions of equality and freedom and their offspring as found in the failure to distinguish equality of opportunity from equality of outcomes and to distinguish freedom as effective freedom from freedom as liberty. The organ transplantation context provides a vivid example of urgency and complexity. In the organ transplantation context, the reality is of dying and death and the reality of the need to respect the transition by way of dying to death. Its language includes (a) a complex set of proposed definitions of death, for example, whole brain death, higher brain death, non-heart beating death, and imminent death – skewed by the expressed urgency to harvest organs; (b) the language of consent as presumed or real, and if real, by whom; (c) the language surrounding the question of ownership of transplantable organs; (d) the reification of bodies and organs; and (e) and maintenance of and timing of removal of those organs. To this last, add the power of social media and the problem is magnified. These problems are exacerbated further by the failure to take hold of the reality of human nature with self-interest as its driving force and to take hold of the central limitations of human life, that is, the reality of human mortality and the inevitability of death.

Many years ago in his Clarke Family Lecture at Notre Dame, Dr. Charles Dougherty presented this analogy to describe health care. He told the story of an airplane pilot and his flight. The pilot came on the intercom and informed the passengers that he had good news and bad news. The bad news was that the plane was in dense fog and had lost its directional controls, but the good news was that it was making great speed (Dougherty, 162). Later, Dr. Todd Whitmore added to the drama by suggesting that the monkeys who had been in the cargo-hold had escaped and were now in the cockpit and were tinkering with the flight instruments. Dr. Whitmore identified the monkeys as various special interest groups such as insurance companies, lobbyists, policymakers, big Pharma, and the ever-present monkey – ordinary human greed – a particular kind of self-interest to be fed perhaps by the magic of "government money" (Whitmore, 186). It is true. We continue to make great speed in health care, but what about the control of our direction? Is the direction the task of just one person – the pilot? Are the other members of the crew inept? Are the passengers to be passive? Can the ground crew offer assistance? And finally, what should be done about the monkeys in the cockpit?

The most significant economic pressure is the rising costs of health care coupled with the ever-increasing demand and ever-increasing cost of the delivery of high-tech medicine. As a percentage of Gross National Product (GNP), health care costs have increased from 4% in 1940 to approaching 18% in 2025. To this, add the steadily increasing cost of insurance, insufficient levels of reimbursement from government and other third-party providers, and the reluctance of patients who now perceive themselves as "fully covered" to pay out of pocket for health care. Compound this by an increase in the number of uninsured half of which, the young and the healthy along with the wealthy, are uninsured by choice. For those who cannot afford health insurance, there is limited access to health care. To this mix, add the demand for ever higher levels of compensation for physicians, especially physician employees, hospital administrators of multiple levels, and health care insurance executives and administrators.

Added to the economic pressures intrinsic to the practice of medicine is the external pressure spawned by the litigious culture within which medicine is practiced. This litigious culture, whatever its origin, has generated numerous lawsuits, some justified and some not, against physicians. Of course, those that are justified ought to result in appropriate and sufficient awards for damages to the injured party, and, if the harm was the result of medical malfeasance, ought to result in appropriate oversight and penalty of the physician, including the penalty of loss of the privilege of practice. Some of the lawsuits, however, have resulted in outrageous financial awards, well beyond reasonable compensation for the economic losses caused by the injury or harm suffered. When to this compensation for economic loss is added outrageous awards for pain and suffering, the disproportion of the financial award redounds through the system, across the professions, and into society. The frequency of lawsuits has resulted in the loss of physician time from practice, the increase in medical tests and procedures ordered for patients to protect physicians and hospitals with the attendant increase in costs for the patients, the increase in malpractice insurance, the decrease in the number of physicians willing to engage in certain specialties or to practice in certain geographical regions, and the rise of a new generation of obscenely wealthy trial lawyers who receive 25%–30% cut of the jury awards. And the downward spiral continues.

Among the political pressures, political as broadly construed, are the competing claims of the efficiency and appropriateness of the federal government as the sole provider of health care as opposed to the similar claims of the free market to provide health care through a variety of mechanisms that range from fee-for-service to for-profit managed care systems.

Among the ethical problems are the just and appropriate use and distribution of medical technological advances, what counts as disease to be ameliorated by medicine, the withdrawal and withholding of treatment that is no longer beneficial, the continuation of treatment that is beneficial, and rationing, precipitated by the overwhelming need in the presence of finite resources, of potentially beneficial services.

(2) Challenges for the Individual

To try to put some order into this complex problem, it is appropriate to begin by addressing the issue on the level of the individual in society, then move to the professions, and then, finally to a consideration of the problem of system. There are several overlapping challenges for the individual consideration of health care. Despite the overlapping, it is helpful to try to dissociate them. They are (a) the conceptual problem, that is, the language of health care; (b) health care as a basic good; (c) the economics of payment for finite goods; (d) the reality of finite resources; (e) the acknowledgment of finitude; and (f) to limit choice in choosing medicine first for medical indications.

(a) The problem of health care as a problem for individual human beings is first a conceptual problem, that is, the problem of understanding the essential nature of health care. Very often the attempt to approach the issue is to locate it in the disjunction which is offered in the following: health care is either a right or a commodity. At the extreme, the rights holder claims health care as a positive right, a welfare right, to be provided by, well, someone. The commodity claimant considers health care as a bit of merchandise, another thing to be purchased by those consumers who have sufficient funds.

This proposed disjunction is a false dilemma. Neither understanding, taken on its own, is correct; however, each has some truth in its claim. So perhaps what is called for is an *Aufhebung*, a higher insight that embraces the truth of each and leaves behind as false the absolute claims of both.

(b) Health Care as a Basic Good

Health care is a basic good. Health care, along with other basic goods such as food, clothing, and shelter, is necessary as an integral part of the necessary conditions for human flourishing. Fulfilling these conditions provides for the common good understood as the set of conditions that are required if human beings are to be capable of leading a good human life. So if health care is a basic good, then it occupies a position similar to other basic goods. But the basic goods are produced by society for the good of society. In this highly individualized environment, human beings often forget the social nature of the production of the basic goods and they often forget the giftedness of the materials that are present in the world to make possible the production of the basic goods. These materials include the raw materials of the earth and the intellectual material of human intelligence that guide the enterprise that fashions the raw materials into goods.

If health care is appropriately considered among the basic goods, then the same principles that are operative in supplying other basic goods should be operative in the distribution of health care. Everyone should have this good. Human beings who are capable participants in the society are responsible to take reasonable means to provide these goods for themselves and for their families. They are free to use their resources to purchase the good; they are limited to using the good appropriately, that is, for medical need. If for some compelling reason, however, there are some people, who, because of infirmity or immaturity or incapacity, are unable to provide this good for themselves and their families, then the basic good needs to be provided for them by society. If this good is not provided, they and society will not flourish. This provision of medical care for those incapable of providing for themselves has two sources. One is philanthropy and the other is governmental distribution through taxation. The role of philanthropy is evident in the names of individuals and of religious organizations on buildings in major hospital centers in the United States. The governmental distribution is evident in the many federal and state programs financed through taxation to serve the medical needs of those requiring such assistance. From this reality, a complex two-tier system, one private and one public, emerges. The two-tier system recognizes the dignity of every human being in their freedom to use their property to purchase goods, here the good of health care, and the dignity of the human being to receive from others necessary medical care as a matter of distributive justice. Every individual as citizen is called to recognize the payment of taxes to support those who cannot purchase the basic good of health care as an investment in the common good. This is a contribution to the flourishing of society. Recognition of this distribution as a social investment requires vigilant oversight in its administration and responsible use by its recipients. (This topic as a political challenge is treated more specifically in Section A-4 of this chapter.)

(c) Payment for Finite Goods

A third problem for the individual human being in regard to health care as a basic good is the understanding of the psychology of payment for limited goods. One of the ways that human beings understand the limited nature of goods is in their real payment for these goods. However, now much of health care is compensated for by third-party payments, private insurance – most often paid for by employers as a benefit and later mandated by the government for businesses of a certain size – and by the government in the Medicare and Medicaid programs. This is a relatively new phenomenon; it came into existence after World War II. Now on its face, that seems like a good and it is a good, but it is not an unproblematic good. The delivery of this new good forgot to take into account human nature. The third-party payment system insulated the individual from the cost and perhaps even knowledge of the cost, therefore the basic good ceased to be understood as a scarce resource. Economists, observing this new arrangement, report that the use of medical resources by patients varies dramatically with the existence of third-party payments. Their conclusion, easily understood when human nature is taken into account, is that the larger the share paid directly by the patient, the smaller the growth in expenditures in medical products and services. Conversely, the smaller the share paid directly by the patient, the larger the growth in expenditures in medical services and products. The growing use of emergency room facilities as centers for primary care evidences this practice.

(d) Finite Resources

A fourth problem for the individual, even the individual who recognizes the limitation of resources, is the best way to use the resources. A reasonably healthy lifestyle contributes to the lessening of the need for the scarce resource. But, inevitably, the day arrives when there is need and what then do we require as medical intervention? The response most often heard is "Do everything." What does "Do everything" mean? It ought to, at least, mean that the medical interventions be appropriate, that is, that the resources used in medical treatment provide a commensurate benefit to the person. This seems the appropriate place to recall and apply the distinction that is part of the Catholic health care tradition between ordinary and extraordinary means in the pursuit of health care and to insert a reminder that only ordinary means are morally obliging. That distinction can be found in the *Ethical and Religious Directives for Catholic Health Care Services* in sections 56 and 57.

> 56. A person has a moral obligation to use ordinary or proportionate means of preserving his or her life. Proportionate means are those that in the judgment of the patient offer a reasonable hope of benefit and do not entail an excessive burden or impose excessive expense on the family or the community.
>
> 57. A person may forgo extraordinary or disproportionate means of preserving life. Disproportionate means are those that in the patient's judgment do not offer a reasonable hope of benefit or entail an excessive burden, or impose excessive expense on the family or the community.

(e) Human Finitude

A fifth problem for the individual human being is the reminder that the power of health care is to provide a limited means to care for a limited life. We are finite beings and the material bodies of our finite sojourn are corruptible. That our lives are lived in such circumstances is gift and limit. Stanley Hauerwas in his works, especially *Practicing Patience*, warns about the danger of ascribing an inordinate power to medicine – "the Promethean presumptions of modern medicine" (Hauerwas, 270). He suggests that the practice of Christian patience by each of us has a great deal to offer to the community in its concern for health care. Through our patient suffering when we are ill, we respond to the call to imitate Christ. Through our patience with each other, we aspire to imitate the patience of God with us. Hauerwas says,

> To be patient when we are sick requires first that we learn how to practice patience when we are not sick. God has given us ample resources for recovering the practice of patience. First and foremost, we have been given our bodies which will not let us do whatever we think we should be able to do. . . We are our bodies and, as such, we are creatures destined to die. The trick is to learn the great good things my body makes possible without hating my body, if for no other reason than the death of my body is also my death. To practice the patience of the body is to be put on the way to holiness as we learn that we are not our own creations.
>
> (Hauerwas, 2009, pp. 295–296)

The patient acceptance of the limits of health care and the patient acceptance of the limits of life prevent our looking to medicine for a salvation that it cannot deliver.

(f) Medical Need Priority

A sixth problem for the individual is the understanding of the appropriate restriction of the limited resources of medicine to medical need. Medical resources have as their primary application to cure illness, to assuage suffering, and to provide compensation for disability. The use of these limited resources for enhancement purposes ought not to be requested by patients, until such time as medical resources are available in sufficient quantity to respond to basic medical needs of the whole community. This requires individuals to be sensitive to the needs of others and to be aware of the requirements of the place of the individual as a member of a particular community whose existence sustains the good life of the individual. An appropriate remedy here might be for the individual, who has the desire and the wherewithal to purchase medical resources for enhancement purposes when they become available, once the basic needs of all have been met, to donate an amount of money equal to the cost of the procedure to a relevant charity.

(3) Challenges for the Profession

To address the problem of the distribution of health care at the level of the medical profession requires that the observations previously indicated, that is, we are all members of a society and medicine is a limited resource, be recalled. The physician as citizen encounters all the same problems as other individuals in society. The physician precisely as a member of the profession assumes greater obligation for proper distribution of the goods of medicine.

(a) Obligations to Society

A consideration of the nature of the profession provides the grounding of the obligations of the profession and sheds some light on how the profession can contribute to the amelioration of the distribution problem and why the profession is obligated to attend that just provision. Membership in a profession is a privileged position whose purpose is to serve the public good. This commitment to serve the public good is paramount, even though the practice of the profession provides the livelihood for the professional. The privilege of membership in a profession confers status to those so admitted and confers obligations upon the professional. Nonetheless, physicians have no proprietary claim over their practices. The physician receives knowledge and power from institutions that the society has put into place to allow the physician entry into the profession. While physicians work very hard for their education and physicians pay a great deal of money, which represents only part of the cost, for that education and physicians have the right to expect a fine level of compensation, they ought not to consider their profession their private property.[2] The institutions, the medical schools, the colleges, and the universities of which they are sons and daughters; the scientists, both the famous and those who labored in relative obscurity who came before them; the teachers, who invested so much in them; the country that sustained peace and offered them the liberty that permitted their course of study, were not created by them. All of these were put into place by society so that some might have the privilege of becoming physicians in order to serve the needs of society. Physicians, by accepting the opportunity to become a member of the medical profession, enter implicitly into a social contract between themselves and society for the purpose of caring for the sick and disabled members of society. Through their practices over a lifetime, they have the opportunity to make this contract explicit. At this difficult time in medicine and in times of real crisis, physicians ought to remember this social contract, reflect on its meaning, and explicitly affirm it by their actions. Having accepted these particular goods of this society, physicians now have certain obligations/certain duties toward it and its members, that is, to use the skills that they have learned and the competencies they have mastered for the good of their patients and for the good of their society. Of course, for physicians whose lives are embedded in the Catholic religious tradition, their obligation is grounded in God who creates, redeems, and sanctifies.

(b) The Success of Medicine

A second problem for physicians lies in the success of medicine. The advancements of medical science in technologies, medicines, antibiotics, and now genomic medicine combined with the advance in medical skill as well as the advance in pain relief medication have opened the door for the safe use of the art of medicine beyond serving the sick. These tools can be used to satisfy human desires whether the desire is to be more beautiful, to look younger, or to be taller. How ought the profession respond to these desires and where ought the line be drawn? There has been in the past 50 years a proliferation of the nonmedical use of medicine. Enhancement plastic surgery is just one example; elective abortion is another. In the past and on the horizon is the possibility of request by patients for the amputation of healthy limbs. If the request is given a name such as body dysmorphic disorder and it is included as a disease in the *Diagnostic and Statistical Manual of Mental Disorders*, ought physicians apply their sophisticated surgical expertise to satisfy the desire? Now just as individuals ought not to use medicine for nonmedical needs until the basic health care needs of all members of society are met, so too physicians ought to reserve the use of their skills for medically indicated procedures. If the basic needs of all in the community are met, then physicians should enjoy the opportunity to satisfy appropriate human desires. An appropriate remedy here might be for the physician who has the expertise, desire, and the time to render such nonmedical service, to donate an equivalent service to sick and/or needy people. The initiation, oversight, and enforcement for this type of distribution should be the task of the profession. Failure to do so risks external control.

(c) Sharing in the Social Contract

A third problem for physicians as a group is the distribution of the goods of the practice across the Nation and across the population. Because the Nation has invested so much in the education of physicians, it has a right to expect a return on that investment. All physicians in the United States should accept a share of Medicare and Medicaid patients. This is part of the social contract. All physicians, because they have invested so much time and energy and money in their education have the right to expect a return on that investment by receiving fair reimbursement for treating patients. This fair reimbursement comes from direct patient payment, and all third-party payers including the government. This, too, is part of the social contract.

(d) Maintaining Competence

A fourth problem for physicians is maintaining their own competence and the competence of the profession. Each physician is required to be competent in the discipline and to maintain the standards of the profession. The maintenance of the standards of the profession requires physicians to oversee their colleagues in the profession. Attention to these related obligations should decrease the level of harm, whether the harm be culpable or not, to patients with a subsequent decrease in the malpractice suits. The intersection of medicine and law at the point of patient harm should be settled not in the courtroom, but before administrative law panels with the expertise and practical wisdom from physicians, attorneys, and ordinary people to render fair judgment and the power to enforce those judgments.

(e) *Limitation of Expertise*

A fifth problem for physicians is the recognition of the limitation of their field of expertise. Their field is medicine and the use of the best tools that contemporary medicine has to cure, to heal, and to ameliorate illness and disease in individual patients and in the domain of public health. Physicians as physicians have no expertise in solving problems of poverty, racism, or food insecurity. They can rightly indicate the effects of poverty, racism, and hunger on health and well-being, but the solution of those problems belongs to others in society. As citizens, physicians can offer that expertise to those whose task it is to address those problems and, as citizens, they can advocate for the kind of change their expertise deems appropriate. Most physicians as physicians have no expertise in spirituality or religion. As physicians, they can be sensitive to those needs in their patients; they can be respectful of their patient's beliefs, even when those beliefs cause the refusal of the proposed medical treatment; and they can refer patients to those with expertise in religion and spirituality. Of course, all the obligations developed here for the medical profession apply *mutates mutandi,* to the legal profession.

(4) *Challenges for the Polity*

(a) *Structuring Health Care*

With all these considerations in place, the next issue is the role of the Republic, a representative democratic polity, in putting into place the necessary structures to serve the health care needs of the citizens. The polity must provide a structure that makes possible a system of health care (1) that serves the medical needs of the community; (2) that respects human dignity and recognizes human limits; (3) that is competent and efficient; (4) that rewards the sacrifices of those who will provide the service; and (5) that will continue the marvelous advances of medicine. Neither a free-market approach by itself nor a welfare-rights approach by itself is adequate. The free-market approach, while protecting the exercise of the liberty of individuals in the use of their property, often neglects the just claims of the needy. The welfare-rights approach, while making just claims on behalf of those in need, is often unmindful of the limits of human nature, the danger of creating a permanently dependent class, and the limits of the resources of medicine. When health care is understood as a basic good, then it follows that the primary obligation falls upon individuals to provide it for themselves and their families.[3] This obligation can be satisfied by direct payment or by the purchase of insurance to mitigate against the fear of economic disaster in the face of catastrophic illness. With the satisfaction of this obligation on the part of the individual comes the right to make choices. However, choice is always limited and, here, should be limited by real medical need. If the individual cannot provide the basic good of health care, then the polity is obliged to provide a basic health care package. The basic package will have to be limited, because the resource is limited. The determination of the contents of that basic package is to be a task undertaken by public participation of all the stakeholders in the presence of the understanding that medicine is a limited resource. The scarceness of the resource will be ameliorated if individuals use only what they need and if physicians restrict their practices to real medical need.

(b) A Tiered System

Because of the economic stratification of society, stratified both because of levels of income and because of levels of medical need, there must be in place a variety of opportunities to purchase health care. Those with abundant resources are free to decide that their wealth is sufficient to purchase their medical care as needed. Those with more modest resources are free to purchase medical insurance in a form that satisfies their anticipated medical needs and is affordable for them. They must be mindful of the limits of that insurance that they and others will most certainly use as well as the nature of the insurance provider as a business. Those who, whether temporarily or permanently, are unable to pay for medical care, directly or indirectly by way of purchased insurance, must be assisted in the provision of medical needs. Hence, a complex tiered system is necessary. The tiered system requires the application of both the principle of solidarity and the principle of subsidiarity. The creation and maintenance of a public system is an obligation, in solidarity, of a society that aspires to justice. Subsidiarity, as the principle that requires that social issues be dealt with at the most local level that is capable of satisfying the need, directs the practical operation of the task.

(c) Provisions of a Public System

Two important questions for the public system are (1) How should it be provided? and (2) What should be provided? In a complex society, those nearest the people to be served and the service to be provided have better knowledge about the need and better control of its delivery. The provision of service should start as locally to the problem as possible. The more distant the provider of service from the problem, the more expensive the delivery of service becomes as the complicated administrative networks increase. Among the potential providers are the extended family, then associations, namely, charitable associations, businesses, unions, and finally, the government. The government, local, state, and federal, should be providers only when the social network is insufficient. The federal government should be the provider of last resort.

Everyone should have this good at a basic level. Once this basic level has been provided, then the scarce resource, the goods of medicine, should be made available for purchase. In a representative democracy, the people – whether directly or through their representatives – decide the direction of public funding for those who need assistance. The people decide (1) how much of the public treasury is to be allocated for medical care; (2) what kinds of medical care provide the most good for the most people within the limits of the financial allocation; and (3) a mechanism for allocation, review, and reallocation. The liberty to purchase the power of medicine for elective goods should not be permitted until the basic good for all is accomplished. Moreover, those who have the power to purchase should, as they recognize the givenness of much of what they have received, exercise justice informed by charity as love in the distribution of medical care toward those less endowed.

(d) The Oregon Plan

Once the necessity of delivering health care through the government is acknowledged, the states can serve as a hinge between the federal government and the individual needing the public good and as laboratories for testing programs of distribution. The state of Oregon provides an example of a method for the distribution of public funds for medical care. Through its Health Evidence Review Commission, Oregon developed, and now maintains, a mechanism – the Oregon Health Plan – that recognized both the limits of funding for medical care and the power of citizens to determine its distribution. The Commission with input from the stakeholders, the citizens of Oregon, develops a priority list of health care services. (The complete list is available at https://www.oregon.gov/oha/hpa/dsi-herc.) The priority list is developed by a consideration of the benefit, both as clinical effectiveness and cost-effectiveness, of the service to the population served.

A ranked list is determined by a prioritization formula which is a computation of health care category, population and individual impact measures, effectiveness, and need for service. The 2020–2021 prioritized list included 662 categories of medical maladies. At its biennial session, the legislature determined the amount of funds to be allocated for medical care. Once the funds were exhausted, the distribution plan was complete for the next two years. Of these 662 categories, those ranked from 1–471 were able to be funded by the allocation of the funds provided by citizens to the legislature. The top five categories were in order: (1) pregnancy, (2) birth of an infant, (3) prevention services with evidence of effectiveness, (4) substance use disorder, and (5) tobacco use disorder. The final unfunded categories 649–662 represented medical issues for which there was no or minimally effective treatment. If the citizens are dissatisfied, they can, through the power of the ballot increase or decrease the biennial allocation of funds and through their participation in the public meetings, determine a new direction of allocation of funds.

(B) The Role and Limits of Catholic Health Care

(1) The Role of Catholic Health Care

(a) Catholic health care institutions as Catholic accept as the core of their identity and directive of their practices the life of Christ and the creative providential action of a loving God. Acceptance of these core notions requires their proclamation and articulation as well as actualization in practice. Their proclamation provides a bold statement of love and commitment in a world groaning in a culture of killing and abandonment. Their proclamation recalls some central truths of human existence including the truth that we are God's creatures fashioned in a particular nature with minds and bodies to know, to love, and to serve God. Failure to make that proclamation is a kind of denial. It is to say with Peter, "I know nothing of the man" (*Matthew* 26: 72). Failure to make the proclamation risks the possibility of forgetfulness that diminishes internal institutional purpose and the loss of the external role that acts, to use the words of Fr. Kevin O'Rourke who was a towering figure in Catholic health care ethics in the U.S.A., as "leaven . . . by offering health care in accord with the example and teaching of Christ" (O'Rourke, p. 2) and acts to penetrate "secular society with the healing spirit of Christ" (O'Rourke, p. 4).

(b) Healing Ministry

The healing ministry of Christ is part of the identity of Catholic health care institutions and they rightly cite that activity of Jesus "to heal as Jesus healed." Some examples found in the scriptures are the healing of the leper, the servant of the centurion, and the mother-in-law of Peter, and the restoration of sight and speech and mobility. Yet, Jesus as healer of physical illness is just one dimension of His healing ministry. His radical healing ministry extended beyond the healing of bodily infirmity. He healed those who suffered from sin as well as those who suffered from physical infirmity. He drove out demons and forgave sinners and condemned hypocrisy. A health care institution worthy of the name Catholic would, through the continuous presence of clergy, as well as a full complement of medical practitioners, keep alive the multidimensional healing that our fallen human nature requires.

(c) Beyond Healing

However, healing of physical illness is not always possible. Furthermore, the exclusive focus on healing is too narrow and too exclusive a center. It is to buy into the myth of modern medicine that offers the promise of human salvation in more and better medicine. Jesus healed but he also suffered and died. Here, Catholic health care institutions have special obligations because of the Jesus revealed in Scripture. Catholic health care institutions must be places of caring for the dying that is inevitable. And here they must offer visible witness to the truth of the finitude and promise of human existence. In His suffering and dying, Jesus, from the depths of His humanity, called out for consolation. In Gethsemane, He asked to be rescued, "My Father . . . take this cup of suffering from me." He revealed to His friends His grief and anguish. He said, "The sorrow in my heart is so great that it almost crushes me." He asked them to stay with Him, and He is sorely disappointed by their failure to remain with Him. He experienced abandonment and, close to the end, He cried out to His heavenly Father, "Eli, Eli, lema sabachthani." Then, at last, He placed Himself into His Father's care. Catholic health care institutions have to be places and have to provide services and spaces within which human beings who are experiencing crushing sorrow, anguish, and abandonment will find in attendance caring people to touch and wash and anoint their bodies; attentive people who do not turn away from them; loving people whose simple presence sustains them; and faithful people who do not abandon them in their dying.

(d) Witness

In healing the sick and caring for the dying, Catholic health care institutions must provide living witness, simultaneously, to respect for the sanctity of human life and acknowledgment of the transcendent end of human life. The direct destruction of innocent nascent human life hidden under such euphemisms as pregnancy termination, selective fetal reduction, or beneficent killing as an aid in dying must remain proscribed. With this forbidding comes the obligation to offer succor to women and accompany the dying. Women are to be cared for in a manner that respects their dignity, their intelligence, and their moral strength, even as they may be experiencing a temporal and particular vulnerability. Rather than leaving her in privacy, she needs to know and to be welcomed into a community of care. When a woman is pregnant, she knows she is with child. If, within the contemporary horizon this truth is being hidden from her, Catholic health care institutions ought to speak this truth publicly and often in order to contribute to the recognition of women as moral agents to whom the truth is owed. The brute fact of more than a million abortions a year in the U.S.A. suggests the societal fabrication of a kind of amnesia in regard to the reality and life of the conceived but unborn human being.

(e) Prohibition of Killing

There may be no direct killing and no prolongation of dying in Catholic health care institutions. The exact and powerful conceptual tools, such as the distinction of extraordinary care from ordinary care, developed in the Catholic philosophical and theological tradition, must be applied with resolute firmness. We need to affirm the goodness of the gift of life and the goodness of its end. It is, perhaps, in our dying that we experience, finally, our nature as created beings. Fr. Richard McCormick, S.J. sketched out a careful path for us here. In his words and in his living to the very end, he reminded us frequently that dependency, whether from age or illness, is a call to cling to the power of God. He, when speaking of physician-assisted suicide as an act of isolation and abandonment, said, "[r] ejection of our dependence means ultimately rejection of our interdependence and eventually of our very mortality" (McCormick, 1991a, p. 1133). When he addressed the issue of the cessation of no longer beneficial nutrition and hydration, he reminded us that we as a people who say we believe in life after death ought to act as if we actually believe that (McCormick, 1992, p. 214). He warned us, too, that failure to attend to these distinctions and failure to use the intellectual tools and concepts of the tradition might force people who desire to hold to the tradition to flee it. He recalled the words of Dr. André Hellegers, who in 1979 just before his own death, warned of the inevitable consequences of the displacement of the traditional caring task by the curing goal. Hellegers said,

> [A]s the caring branches of medicine were gradually pushed aside by the curing ones, there seemed to be less use for the Christian virtues. I think that shortly the need of those old Christian virtues will return and once again be at a premium. Our patients will need a helping hand and not a

> helping knife. . . . We must either recapture the Christian virtues of care or we shall be screaming to be induced into death to reach the discomfort free society.
>
> (Hellegers, p. 101)

(f) Clarifying Issues

On the two issues of elective abortion and mercy killing, Catholic health care institutions ought to continue their powerful witness and absolute prohibition. The direct destruction of innocent human life is forbidden. At its core, this is a civil rights issue. Catholics and Catholic Health Care will find many allies, if they are willing to disturb the false peace fashioned by the euphemisms of compassionate killing or aid in dying or protecting the reproductive rights of women. They and their allies may be the agents in the reversal of the culture of death by faithful, prayerful, patient building brick-by-brick, truth by truth, witness by witness of communities who strive to love each other as God loves us.

(g) The Authority of the Church

The Catholic identity of health care institutions is tied to the authority of the Church in its teachers and its doctrines. The hierarchy has an authority, bequeathed to it by Christ, to guide the faithful. Catholic health care institutions have strong responsibilities to operate within the ambit of that authority. Nonetheless, as health care institutions, Catholic health care institutions are subject to other authorities, among the most significant are the authority found in the art and practice of the profession of medicine and governmental regulations. Authority exercised rightly recognizes the power of the dialectical tension between theory and practice in the pursuit of the truth. Authority is not exercised for its own sake or for the sake of power but for the sake of truth (McCormick, 1996, pp. 12–17). Both domains of authority, medicine and church, are capable of incredible hubris and authoritarianism. Nonetheless, there are remarkable examples of the cooperation of the authority of the Church and the authority of medicine in the service of the good of God's people in health care. Results of that cooperation can be found in the ongoing work in the *Ethical and Religious Directives for Catholic Health Care Services*. One particular example of this cooperation is evident in Directive 58 which asserts a presumption in favor of providing food and water to patients so long as the food and water provide a benefit for that patient. Directive 58 was accomplished by the careful testimony of physicians, theologians, and philosophers. The physicians offered their medical judgment that there are some conditions of illness and decline in which food and water no longer benefit the person. Philosophers and theologians offered their expertise in the careful application of the distinction between ordinary and extraordinary means of preserving human life of the person, in their affirmation of life as a fundamental, not an absolute, value, and in the distinguishing of physical continuation from human existence. Directive 58 affirms:

> 58. In principle, there is an obligation to provide patients with food and water, including medically assisted nutrition and hydration for those who cannot take food orally. This obligation extends to patients in chronic and presumably irreversible conditions (e.g., the "persistent vegetative state") who can reasonably be expected to live indefinitely if given such care.[40] Medically assisted nutrition and hydration become morally optional when they cannot reasonably be expected to prolong life or when they would be "excessively burdensome for the patient or [would] cause significant physical discomfort, for example resulting from complications in the use of the means employed."[41] For instance, as a patient draws close to inevitable death from an underlying progressive and fatal condition, certain measures to provide nutrition and hydration may become excessively burdensome and therefore not obligatory in light of their very limited ability to prolong life or provide comfort.

(b) Special Concerns

There are, within the contemporary horizon, two issues requiring serious attention in Catholic hospitals. These two issues require careful attention on the part of the authorities of medicine and church. One is found in the distinction between withdrawing and withholding of treatment; the other is the question of the care appropriate to certain children who have conditions incompatible with life. In regard to the distinction between withdrawing and withholding of treatment, theologians and philosophers are now, for the most part, quite content to say that the ethical assessment of withdrawing and withholding is entirely dependent on benefit to the patient. If there is no benefit, withdrawing and withholding are morally equivalent. Some physicians, on the other hand, persist in maintaining that withdrawing treatment feels different, for them, from withholding. In their professional experience, these actions are not the same. Philosophers and theologians need to listen attentively to this testimony by physicians. There needs to be a reopening and a continuation of that conversation.

The appropriate care of children who suffer conditions incompatible with life has become a more sensitive and pressing issue with the advance of technologies surrounding pregnancy and prenatal care. Once the diagnosis of a condition incompatible with life has been confirmed, how do we care for the two human beings, mother and child, in this sad and temporarily devastating situation? This issue is dealt with in Chapter 8 – Special Relations.

(2) *The Limits of Catholic Health Care – What Is Forbidden*

(a) *Catholic Health Care Within a Particular Political Structure*

The capacious goals of Catholic medical care are not without limit. The most obvious internal limits, of course, have to do with the direct taking of human life in elective abortion and assisted suicide. Catholic health care institutions have been consistent and clear that those practices are forbidden and, for the time being, they are protected by law from their having to perform these acts. Nevertheless, Catholic health care institutions have been challenged. Recall that in the wake of *Roe v. Wade* in 1973, the first challenge heard by the U.S. Supreme Court was one that questioned the right of two Catholic hospitals, Saint Vincent and Saint Mary, in Green Bay Wisconsin to refuse to perform elective abortions. The refusal of the hospitals was protected by the Court as an exercise of the religious freedom guarantee of the First Amendment.

Religious institutions including hospitals have enjoyed this freedom of religion for its institutions not only to operate but to flourish. Moreover, this free exercise has served the good of this nation. Religious institutions, in the exercise of spiritual and corporal works of mercy, have directed their resources to moral and spiritual development of their members and, as well, to education, both moral and secular, and to caring for the vulnerable including the sick, poor, frail, and elderly without regard for religious affiliation. This free exercise has enhanced the life of the nation and supplied stabilizing mediating structures. Similarly, throughout the history of this nation, its legal institutions have fashioned a variety of remedies and accommodations to keep the tension between non-establishment and free exercise appropriate to the ordering of the polity and the rights of citizens. Legal history provides ample testimony to the ongoing struggle in the complex growth of this nation; and more recent history has witnessed development as the courts and legislatures have addressed the issue. The Supreme Court decision in *Smith v. Oregon*, and the response of the U.S. Congress in the *Restoration of Freedom of Religion Act* (RFRA) in 1993 and *Religious Land Use and Institutionalized Persons Act* (RLUIPA) in 2000, are recent attempts to provide broad protection for religious freedom. Together, RFRA and RLUIA prohibit the federal government from:

> [S]ubstantially burden[ing] a person's exercise of religion even if the burden results from a rule of general applicability unless the Government "demonstrates that application of the burden to the person – (1) is in

furtherance of a compelling governmental interest; and (2) is the least restrictive means of furthering that compelling governmental interest." 42 U.S.C.§§2000bbb-1(a), (b). As amended by the Religious Land Use and Institutionalized Persons Act of 2000 (RLUIPA), RFRA covers "any exercise of religion, whether or not compelled by or central to, a system of religious belief" §2000cc-5(7)(A).

There are several important points worth noting. The first is the centrality of free exercise of religion even in the presence of a law of general applicability. The second permits the federal government to limit free exercise only if the government can demonstrate that (a) there is a compelling governmental interest at hand and (b) only if the means proposed by the government are the least restrictive means available to accomplish that governmental interest. The third is the broadening of the notion of exercise of religion beyond those actions which are "compelled by or central to a system of religious belief." Clearly these decisions incline toward freedom for religion.

Confirmation of this inclination toward freedom for religion can be found in recent Supreme Court decisions (573 U. S. 682 (2014)), such as *Burwell v. Hobby Lobby Stores, Inc.* (13–354) and *Conestoga Wood Specialties, Inc.* (13–356), and in the vacating and remanding of the case of the *University of Notre Dame v. Burwell, Sec. of Health and Human Services* et al. (14–392) to the Court of Appeals in the Seventh Circuit for reconsideration in light of the parameters set forth in *Hobby Lobby* and *Conestoga Wood*. In each of these cases, the Supreme Court reaffirmed the importance of religious liberty for Hobby Lobby's Green family as Pentecostal Christians, for Conestoga Wood's Hahn family as Mennonite Christians, and for the University of Notre Dame as a Roman Catholic institution to operate within the framework defined by the teachings of those traditions. Despite the appearance of a perceptible inclination in the rulings of the Court there are many issues yet to be decided. Among them are (1) who counts as a "person" guaranteed free exercise of religion – natural persons surely and perhaps some artificial persons, including closely held corporations; (2) what counts as a "religious institution" – places of worship surely and perhaps affiliated religious organizations such as hospitals, schools, groups which dispense charity under the umbrella of a religious organization; (3) what counts as a "compelling governmental interest" and what are the limits of the government's entanglement in the operation of religious institutions; and (4) what other options are readily available.

While there is history of respect for religious freedom, it is to be expected that the religious institutions requesting the free exercise exception would defend their positions in a way that is not destructive of the order of the polity and in such a way as to garner respect from the members of the polity. It seems appropriate for those who speak for the tradition claiming a free exercise exemption to indicate not only that the required services might be available elsewhere – hence the mandated service can be provided by someone else and need not involve the religious institution – but also to explain that there are compelling reasons for refusal to provide or to cooperate in provision of the service.

(b) Contemporary Challenge

More recently, Catholic health care institutions have been challenged to cooperate in practices, which although at a distance from the taking of human life, can be seen as instances of cooperation with evil. Catholic health care institutions face serious challenges to the exercise of their religious freedom with the implementation of the mandated provisions for the purchase of health care in the federal Affordable Care Act (ACA) and the approved replacement policies including those provided by employers. The challenges require participation by way of cooperation in actions, such as elective abortion and contraception, deemed immoral in the Catholic tradition, which holds these practices to be damaging to individuals, to the institution of marriage, and to the polity. An understanding of the principles that guide cooperation in complex human acts where the cooperation can be seen as cooperation in evil and an application of these principles to the issues of elective abortion and contraception identifies the possible harms. Cooperation in these acts by Catholic institutions forces them to lie down in a Procrustean bed wherein acquiescence to these objectionable government-mandated services in the name of toleration in a pluralistic polity forces a damaging or perhaps even fatal encounter with this contemporaneous Procrustes. Recall that those who were forced to lie down on the bed of Procrustes suffered alteration so as to conform their bodies to the size of the bed. Those of shorter stature were stretched until their bodies accommodated the length of the bed. Those of longer stature had limbs lopped off to conform to the limits of the bed. Both accommodations – racking or hacking – can be debilitating. The stretching of the limbs by cooperating in forbidden practices might result in permanent weakness; the amputation of limbs by embracing forbidden practices might prove fatal.

(c) The Catholic tradition understands its opposition to elective abortion and its opposition to contraception to serve the good of the polity, as well as the good of its own adherents. The use of the term "elective" or "direct" abortion is meant to indicate that the act, whether accomplished by chemical means or surgical means, is chosen to bring about the death of the human being developing within the body of the woman. It is an act without medical necessity, an act without medical indication, and an intervention that ameliorates no medical condition. This opposition to elective abortion is considered a service to the common good so as to make the exercise of effective freedom – freedom to choose the good – possible. Opposition to elective abortion is viewed as a political good inasmuch as, in the narrow sense, it protects innocent human life, the life of the preborn child, from direct destruction and thereby allows for the possibility that this human being might achieve other goods, including the good of liberty, as well in the broader sense by restraining society from acquiescence to direct killing as a solution to human problems.

Opposition to contraception is considered a political good inasmuch as the Catholic tradition views it as protecting the institution of marriage, the hinge institution that serves the stability of society, and protection of individuals inasmuch as prohibition of the use of contraceptive drugs and devices might serve as a contribution to the ordering of the passions and an occasion for human flourishing.

The focus on the good intended by the Catholic tradition then, rather than first focusing on permissible cooperation, provides the starting points for discussing the appropriate response to the requirements set forth in the Affordable Care Act (ACA). When these starting points are clearly defined and reasonably defended, the issues at hand can be properly understood as civil rights issues with a proper place in the public domain. But before attending these very different issues, that is, elective abortion and contraception, there are two brief caveats that require attention. The first caveat is that, when treating the issue of abortion, the focus is on elective abortion and not special cases in which abortion might be considered justified as a form of indirect killing. The second caveat is that the conjunction of these two terms contraception and abortion seems to suggest they are the same type of act. They are not and their conjunction can cause confusion within the Catholic community and in the public arena. The precise distinction between abortion and contraception and between contraceptives that prevent egg and sperm fusion and contraceptives that are abortifacient needs to be made carefully in every discussion.

Catholic opposition to elective abortion as both a grave harm to society and a grave sin has its foundation and defense in two separate domains. One is science and the other is Catholic moral tradition. The Church turns to science for information on when human life begins and how it develops. If the developmental sciences report that individual human life begins with the union of egg and sperm, then the direct destruction of that life at any point in its developmental trajectory is a question of killing a human being. The Catholic moral position, informed by Scripture and tradition, holds that human life from its beginning to its end is a gift from God. This gift, fashioned in the image and likeness of God who is creator and steward of life, is to be cherished and protected. Hence, the direct destruction of innocent human life is assessed as an objectively evil act. (The issue of the ontological status of the preborn human being is treated in Chapter 4.)

Elective abortion, as it is understood within the matrix defined by science and Catholic moral tradition, is the direct destruction of innocent human life. It is thus a violation of the first protection, that of human life, that must be secured by government and is an objectively evil act. Other possible instances of abortion, such as those where the life of the woman is at risk, require careful analysis within the understanding of the two lives joined within and sharing, for a time, the body of the woman and the moral and legal requirement of her protection from aggression whether that aggression be a material or formal injustice. (The potential conflict within the physical and moral union of mother and child in pregnancy is treated in Chapter 8.)

Catholic concern with contraception is to be situated within the Church's understanding of marriage and the marriage act, as well as its understanding of the role of marriage within the polity. This understanding is considered a political good inasmuch as the tradition views it as protecting the institution of marriage that serves the stability of society and the flourishing of individuals. Marriage is a natural social institution, not a conventional institution fashioned by government. The government can make laws protective of the institution of marriage, but it cannot define the essential nature of marriage. According to the Catholic tradition, marriage is the union between a man and a woman and it is marked by two signs. One is the sign that signifies the marriage; that is the union of Christ and the Church. The other is the sign that signifies and contains the reality of marriage. That sign is the marriage act: conjugal intercourse. As the marriage act, its expression is normatively limited to the marriage union. The marriage act has many ends that are to be accomplished and ordered within marriage, including (1) nurturing and satisfaction of the sexual drive, (2) procreation and nurturing of offspring, if there are to be offspring of this marriage, and (3) the union of the man and the woman. St. Alphonsus Liguori (1986, §6.882) designated (1) and (2) as intrinsic contingent ends of marriage – they are to be accomplished within marriage under the guidance of reason. He designated (3) as the intrinsic necessary end of marriage – it is to be accomplished only within marriage and its possibility is a necessary condition for marriage. Bernard Lonergan (1967, p. 16ff) ordered those same ends within the complexity of human nature as hierarchically physical, rational, and spiritual – that is, the lower disposes to the higher. In that understanding, the physical union of husband and wife in sexual intercourse and the pleasure experienced in that act exercises an upward dispositive thrust toward friendship that is rational and, ultimately, to love that is spiritual. (This topic is developed in Chapter 5.)

If what the Catholic tradition holds – that procreation is inseparable from every act of marital intercourse rather than inseparable from the totality of the marriage – is the case, then contraception would be understood as a sin inasmuch as it is deliberately chosen failure to accomplish one of the intrinsic ends of marriage. But, there is the possibility of development within the tradition. Moreover, the tradition acknowledges that not all sin is a fit subject of law. So, what of contraceptive practices and the good of the political order? The availability and use of contraceptive drugs and devices by those who are not married has witnessed wide engagement in sexual intercourse outside of marriage. The structures of the natural world, including marriage as a natural social institution and the differentiation and ordination of the sexes toward each other, were set aside and ignored. The powerful drive of an individual's seeking the exquisite pleasure of sex has been removed from the structures that guided its actualization in the service of individual and societal goods. The consequences for the polity include the degradation of the culture and the structures that direct and stabilize its evolution. The consequence for individuals is the disruption of the ordering of their passions with consequences that range from physical to emotional to spiritual.

(d) Principles of Cooperation

The possibility of participation by Catholic institutions and their agents in these acts warrants careful attention to the nature of the act in question and the degree of participation required in the act. Degrees of participation, as required by the complexity of human actions, are developed as categories of cooperation, used to discern the nature and degree of involvement in the objectively evil action of another. It is important to note that the principles of cooperation are limiting principles, that is, they serve to justify action in complex moral situations while still recognizing the evil of the act of the principle agent.

The first distinction to be made is between (I) formal and (II) material cooperation. Cooperation is formal when one "concurs in the bad will of another." Cooperation is material when one "concurs only in the bad action of another apart from the intention of the cooperator" (Liguori, *Theologia moralis*, II, §63).[4] There are two critical notions here: intent and the evil act. For an instance to be one of formal cooperation there are two conditions required: (A) the act must be objectively wrong and (B) the act must be intended – willed – by the cooperator. The intending of formal cooperation can be (1) explicit or (2) implicit. Formal cooperation is explicit when the cooperation is directly intended; it is implicit when the cooperation is intended, not for the end of the intrinsically evil action, but directed to some other good which might be accomplished concurrently with the unintended end.

For an instance to be one of material cooperation only, the evil act must never be intended by the cooperator and the assistance provided by the cooperator must be assessed. In assessing the possibility of material cooperation, it is critical to remember that, because it is cooperation with evil, there exists a presumption against cooperation that must be overcome. It is also important to remember the reach of the cooperation; it extends to the person or entity that receives the cooperation, the person or entity that cooperates, and all who witness or are recipients of the cooperation. Material cooperation is susceptible of varying degrees and hence degrees of culpability. It can involve supplying the means, facilitating the act, or failing to prevent the act. It can be called for because of duress of varying degrees or because of special technical or vocational roles. It can be called for on account of proportionately grave reasons. Navigating this complexity of moral activity requires the further development of categories of material cooperation as (A) immediate and (B) mediate. Immediate material cooperation in an intrinsically evil act occurs when the cooperation is essential to the commission of the act, that is, the act could not occur without the cooperation. Mediate material cooperation in an intrinsically evil act occurs when the circumstances are such that the cooperation is not essential to the commission of the act, that is, the act will happen even without the cooperation. In considering mediate material cooperation, elements that require attention include (1) proportionality and (2) causal influence. The judgment that the cooperation is proportionate requires examining the gravity of the evil to be done as measured against the good protected or evil avoided. Causal influence can be direct or indirect. Direct causal influence is considered (a) proximate; indirect causal influence is considered (b) remote. Finally, the possibility of scandal must be examined. Scandal, as a theological category, is the possibility of causing sin in another, that is, the cooperation might cause another to engage in the intrinsically evil act, engage in similar acts, or cause another to now consider the act morally permissible. Explicit formal cooperation in an evil act is always forbidden. All forms of cooperation require a judgment of practical reason, which requires weighing and assessing all the elements that are involved in the particular act under consideration. Consequentially, there can be no bare algorithmic formula the application of which resolves the issue. Nonetheless, thoughtful consideration of the distinctions attending the notion of cooperation in the presence of a clear recognition of the objective evil that the cooperation would enable can facilitate and guide prudential judgment.[5] Thomas Aquinas cautions, however, that the movement from general principles to particular actions is fraught with difficulty:

> The practical reason . . . is busied with contingent matters, about which human actions are concerned: and consequently, although there is necessity in the general principles, the more we descend to matters of detail, the more we encounter defects.
>
> (*Summa theologica*, Ia-IIae, Q. 94, a. 4)

(e) Application of the Principles of Cooperation

The act of cooperation to be examined here is the purchasing of health insurance by employers that would permit employees to engage in practices that the employer judges, reasonably and publicly, to be objectively evil and hence harmful to persons who engage in such acts and damaging to social structures that serve the common good. The complexity of the issue at hand is the result of at least three goods enunciated by parties to the dispute: (1) the purchase of health care for employees as part of their compensation; (2) the stability of the polity that might be served by toleration of, expressed by compliance with, laws with which one disagrees; and (3) the freedom of religious groups from entanglement of the government in their activities. The provision of health insurance for employees is a morally good act where the intended end is the health of the insured. Respect for the law by conformity with its just requirements is a good, provided the essential conditions of law are met. Elective abortion is not a service rendered to ensure the health of the woman and, furthermore, it destroys the child *en ventra sa mere*. There can be no cooperation – neither formal nor material – with elective abortion understood as the direct destruction of innocent human life. Such cooperation would be a direct and public repudiation of the Catholic magisterial tradition. Such cooperation would be a repudiation of the obligation of government to protect human life and an intrusion of the government into the activities of a religious entity. The sheer magnitude of the performance of elective abortion when viewed in terms of both the nature of the act and the quantity of lives destroyed beggars the imagination.

Occasionally, an analogy has been developed using the permissibility of prostitution as an appropriate model for dealing with the diversity of values within the polity on the elective abortion issue. There are two points to be made in response. The first is that a more appropriate analogy might be war in which (a) the choice to wage war in the absence of the determination of the *jus ad bellum* conditions and in which the destruction of one million innocent human lives a year were a directly chosen end and (b) the choice to carry out war in which a judgment of proportionality – a requirement of *jus in bello* – is absent from consideration. The second is that no cooperation with these objectively evil acts so construed would be countenanced. Hence, explicit formal cooperation with elective abortion is impermissible.

The argument that implicit formal cooperation might be acceptable fails in the face of the inability to frame a good concurrent with and proportionate to the gravity of the objective evil of elective abortion. The possibility of material cooperation that is either immediate or mediate is not permitted because, without this cooperation, the objectively evil act will more likely not occur or will occur with less frequency. Evidence for this assessment can be found in two sources: (1) in the number of abortions performed before and after its easy availability as an elective procedure became legally permissible and (2) the pedagogical effect of the law, as it exercises both its limiting role in practice and its directing role in teaching. Refusal of cooperation by the Catholic tradition provides public witness to the value of respecting human life. The impermissibility of mediate and immediate cooperation renders the issue of causal intentional proximate cooperation moot. The issue of remote mediate cooperation – the "Pontius Pilate solution" of hand-washing by directing payment by third parties, including governmental agencies and insurance fund administrators – is impermissible, first, because of the gravity of the evil and, second, because of the possibility of scandal.[6] The more the public prestige and dignity of the agent of the cooperation – university president, hospital administrator, public official – the greater would be the possibility of scandal. All cooperation with elective abortion would risk a fatal fit on a Procrustean bed. Cooperation in objectively evil acts in the name of toleration is damaging to the agent of cooperation as well as the agent of the action. Moreover, in the case of elective abortion, cooperation would be destructive of the very fabric of the civil community. Finally, the intrusion of the government in the health care benefit plans offered by employers holding particular religious views is an unnecessary entanglement of government in the affairs of the employers and a failure to abide by the government's own least restrictive requirements.

Cooperation by means of payment of health insurance premiums to provide contraceptive services, whether pharmaceuticals or devices, is similarly a complex matter. As in the examination of elective abortion, it is acknowledged that the provision of health insurance for employees is a morally good act where the end of the insurance is truly the health of the insured. And, as differentiated from elective abortion, contraception, while an objectively evil act, appears at first glance not to have the same gravity as abortion. Nonetheless, it is remarkable to note that what was considered a liberty claim, that is, a right free of governmental interference, some 50 years ago in *Griswold v. Connecticut* is now considered a positive right – a right to be provided by others under the coercive power of the government. The consideration of cooperation in providing health care coverage as contraceptive drugs and devices to those engaging in sexual intercourse outside the union of marriage will be considered first, and then cooperation in providing those means to the partners in marriage will be considered.

(i) Cooperation in contraceptive coverage outside of marriage

The Catholic tradition holds that engaging in sexual intercourse outside of marriage violates the necessary intrinsic end of marriage as a union between one man and one woman. Sexual intercourse and its attendant sexual pleasures are oriented to nourishing the good of the marital union. Engaging in those activities outside of marriage – whether the activity is adultery or fornication – is considered in both cases an instance of lust, and in some cases injustice. Injustice arises when the act is adultery and that which owed to one partner of marriage is given to someone outside the marriage. Lust arises when the pursuit of sexual pleasure is not properly integrated into an ordered life as directed by right reason. The easy availability of contraceptives has modified the relations and responsibilities of men and women toward each other, and has recast the understanding of marriage and its ends. This newly found liberty to engage in sexual intercourse free of the possibility of procreation – an intrinsic contingent good of marriage – provides the means for some women to engage in the pleasures of sexual intercourse as do some men – that is, outside the commitment of marriage. Fornication or adultery has become, for some, an expectation as part of casual dating rituals and casual relationships. Of course, they are no longer called fornication or adultery. They have become "just sex" – as casual as a handshake or a slap on the back or even a matter of a market exchange – sex as the coin for dinner or the consummation of a business encounter. Sex as a noun was emptied of content as a particular way of human being in the world. Sex as a verb was deprived of its meaning as the marriage act – an intimate act between husband and wife that signified and contained the reality of their bodily, emotional, and spiritual union; an act that, in the presence of appropriate conditions, made procreation possible; and an act that disposed and ordered the lives of the spouses to their final end – union with God.

Again the act of cooperation to be examined here is the purchasing of health insurance by employers that would permit employees to engage in practices, namely, the use of contraceptive devices and drugs by those engaging in sexual intercourse outside of marriage – that the employer judges, reasonably and publicly, to be harmful to the polity and objectively evil, and hence harmful to persons who engage in such acts. Formal explicit cooperation is impermissible. The possibility of formal implicit cooperation requires the identification of a good that might be accomplished concurrently with the unintended end of the cooperation and proportionate to the gravity of the attendant objective evil. The putative objective good that is often identified is the prevention of conception. The objective evil that is consistently ignored is the damage to women and men in the seeming permission granted by easy access to contraceptive devices and drugs to engage in sexual intercourse outside of marriage. The right of everyone to orgasm and the required freedom from sexual restraint can be accomplished because there is no longer the danger of entanglements – of children, of men and women to each other, of women to the children of whom they are mothers, and of men to the children of whom they are fathers. Absent from the consideration is the possibility of harm, both as physical damage in disease and emotional damage to the character of the individuals engaged in such activities outside of marriage in the disordering of their passions and the consequent effect of this disordering on effective freedom. Evidence for the understanding of this evil stems from antiquity to the present. An example of this understanding in antiquity can be found in Plato's *Republic* where Socrates describes for the young Glaucon the composite animal whose rational, spirited, and appetitive powers are symbolized by, respectively, man, lion, and multiheaded beast (*Republic* 588b – 589d). The gorging of the multiheaded beast, seat of the appetites for food, drink, and sex, strengthens the beast and threatens the enslavement of the man. Evidence of the deleterious effects of pre- and extramarital sex on individuals so engaged and on third parties, including spouses and children, marriage as an institution, and society, while widely documented and known by studies from institutions that range from the Family Research Council to Harvard University, is widely ignored in the calculation by those pressing for cooperation. The gravity of the harm outweighs the putative good; hence, there can be no formal implicit cooperation.

Material cooperation as either immediate or mediate is impermissible because (a) the putative good to be accomplished by the use of contraceptive drugs and devices – the prevention of conception – will more likely occur if there is no sexual intercourse outside of marriage as the tradition teaches and (b) the gravity of an increase in harmful consequences that might occur in the presence of the appearance of permission to engage in extramarital intercourse that such cooperation might indicate. The same danger would be present in the causal influence exercised by any proximate or remote cooperation. Cooperation with the distribution of contraceptive devices – even the arms-length participation provided by insurance carriers and administrators – for the purpose of engaging in sexual intercourse outside of marriage would risk a disabling fit on a Procrustean bed. This disabling would mute the voice of the tradition and hinder its prophetic role in the transformation of culture.

(ii) Cooperation in contraceptive coverage within marriage

Finally, the question of cooperation by means of the use of insurance benefits to provide contraceptive drugs and devices for those who are married is to be attended. As long as the Catholic magisterial tradition holds that procreation is inseparable from every act of marital intercourse, there can be no cooperation. Catholic institutions should refrain from including such coverage in their insurance packages. Furthermore, people who work in Catholic institutions should know and understand the commitments of the tradition, which claims several possible evils that might occur. These evils may include the failure to fulfill the procreative end of marriage; the possibility of the marital partners' objectifying each other as mere means of sexual gratification; the possible loss of sexual appetite for either or both spouses because of the side effects of the pharmaceuticals; and the potential physical damage to women from the use of contraceptive drugs. Against these evils, the good of the regulation of procreation by natural family planning as the control and mastery of sexual appetites by reason is presented. Natural family planning is claimed to contribute to the strengthening of marriage and growth in respect for the spouses. Both contributions are social goods. And here the argument is joined.

(f) Special Concerns

Of course, this position is not unproblematic either within the Catholic Church or within society. In the face of a general lack of acceptance of the Church's teaching on contraception, the institutional Church, if it is to be credible, must attend to the issue. That many Catholics are using artificial contraception is evidenced not only by the Guttmacher Institute's findings repeated over many years, but also by findings of those such as Dr. Richard Fehring of Marquette University who has studied the issue from a Catholic perspective. Few Catholic couples, perhaps as few as 2–3%, practice natural family planning (Fehring, 177). There are at least two ways that the Church can attend to this issue: first, to call the faithful to be faithful; second, to reexamine the issue. Included in both possible approaches are a reflection on the Cross and a reminder that we are called upon to serve the Lord with our minds as well as our obedience. Both would require not only the intentional direction of the resources of the Church but also attentive and respectful study. (See Chapter 5 and its endnotes for treatment of this issue and the debates surrounding this issue.)

In considering the question of cooperation with objectively evil acts, it is good to recall the conversation, as written by Robert Bolt in *A Man for All Seasons* between Thomas More and the Duke of Norfolk as the Duke tried to encourage More to cooperate with the King by signing the Act of Supremacy:

> **Norfolk suggested:** Oh, confound all this . . . . I'm not a scholar, as Master Cromwell never tires of pointing out, and frankly I don't know whether the marriage was lawful or not. But damn it, Thomas, look at those names . . . . You know those men! Can't you do what I did, and come with us, for fellowship? **More responded:** And when we stand before God, and you are sent to Paradise for doing according to your conscience, and I am damned for not doing according to mine, will you come with me, for fellowship?
>
> (Bolt, p. 78)

(C) Scarcity and Extreme Measures in Ordinary and Extraordinary Times

(1) Scarcity in Ordinary Times – Organ Donation

Marvelous technological advances have brought with them the possibility of the transplantation of life-sustaining organs to patients whose organs failed. With the advent of drugs to prevent rejection of the transplanted organ as a foreign body, a new era of medicine emerged. Because of the limit of available organs, the importance of transplantable organs, and the sensitivity of organ sharing, there are regulations to guide organ donation and use. In the United States organ procurement and transplantation policies are directed by the federal government through the Department of Health and Human Services (HHS) and its Organ Procurement and Transplantation Network (OPTN) which was established in 1984 through the National Organ Transplant Act. In 2000 the regulatory framework for the structure and operations of OPTN was established by HHS. OPTN contracts with the private, nonprofit agency, United Network for Organ Sharing (UNOS), to manage the donation, procurement, and distribution of organs in a public-private relationship.

There are several general principles that guide the donation and use of life-sustaining organs in the United States. The first is the allocation should be fair, that is, the distribution should be open to all. A second is that objective medical criteria should be determinant. Here, the probability of success in the recipient is controlled. Factors that contribute to this determination are tissue and blood type, urgency for the patient, and distance of the recipient from the donor. A third is that the process be transparent, that is open to public scrutiny. A fourth is the necessity of informed consent. There is one absolute rule in governing the donation of life-sustaining organs; that is the "dead donor" rule (DDR). This rule forbids killing to remove a vital organ. There must be sufficient certitude that a patient is dead before vital organs are removed.

(a) Catholic Teaching on Organ Donation

In the Catholic religious tradition, organ donation, whether living donation or cadaveric donation, can be seen not only as a good but as an act of charity provided certain protections are in place to protect the donor as well as the recipient. In the modern era, many of the Popes addressed favorably the appropriateness of organ donation as an act of charity. Statements of the recent Pontiffs and the American Bishops in their *Ethical and Religious Directives for Health Care Services* (ERDs) on this medical advance attest to the good of organ donation.[7] Pope John Paul II addressed the issue of organ donation as a heroic gift of self in his encyclical *Evangelium vitae* in the following:

> It is in this context, so humanly rich and filled with love, that heroic actions too are born. These are the most solemn celebration of the Gospel of life, for they proclaim it by the total gift of self. They are the radiant manifestation of the highest degree of love, which is to give one's life for the person loved (cf. Jn 15:13). They are a sharing in the mystery of the Cross, in which Jesus reveals the value of every person, and how life attains its fullness in the sincere gift of self. Over and above such outstanding moments, there is an everyday heroism, made up of gestures of sharing, big or small, which build up an authentic culture of life. A particularly praiseworthy example of such gestures is the donation of organs, performed in an ethically acceptable manner, with a view to offering a chance of health and even of life itself to the sick who sometimes have no other hope.
>
> (*Evangelium vitae*, §86)

Pope Francis in his April 13, 2019 address to the Association of Organ Donors acknowledged the need for organ donation and encouraged donation as an instance of generous solidarity. He said,

> Developments in transplant medicine have made it possible to donate organs after death, and in certain cases even while living (in the case of kidneys, for example), in order to save other human lives; to preserve, recover and even improve the health status of many sick people who have no other alternative. Organ donation responds to a social necessity because, notwithstanding the development of many medical treatments, the need for organs is still great. However, the significance of the donation for the donor, for the recipient and for society is never exhausted in its "utility", as it relates to profound human experiences filled with love and altruism. Donation means looking and going beyond oneself, beyond individual needs, and generously opening oneself to a broader good. In this perspective, organ donation is proposed not only as an act of social responsibility, but as the expression of universal fraternity that binds all men and women.
>
> (Pope Francis April 13, 2019)

The American Bishops address organ donation through the *Ethical and Religious Directives for Catholic Health Care Services* which are updated as needed and issued regularly. Directive 30 of the ERDs addresses the issue of living donation of organs and states:

> 30. The transplantation of organs from living donors is morally permissible when such a donation will not sacrifice or seriously impair any essential bodily function and the anticipated benefit to the recipient is proportionate to the harm done to the donor. Furthermore, the freedom of the prospective donor must be respected, and economic advantages should not accrue to the donor.

The important points to note about living donation are (1) it must not impair the bodily integrity of the donor; (2) it must flow from the donor's informed consent which requires sufficient knowledge and freedom; (3) there must be a proportionate relationship – more good than harm – between the potential harm to the donor and the potential benefit to the recipient; and (4) the donation must be a gift.

The issue of donation of organs after death is addressed in Directives 63 and 64 which state:

> 63. Catholic health care institutions should encourage and provide the means whereby those who wish to do so may arrange for the donation of their organs and bodily tissue, for ethically legitimate purposes, so that they may be used for donation and research after death.
>
> 64. Such organs should not be removed until it has been medically determined that the patient has died. In order to prevent any conflict of interest, the physician who determines death should not be a member of the transplant team.

The important points to note about cadaveric donation are the following: (1) donation is encouraged by the Church; (2) the organs may be donated for use in the living and/or for medical research; (3) a determination of death must be made before organs are removed; (4) the determination of death must be made by a physician who is not associated with the team responsible for transplantation of the organs; and (5) the determination of death is a matter of medical expertise. The Popes from Pius XII to John Paul II recognized the specific role of medicine and science here. As Pope Pius XII clearly stated, "It is for the doctor . . . to give a clear, precise definition of death and of the moment of death." Furthermore, John Paul II as Pope maintained that it is the task of "scientists, analysts and scholars" [to] "continue their research and their studies to determine in the most precise way possible the exact moment and the irrefutable sign of death." In his August 29, 2000 address the Italian Association for the Donation of Organs, Tissues and Cells, Pope John Paul II addressed the necessity of the determination of death before organ removal. He was precise in distinguishing the death of a person – "the total disintegration of that unitary and integrated whole that is the personal self" – from the biological signs that follow death. The latter determination lies in the provenance of physicians and scientists. The Holy Father said:

> Acknowledgement of the unique dignity of the human person has a further underlying consequence: *vital organs which occur singly in the body can be removed only after death*, that is from the body of someone who is certainly dead. This requirement is self-evident, since to act otherwise would mean intentionally to cause the death of the donor in disposing of his organs. This gives rise to one of the most debated issues in contemporary bioethics, as well as to serious concerns in the minds of ordinary people. I refer to the problem of *ascertaining the fact of death*. When can a person be considered dead with complete certainty?
>
> In this regard, it is helpful to recall that *the death of the person* is a single event, consisting in the total disintegration of that unitary and integrated whole that is the personal self. It results from the separation of the life-principle (or soul) from the corporal reality of the person. The death of the person, understood in this primary sense, is an event which *no scientific technique or empirical method can identify directly*.
>
> Yet human experience shows that once death occurs *certain biological signs inevitably follow*, which medicine has learnt to recognize with increasing precision. In this sense, the "criteria" for ascertaining death used by medicine today should not be understood as the technical-scientific determination of the *exact moment* of a person's death, but as a scientifically secure means of identifying *the biological signs that a person has indeed died*.
>
> (John Paul II, 2000, n. 4)

(b) Complexity of Organ Transplantation

That there is a real and pressing need for organs is indisputable. The possibility of success requires a sufficient supply of organs. And it appears that the organ donation system in the U.S.A. does not have access to a sufficient supply of the necessary organs. Possible solutions range from the improvement of the donation system (whether living or cadaveric donor) to sale of organs from both live and cadaveric donors, to the payment of a set fee, a kind of user fee, to the donor or the family, from presumed donation to conscription of cadaveric organs, and from the possible generation of new organs from the adult stem cells – reversed and induced into pluripotent stem cells – of the patient. Each has a set of problems. Among them are the following: first, the characterization of organs as property and the consequences of that characterization in regard to the transfer of organs; second, the determination of death and the permissible removal of organs; third, the nature of consent; and fourth, a distribution plan.[8]

(c) Characterization of Organs

Organs are not property. While it might be possible to construe, for the sake of an argument, an analogy between the dominion/possession/ownership of things and the dominion/possession/ownership of body parts, it remains an analogy not an equivalence statement. Body parts are not things; they cannot be reified. They are elements of an integrated system. When they are healthy, they contribute to the good of the whole of the person. They may be excised when they threaten the good of the whole. They are not things in the sense of objects to be bartered, bought, and sold. They are received; they have been given to us whether the source be – to use Jeffersonian language – given by Nature or Nature's God. Because they are given, they may be re-given, in certain circumstances with limitations. They may be given out of the spirit of charity as a love which removes any sinfulness from the mutilation. The principle guiding the giving is the principle of totality with its careful distinguishing of the whole as a physical whole or a moral whole and a consequent limitation of action. A human being as an individual is physical whole and may have a body part removed to protect health and life. A human being as a member of society is part of a moral entity – a part of a whole – which may demand the activities, and only the activities, of the individual to serve the good of society. Except in extraordinary circumstances such as a just war, society cannot ask the individual to sacrifice life.

Living organ donation falls between these. A human being may, as an act of charity, give part of the body to serve or save the life of another human being provided that the integral goodness of the human being is protected and the part is used by the recipient for a good. (The principle of totality is treated in Chapter 2, Section D-7.) The consideration of the possibility of alienation of our organs from ourselves, as would be the case in the sale of organs, as an appropriate descriptor of relationship of organs to the person suggests a kind of Gnostic dualism. We are embodied beings; we are ensouled beings – human life is body, soul, and spirit as a unified whole. The dissociation of the self from the body and its organs is a stretch too far and not even claims of privacy and forbearance can be used to shore up the dissociation. The laws protecting privacy rights are held usually against an external agent and even they are limited by the possibility of our doing harm to ourselves.

(d) Cadaveric Donation and Determination of Death

Organs such as the heart and lungs and liver and pancreas and kidneys may be removed from cadaveric donors provided they are really cadavers. To paraphrase a famous coroner the patient must be "not only merely dead but really most sincerely dead" (Coroner in the *Wizard of Oz*). The word sincerely, from its Latin roots *sine cere*, means without wax. It was used to describe a piece of marble sculpture whose flaws were not filled in by wax. So until a determination is made that the patient died, that is, "the patient is most sincerely dead" and the organ procurement officer is not just making this up to get the organs, there can be no removal of organs.[9]

An accurate determination of death is essential for the success, both publicly and morally, in the organ transplant program. The controversy over the determination of death as irreversible coma, since it was first proposed in 1968 in the *Report of the Ad Hoc Committee of the Harvard Medical School to Examine the Definition of Brain Death*, continues. The Report maintained that there were two reasons for the necessity of a new definition. The first was the relief of the patient, the family, and the medical institution from the burdens of an indefinitely prolonged coma. The second was the removal of the controversy on obtaining organs for transplantation. The first is not problematic; the second becomes problematic when it drives the determination of death for utilitarian reasons. Diagnosis of irreversible coma indicates that medicine can do no more for this person. Concern about this second motivation was articulated from the very beginning in response to the language of Dr. Henry K. Beecher who said, "Can society afford to discard the tissues and organs of the hopelessly unconscious patient when they could be used to restore the hopelessly ill, but still salvageable individual?" In response, Hans Jonas wrote,

> Society . . . cannot afford a single miscarriage of justice, a single inequity in the dispensation of its laws, the violation of the rights of even the tiniest minority, because these undermine the moral basis on which society's existence rests.
>
> (Jonas, 1980b, p. 115)

In the more distant past, the declaration of death was made on the basis of cardio-pulmonary criteria, that is, the failure of the heart and the lungs to sustain life. The brain death determination is a more recent addition. Here, the declaration of death is made on a determination that the whole brain, cerebral cortex, cerebellum, and brain stem have ceased to function in the regulation of the vital functions of the body. More recently, other determinations of death within the context of salvaging organs have been offered including higher brain death and donation after controlled cardiac death (controlled DCD). Higher brain death is the determination of death based on the destruction of function of the cerebral cortex understood as the necessary material matrix for rational thought. Donation after controlled cardiac death is the determination of death within a hospital setting based on the occurrence of the cessation of heartbeat and respiration without evidence of cessation of whole brain function. While these last two have been offered with the same dual purposes in mind, namely, the relief of the patient, family, and medical resources and the procurement of relatively healthy organs for transplantation, the strong emphasis on the procurement of healthy organs for transplantation appears to drive the declaration of death. The first two sets of criteria, traditional cardio-pulmonary cessation and whole brain failure, provide sufficient moral certainty to permit removal of vital organs for transplantation. The second two sets, higher brain death and controlled donation after cardiac death DCD, do not enjoy that same moral certitude.

Controlled donation after cardiac death in a hospital-initiated process is begun when a determination is made that life support mechanisms in place no longer serve to benefit the patient and the patient or surrogate has agreed to the removal of the life support mechanism and to the retrieval of the vital organs. The process includes (1) removing life support from a patient who no longer benefits from that support; (2) waiting for the occurrence of asystole, that is, the cessation of electrical activity of the heart tissue with the consequence of the cessation of circulatory function; (3) the declaration of death; and (4) the removal of vital organs. The process of controlled donation after cardiac death requires further specification. As with all organ donation consent is required. The consent may be the prior informed consent of the donor or the appropriate surrogate. The life support is removed because it no longer benefits or is excessively burdensome for this patient. The patient is given appropriate comfort care. The occurrence of asystole is judged as truly present and perceived irreversible in this patient. This requires appropriate waiting time. The critical determination is the assessment of how much time is enough to be certain that the putative donor is beyond repair and how much time is too long for the successful harvesting of usable organs. The measure of waiting time varies from 75 seconds to 10 minutes by institutional practice. The longer the waiting time the greater the possibility of organ damage and loss of quality for transplantation. The Institute of Medicine in the United States recommends no less than a five-minute waiting time as the sufficient time to be morally certain that the heart in the potential donor would not restart in that donor (IOM, 2000, p. 39). The declaration of death is required of the attending health care team, not the transplant team. Only after that declaration may vital organs be removed by the transplant team. The roles of attending physician and transplant physician must remain separate. Controlled donation after cardiac death seems to serve two goods: (1) on the part of the donor the good of the charitable intention of the donor to serve the life of another is protected and (2) on the part of the recipient the good of the use of the vital organs sustain life or improve quality of life. The major problems in the controlled organ donation situation are careful adherence to the wait time for asystole and the use of certain drugs administered to preserve the vital organs targeted for transplant. If the drugs, phentolamine and heparin, currently in use in some transplant centers to preserve the vital organs are administered at the time of removal of life support and they hasten dying in the donor, they may not be used. If it can be shown that these drugs do not hasten death, they may be used as a good in preserving the vital organs for use in the recipient. At this time there is no single consistent official policy regarding controlled donation after cardiac death in the United States. Some transplant centers, for example, the University of Pittsburgh Medical Center, proscribe the use of phentolamine and heparin. Others claim that the intention of preserving organs not hastening death permits the use of these drugs.

Higher brain death is the determination of death based on the destruction of function of the cerebral cortex understood as the necessary material matrix for rational thought. A patient diagnosed as having suffered higher brain death has lost cerebral cortical function including the ability to communicate, to think, or to initiate purposeful movement. The patient retains, without artificial support, brain stem functions including breathing, circulation, and hemodynamic stability. The patient often evidences noncognitive activities such as normal sleep and awake patterns, eye opening, and spontaneous nonpurposeful movements. Bowel and bladder control are lost. The maintenance of the patient in this state requires assisted nutrition and hydration. A consensus has developed on the observable criteria in patients for the designation of permanent vegetative state. They are the following:

1. No evidence of awareness of self or environment; no interaction with others.
2. No evidence of sustained, reproducible, purposeful, or voluntary behavioral responses to visual, auditory, tactile, or noxious stimuli.
3. No evidence of language comprehension or expression.
4. Return of sleep-wake cycles, arousal, even smiling, frowning, yawning.
5. Sufficient hypothalamic and brainstem autonomic functions to survive if given medical or nursing care.
6. Bowel and bladder incontinence.
7. Variably preserved cranial nerve and spinal reflexes.

(*New England Journal of Medicine*, 1994, p. 1500)

After four weeks of a patient in this condition, the designation of the patient changes to a persistent vegetative state. When the condition continues – 3 months after a nontraumatic brain injury in many states and 12 months after a traumatic brain injury in other states – the patient is classified as being in a permanent vegetative state. Because of the medical uncertainty about the status of persons in this condition, they are not candidates for organ harvesting.[10] They cannot be declared dead by either the whole brain death standard or the cardio-pulmonary standard. The removal of artificial nutrition and hydration from a patient diagnosed as suffering from PVS syndrome requires Court petition in most jurisdictions.[11] When nutrition and hydration are removed the occurrence of death varies from hours to days to weeks. The time passage from removal of nutrition and hydration to declaration of death generally renders the vital organs unusable for transplantation. This coupled with the medical uncertainty about the state of these patients requires their protection rather than their use. Harvesting organs from a person whose circulatory and pulmonary systems appear to be functioning without medical or artificial assistance is an affront to medicine.

(e) Consent and Organ Donation

Organ donation after death requires consent. In the best of circumstances, the consent originates with the donor whose prior choice directs the donation. This is designated the opt-in decision for organ donation. Nonetheless, final consent to cadaveric organ donation frequently falls to the family after the death of the person, even when it is the case that the person, while alive, signified a willingness to be an organ donor. This issue often arises in the midst of family grief. To forestall cadaveric organ donation from becoming an issue, the family needs to be part of the decision process earlier. Just as families have discussions about estate planning, end-of-life care, and even funeral planning, they need to have discussions about organ donation. This discussion might be facilitated through the primary care physician and through the houses of worship in appropriate seasons.

It is a fact that there remains a perennial shortage of organs suitable for donation despite its characterization as an altruistic act, an act of charity, an act of self-gift, a noble act, and its wide advertisement in those terms. A movement from the opt-in to an opt-out structure has been suggested to increase the number of suitable organs. The opt-out structure operates from the presumption that since most people are motivated to perform charitable acts and would do so if asked and since, now dead, their organs are of no use to them, it is acceptable to remove their organs to save the lives of others. The opt-out strategy presumes that if the person did not want their organs so used, they would have made that choice known. This presumption, while it might serve the good of increased availability of organs, operates in the presence of a diminishment of informed consent with the resultant loss of respect for the putative organ donor. The opt-out presumption has similarities in execution to conscription. Another option as an attempt to increase organ availability is the mandated choice structure in which a person is forced to choose opt-in or opt-out when filing an important legal document. This choice can be made in a variety of seemingly noncoercive situations such as applying for a driver's license, registering to vote, and filing taxes. While this option may have an element of coercion, it provides a degree of respect for the dignity of the donor as making a free choice.

The consent to living organ donation is more problematic. Hence, there are some lines to be drawn here. There seems to be no moral issues with the donation of blood. The donation of sperm or ova is problematic when the finality of the donation is directed to progeny outside the commitment to progeny and outside of marriage. The donation of a kidney is problematic, if the requirements of informed consent are not rigorously applied. The knowledge component is lacking if the donor is not sufficiently informed of the risks. The prospective donor must be made aware of the fact that the mortality rate in kidney donation is 3 in 10,000; that the single remaining kidney operates at an efficiency slightly reduced from (80%) the operation of the paired kidneys; that there is an increased incidence of End State Renal Disease (ESRD) in kidney donors 15 years after donation (the cumulative incidence of ESRD was 30.8 per 10,00 donors and 3.9 per 10,000 for healthy non-donors); and that there is an increased lifetime risk of ESRD by age 80 (90 per 10,000 for kidney donors and 3.9 per 10,00 for healthy non-donors.) These data are taken from the February 13, 2014 report of the Johns Hopkins School of Medicine which analyzed the incidence of ESRD in 96,217 individuals in the U.S.A. who donated a kidney and compared this with data from the Third National Health and Nutrition Examination Survey (NHANES III). These new data require a deeper reflection on the claim that one kidney of a pair is redundant and the claim that the refusal to allow the poor to sell a kidney is another kind of exploitation which separates the poor from participation in an upward economic activity which might serve to their leading a better life.

(f) Distribution Issues

Given the fact of asymmetry between the availability of organs for transplantation and the need of patients, a distribution scheme is necessary and appropriate. The distribution of organs has been assigned to the United Network for Organ Sharing (UNOS) under the direction of the Organ Procurement and Transplant Network (OPTN). Together with the transplant community, physicians, other health care providers, organ donors and recipients, the Board of Directors of OPTN develops policies to guide and direct the provision of organs in the U.S.A. These policies are open to development as new clinical information becomes available. These policies are open in the sense that they are transparent. This customary practice policy, while not perfect, has gained social acceptance and it avoids some of the problems inherent in other suggested practices such as a market approach or a lottery. The social grounding and social acceptance of the guidelines is an acknowledgment of long-term public funding of transplant technologies. Both the market approach and the lottery approach offend human dignity. The market approach offends because it puts a price on human life and the lottery approach because in treating all as equal it does not distinguish significant differences in potential medical success for particular individuals. The market approach puts too low a value on equal dignity; the lottery approach puts too high a value on equal access.

UNOS has created a computerized program to match organs with potential organ recipients. Medical and logistical factors frame the process. UNOS asserts that there are no social criteria. As with all distribution programs of limited resources, there are exclusion criteria and inclusion criteria. The first exclusionary criterion is medical suitability, that is, can this particular organ be successfully transplanted into this particular person who will then be restored to a functional level of living. A second criterion measures the distance of the available organ from the potential recipient, that is, is the available organ physically close enough to the potential recipient so that the organ remains functional. Negative answers to these questions are sufficient for exclusion. A third criterion is social sustainability, that is, is this person so situated as to be able to maintain the level of treatment necessary to sustain life with the transplanted organ or are there support structures in place to provide this care for them. Once the list of potential included recipients is complete, the inclusion factors which are specific for particular organs are added to the recipients' profile. A computerized program then generates a ranked list of appropriate recipients.

For the four most frequent transplant organs – kidney, lungs, liver, and heart – the factors weighted include distance of the donor hospital from the recipient hospital, medical urgency, and likelihood of survival. Distance of the donor hospital from the recipient hospital is an important and variable factor because of the fragility of the different organs in transport. Kidneys are the most durable; hearts and lungs are the least durable. Kidney and lung transplants add waiting time on the transplant list as a factor. The kidney transplant list adds prior living donor status as a favorable factor in the calculation of rank on the list. All the organs have specific pediatric criteria.

While there is general acceptance of these developed guidelines in the U.S.A., occasionally a family, out of understandable anxiety, attempts to operate outside the guidelines by a direct appeal to the public and to the courts. Because of the great emotional impact of the issue, especially when it involves a child being denied an organ, media, whether print or electronic, get involved. The courts have been used to grant injunctive relief to the enforcement of guidelines and to force an exception to the rules. It is wise to recall that when one child receives an organ another does not.

(2) *Scarcity in Extraordinary Times – Rationing*

The specter of a national emergency or a local emergency, which would require the immediate, albeit temporary, rationing of currently available health care resources, has been addressed in recent times by public health agencies throughout the United States. Using a modification of the triage scenario – the choice scenario – employed by the military but appropriate to civilian circumstances, most localities, while hoping to never have to implement them, have developed a set of guidelines to sort patients for treatment. These guidelines include exclusion and inclusion criteria.

(a) *Exclusion Criteria – Medical Prognosis*

The exclusion criteria determine those who will not receive life-sustaining interventions. The excluded are those for whom there is no possible positive medical intervention and those whose injuries or condition are judged minor and can wait. For the latter, the judgment is made that waiting does them no harm. For the former, the medical judgment is made that treatment is ineffective entirely or ineffective in the available time frame. Treatment of patients not automatically excluded or included – those whose prognosis is uncertain – depends on the judgment of the availability of the scarce resource. Palliation, if available, as comfort care should be provided for those excluded patients who will most likely die without treatment.

Guidelines for the judgment of exclusion are usually the task of a committee within the institutions or agencies. Members of the committee should have no direct responsibilities for the care of individual patients. This should permit the committee to be free from bias and to be perceived as impartial. The operative principles that guide the committee should be (1) based on clinical judgment, (2) applied consistently, (3) transparent, and (4) open to review. The task of the committee is to determine the particular set of guidelines appropriate to the emergency at hand and to serve as the agent that determines that the guidelines apply to the individual patient. The committee provides a buffer for the clinical team. Furthermore, the judgment of exclusion comes from a committee rather than a single person allowing for a sharing of the burden. This situation is quite different from the process of withdrawal of life-sustaining treatment that occurs by the attending physician in consultation with family and colleagues once the determination is made that treatment no longer benefits a particular person. In the triage situation, the attending physician forwards the appropriate clinical information to the triage committee. Despite the appearance of a strict mechanism in place, there is a need, if the situation permits, for appeal from exclusion. The appeal would be initiated by the attending physician's clinical assessment which might include pertinent information from the family.

(b) Inclusion Criteria – Medical Prognosis

The initial inclusion criteria result from the combination of two factors. They are medical prognosis and essential social function. Medical prognosis, while never perfect, is the reasonable judgment of the medical team. While there may be an initial judgment for inclusion, subsequent medical assessment of the patient may move to exclusion. Creating a set of decision guidelines is both a difficult and an imperfect task. It is difficult since denial of a particular modality of treatment such as a ventilator may mean death. It is imperfect because it is always attended by a degree of uncertainty. Inclusion requires an assessment of potential benefit here and now. Assessing the benefit requires processing data on prognosis from past patient experiences and from sufficiently large sets from current patients to determine prognosis in a particular patient. In the presence of knowledge about the course of a particular disease the presence of underlying comorbidities and relevant circumstances such as age and disability factor into the assessment.[12]

A number of clinically relevant sets of criteria are available to produce algorithms to assist in the assessment of mortality. They are the Sequential Organ Failure Assessment score (SOFA and mSOFA), the Acute Physiologic Assessment and Chronic Health Evaluation score (APACHE I – IV), and the Laboratory Acute Physiology Score (LAPS2). The SOFA score is the calculation of mortality risk based on the degree of organ dysfunction. The score measures the rate of organ failure by assigning a value to objective measurements of six functions: (1) respiratory, (2) cardiovascular, (3) renal, (4) neurological, (5) hepatic, and (6) coagulation. The mSOFA score adds the Glasgow Coma Score. The APACHE score (now in its 4th iteration) is a calculation based on a combination of factors including age, sex, dates of admission, systolic and diastolic blood pressure, body temperature, heart rate, respiratory rate, glucose, blood urea nitrogen, serum sodium, creatinine, blood hematocrit, white blood cells, serum albumin and bilirubin, urine output, comorbidities, and the Glasgow Coma Score (GCS).

The GCS is a measure of levels of eye-opening response, verbal response, and motor response. The LAPS2 score is an algorithm that results from a two-stage process. The first stage uses selected variables such as age, sex, blood urea nitrogen, serum creatinine, and serum sodium to separate patients into high and low mortality risks. The second stage adds vital signs and additional laboratory values. The LAPS2 score is often used as a variable in a model that includes other patient characteristics such as demographics, comorbidities, and the Glasgow Coma Score. The process of assessing the condition of an individual patient to generate a relevant score is a time-consuming task. In a mass crisis event, the assistance of computer-generated and implemented algorithms for the preferred scoring tool would assist physician judgment. The effectiveness and accuracy of the tool depend on the accuracy of the input data. The score alone cannot be a substitute for clinical judgment.

(c) Inclusion Criteria – Social Function

Essential social function seems the more elastic of the two inclusion criteria and its determination will vary according to the situation. Designating some people as more essential than others flies in the face of equality claims that are central to a democratic republic and to a religious tradition that holds that all are equal before God. However, it is, a matter of fact, that in the face of a disaster, some are more essential for the maintenance and flourishing of the social order than others. Physicians and other health care providers are essential in times of widespread or epidemic disease if the treatment in question protects them, such as a preventative vaccine, so that they are free to care for the sick. Physicians and health care workers would not seem to have priority for the use of ventilators in an illness that requires the use of a ventilator and lengthy recovery time from the illness. This situation renders their ability to serve the sick in the immediate future doubtful. Members of the military are more essential in times of war. Community leaders are essential to maintain order in time of peace and in times of war. Neither the elderly nor the disabled are automatically excluded by age or impairment. They are protected by law in the United States – the elderly at 45CFR§91.11and the handicapped at 29USC§794.

> **45CFR§91.11 Rules against *age* discrimination.**
>
> The rules stated in this section are limited by the exceptions contained in *§§ 91.13* and 91.14 of these regulations.
>
> (a) General rule: No person in the *United States* shall, on the basis of *age*, be excluded from participation in, be denied the benefits of, or

be subjected to discrimination under, any *program or activity* receiving *Federal financial assistance.*

(b) Specific rules: A *recipient* may not, in any *program or activity* receiving *Federal financial assistance*, directly or through contractual licensing, or other arrangements, use *age distinctions* or take any other *actions* which have the effect, on the basis of *age*, of:

    (1) Excluding individuals from, denying them the benefits of, or subjecting them to discrimination under, a *program or activity* receiving *Federal financial assistance*; or
    (2) Denying or limiting individuals in their opportunity to participate in any *program or activity* receiving *Federal financial assistance.*

(c) The specific forms of *age* discrimination listed in *paragraph (b)* of this section do not necessarily constitute a complete list.

29USC§794 Rules against discrimination based on disability

(A) Promulgation of Rules and Regulations

No otherwise qualified individual with a disability in the United States, as defined in *section 705(20) of this title*, shall, solely by reason of her or his disability, be excluded from the participation in, be denied the benefits of, or be subjected to discrimination under any *program or activity* receiving Federal financial assistance or under any *program or activity* conducted by any Executive agency or by the United States Postal Service.

But, the elderly and the disabled are not automatically included either. Age is one factor among many others in scoring mortality risk. Both the APACHE score and the LAPS2 score include age as a variable with increasing age considered an increase in mortality risk. There are often significant underlying conditions such as chronic cardiopulmonary disease (COPD), a compromised immune system, or cancer that combined with age or disability make the elderly or the disabled poor candidates for the putative benefits of the scarce treatment for the current disease.

(d) Informed Consent

The initiation or withdrawal of medical treatment usually requires informed consent. The same rules govern both implementation and withdrawal of a treatment modality. In a mass crisis situation, every effort must be made to respect human dignity by assuring the informed consent of the patient. Even in cases where the patient is excluded from life-sustaining treatment, the patient, if conscious, must be informed of the exclusion and of the reasons for the exclusion. If the patient is not conscious, a living will, advance directive, or POLST document can supply direction. When informed consent is impossible because of the condition of the patient and the limits of time, substituted judgment or best interest judgment can be used in its place. Substituted judgment is the replacement of informed consent by using the expressed or lived values of the incapacitated patient to inform the decision. The values of the patient are supplied usually by the family, a member of the family, or a close friend. If substituted judgment is impossible because of the mass crisis situation, then a best interest judgment is made. The best interest judgment is that which a reasonable person of a character and type similar to the incapacitated patient most likely would have decided in the situation at hand. The attending physician, with appropriate consultation when possible, assumes the burden of applying the best interest judgment. While there cannot be absolute certainty that the application of the substituted judgment or the best interest standard represents the real informed consent that the patient might have exercised in this situation, there must be at least moral certainty that this is the case. Moral certainty here is both a limit and a consolation.

(e) Triage Example – New York State Task Force Report on Ventilator Allocation

An example and a significant, helpful guide to the allocation of scarce resources was developed by The New York State Task Force on Life and the Law in its set of guidelines for ventilator allocation published in 2015. The Task Force has been in existence since 1985 under the direction of the New York State Department of Health. The work of the Task Force is to develop public policy at the intersection of medicine, law, and ethics. To date it has issued 23 reports including: withholding and withdrawing of life-sustaining treatment; the treatment of impaired newborns; assisted reproductive technologies; organ transplantation; assisted suicide; and genetic testing. The Task Force is chaired by the New York State Commissioner of Health who is joined by governor-appointed volunteer members. The members have expertise in the fields of medicine, law, philosophy, religion, and bioethics.

The work on the allocation of ventilators as a scarce resource was begun with the circulation of a draft document in 2007. This document was distributed widely and commented on extensively. The committee on this particular issue was convened in 2009 to receive the comments of the outreach draft and to begin their work of analysis. The new draft document was completed in 2011 and the public comment phase was opened. Focus groups were created throughout the State. Upon completion of the public input, the committee returned to its work. In 2015, the committee finished its work and published its report. The Report contains separate sections on the allocation of ventilators to adults, to children in the pediatric setting, and to children in the neonatal setting.

The Task Force set its recommendations within an ethical framework that included the following components: (1) the duty to care which is primarily the task of health care providers; (2) the duty to steward resources which is primarily an institutional duty; (3) the duty to plan responsibly which is primarily a duty of governmental entities; (4) the duty to distribute the treatment modality justly – here the principle of distributive justice is operative; and (5) the duty to be transparent. The Task Force recommended a three-step process based on the assessment of clinical factors. The three-step process included (1) exclusion criteria; (2) assessment of mortality risk; and (3) time trials. The Task Force recommended that social criteria not be used. In its concern for significantly different populations to be served by ventilator allocation, the Task Force distinguished three specific populations: (1) adults – 18 years and older; (2) pediatric patients – those younger than 17; and (3) neonatal patients – those 28 days and younger. Physiological differences in these groups require differences in the assessment of mortality risk. The process for adult assessment of mortality risk utilized the SOFA score. Because there is no one fully validated score mechanism, that is, no evidence-based data tool for determining mortality risk, for children, the Task Force recommended that the clinical judgment of those experienced in pediatric and neonatal care determine mortality risk. Time trials to reassess mortality risk, to be repeated at 48 and 120 hours, were recommended for all three categories. The Task Force developed Figure 9.1 to guide the allocation of ventilators when there are not enough for all who need them. A similar pattern, but with appropriate clinical criteria and measures, was developed for children.

While requiring that the allocation of ventilators be determined by clinical criteria only, the Task Force did recognize the possible situation of multiple patients at the same level of mortality risk, for example, all are code red, needing the only available ventilator. In general, the rule is all patients at the same code level are the same and are to be treated as equals. The recipient of the ventilator is to be chosen by a randomization process. In a situation where multiple adults all have equal likelihoods of survival, for example, all are code red, the Task Force recommended that the decision to receive or continue on a ventilator be based on a lottery. Those denied the ventilator are to receive alternative care and/or palliative care. In a situation where adult and pediatric patients all have equal likelihoods of survival, the Task Force determined that young age may play a tie-breaking role in determining which patient receives or continues with ventilator treatment. This determination in favor of the child is based on a cultural understanding that a child has a potential lifetime to be experienced and

Step 2 – Mortality Risk Assessment Using SOFA[1]	
Color Code and Level of Access	**Assessment of Mortality Risk/ Organ Failure**
Blue No ventilator provided. Use alternative forms of medical intervention and/or palliative care or discharge. Reassess if ventilators become available.	Exclusion criterion OR SOFA > 11
Red Highest Use ventilators as available	SOFA < 7 OR Single organ failure[2]
Yellow Intermediate Use ventilators as available	SOFA 8 – 11
Green Use alternative forms of medical intervention or defer or discharge. Reassess as needed.	No significant organ failure AND/OR No requirement for lifesaving resources

Figure 9.1 New York State Task Force Report: Guide to Ventilator Allocation, 2015, p. 59

the cultural value that children have a stronger claim on society for care. Here the child, 17 years old and younger, receives or continues with ventilator treatment and the adult receives alternative forms of medical intervention and/or palliative care. Neonatal patients remain in the category of children. Therefore, if a neonatal patient and a pediatric patient have equal likelihoods of survival a randomization process is used to determine the recipient or the continuation of the ventilator.

Hans Jonas noted the difficulty in the distribution of scarce resources in an emergency and the appropriate disposition in the face of that difficulty in the following:

> Practicality and necessity, combined with medical judgment, are determinants as to who should be the recipient of a scarce resource. Practical judgment should be made as to the prospect of a good medical outcome. While practical judgment is fraught with a degree of uncertainty, this is not a waiving of rules. It is the acknowledgment that it is impossible to devise exact rules for waiving rules. What is allowable under the conditions of emergency and uncertainty may be later passed over in silence – a unique dispensation that suspends in some non-specifiable way the structures of normal practice
>
> (Jonas 1980b, pp.124–125).

(D) Afterword

If Catholic health care is to flourish in the U.S.A., if it is to serve as leaven, witnessing the life and love of an incarnate God, then it must be prepared to act as light and salt too. Its mission must be clear and it must be open to the appropriation of the developments of medical science advances and the development of understanding of Catholic teaching. Catholic health care must reflect on its identity and teach its mission. It must be a visible reproof to a kind of contemporary medicine which prescribes killing as a remedy for pressing social ills. The continuation of the mission of Catholic health care, as leaven and light and salt, requires the continuous sacrificial commitment of Catholics – lay and religious, health care professionals and business professionals – to accept and contribute to that mission. Catholic Health Care Institutions have a particular witness role to play in the contemporary world. If for economic reasons and practical reasons, it chooses or must withdraw from its extensive involvement in medicine, then Catholic Health Care Institutions should provide services where those services will have the greatest impact for the values it holds and the values it would witness. The locus of Catholic Health Care may shift to issues at the beginning of life – the care of pregnant women and their children – and issues at the end of life – the care of the dying. In their refusal to kill they may, by their witness, initiate the transformation of the culture of death, a culture that embraces killing as a solution to problems, into a new culture of life. That there are few Catholic health care institutions and that their range of service would be rather limited should not appear to be overwhelming obstacles in a tradition that once numbered twelve and the twelve had very limited resources.

In regard to the distribution of health care, do we continue to wring our hands to sound the death knell for the possibility of an excellent health care system that can deliver its goods justly and appropriately? What about Catholic health care in the U.S.A.? Shall we wash our hands of it or do we have the courage to begin anew? A starting point might be found in reflecting on the truths of our shared traditions, both our religious tradition and our civic tradition, and the practices that these traditions nurture. From within this reflection, policies, practices, and institutions that affirm life and its natural beginning and end might emerge. Can the truths of our religious and civic traditions and the witness of our practices provide a framework for institutions to move forward? In regard to organ transplantation do we turn a deaf ear and a hard heart to those whose organs are so damaged that the organs cannot sustain life and its promises or do we allow our hearts, clouded by emotion and untethered from reason, reify what cannot be reified or cross a boundary whose outline remains uncertain so as to increase the supply of organs available for transplantation? Or can we find a place, both in our hearts and in a physical space, where the integrity of the body is respected; where the giftedness of the human giving, even of our organs, is generous; and where the dying of each person remains sacred?

The story of our civic tradition and the values that enliven that tradition is a rich story and a robust tradition marked by sets of values which when held in appropriate tension produced, and can continue to produce, a citizenry and nation capable of extraordinary accomplishments. Here are some of those related sets: rights and responsibilities; the individual in the community and the community as sustaining the individual; independence and self-discipline; freedom and order; present needs ordered to future needs; and self-sufficiency. To cast the people of the nation only as rights-bearing autonomous independent, self-sufficient, free persons is to tell only part of the story and as partial is inaccurate and dangerous. While some may claim these qualities, they, having gained this condition from the work of others, do so only contingently and temporarily. To cast the people of the nation only as dependent, irresponsible, absorbed by the society, focusing on present needs and ignoring future needs, and receiving sufficiency only from the work of others is also partial, inaccurate, and dangerous. While some may be in that condition and be there permanently, many are so only temporarily and they need to have the hope and opportunity for upward movement. The former need our constant, compassionate care; the latter need our encouragement.

The story of our religious tradition is also a rich tradition whose robustness and credibility are challenged both internally and externally in the contemporary world. Nonetheless, we are, as Chesterton reminded us in *The Everlasting Man,* a Resurrection people. Recall that Chesterton recounts five historical moments in which Christianity appeared to be a lost cause only to rise anew and renewed. It is good to be reminded now and then what our religious tradition says about these troublesome marvelous issues of health care in the contemporary world. *The Ethical and Religious Directives for Catholic Health Care Services* (ERDs) offer as the Christo-centric driving force in the following:

> The mystery of Christ casts light on every facet of Catholic health care; to see Christian love as the animating principle of health care; to see healing and compassion as a continuation of Christ's mission; to see suffering as a participation in the redemptive power of Christ's passion, death and resurrection; and to see death, transformed by the resurrection, as an opportunity for a final act of communion with Christ.
>
> (ERDs, Introduction)

Questions for Reflection

1. Read Luke 14:13. What does the text have to say about health care in the Catholic tradition?
2. What are some of the most important challenges to the delivery of health care? Include in the discussion economic, legal, political, medical, and ethical challenges.
3. In discussions of the delivery of health care, the question as to whether health care ought to be regarded as a right or as a commodity is often raised. Assess the proffered disjunction and offer an appropriate approach to the distribution of health care.
4. If health care is a scarce or limited resource, how, given human nature, can its limitations best be handled?
5. Return to the distinction between ordinary care and extraordinary care found in Directives 56 and 57 in Part Five, "Issues in Care for the Dying," of the *Ethical and Religious Directives for Catholic Health Care Services*. How does this distinction serve to guide the use of medical interventions?
6. Medical resources have as their primary application (a) to cure illness, (b) to assuage suffering, and (c) to compensate for disability. Assess the restrictions that ought to apply to both individuals and to the medical profession in the use of the limited resources of medicine.
7. How ought individuals and the medical profession respond to the use of the art of medicine to serve the desire for human enhancement?
8. What considerations are significant in order to put into place appropriate structures to serve the health care needs of citizens?
9. Read *Catholic Health Care Institutions: Dinosaurs Awaiting Extinction or Safe Refuge in a Culture of Death*. What significant points are made as to how Catholic health care can provide witness to the values it holds in the contemporary world?

Notes

1 If one reads *The Founding Mothers*, or considers the lives of the Founding Fathers, one is well aware of the frequency of the death of children in infancy and/or their mothers in childbirth.

2 In accordance with Catholic social teaching private property is a limited claim. It must serve the universal destination of goods. For the precise relation between private property and the universal declaration of goods see *Catechism of the Catholic Church*, 2403–2406.

3 To describe health care as a basic good is to invite debate. Health care has been designated a private good, a public good, a social good, and a requirement of the common good. It has been considered by some a positive right – a claim against others to deliver. It has been considered by still others as a negative right – a right to be protected from interference. In *Health care as a social good*.

Georgetown University Press, 2014; David Craig designates health care as a social good. Craig claims that "A good becomes a *social good* when it is valued so highly by the members of a society that they share it and pay for it together through extensive and coordinated social investment" (p. 86). The extensive investments of the citizens of the United States in health care from research to education to delivery constitute it as a social good.

4 Examinations of the principle of cooperation abound. See Kevin Flannery's *Cooperation with Evil: Thomistic Tools of Analysis* (Washington D.C.: Catholic University Press). Flannery examines the treatment of the principle of cooperation in the writing of Alphonsus Liguori and its application to contemporary issues. He suggests that there are more effective tools for that analysis in the writings of Thomas Aquinas.

5 Benedict Ashley in *Living the Truth in Love: A Biblical Introduction to Moral Theology* (p. 143) offers the following to assist in the determination of the permissibility of material cooperation.

1. One intends and does only what is morally good in the cooperative action, and disapproves and even attempts, if possible, to prevent what is evil.
2. One does not formally cooperate with the evil action of another by directly assisting it, advising it, or approving it.
3. One's material cooperation with this evil action is proportionately more remote the greater the evil of the other's action in relation to the good one hopes to achieve by the cooperation or harm that would result from noncooperation, taking also into account possible scandal, that is, the appearance of formal cooperation that might be a cause of temptation to others.

6 It is important to note that many Catholic health care programs, even when administered by a third party, are self-funded, so cooperation here would actually become an instance of direct cooperation.

7 Within the ambit of Saint John Paul II's *Theology of the Body* organ donation can be understood as a particular form of imitation of Christ's self-gift on the Cross and in the Eucharist.

8 Cherry, M. J. (2005). *Kidney for sale by owner: Human organs, transplantation, and the market.* Georgetown University Press, advocates for a market solution as a more efficient means to distribute resources including body parts.

9 In "Are brain dead individuals dead: Grounds for reasonable doubt," *Journal of Medicine and Philosophy*, 2016, *41*(3), 329–350, E. Christian Brugger argues that as long as there remains reasonable doubt that the human body has lost its capacity to holistically organize itself, there remains the obligation to treat brain dead individuals as if they are living human beings.

10 Fins, J. (2015) *Rights come to mind: Brain injury, ethics, and the struggle for consciousness.* Cambridge University Press, distinguished between individuals in a permanent vegetative state (PVS) and individuals in a minimally conscious state (MCS). The latter can display intention, attention, and memory, while the former cannot. Dr. Fins maintains that this clinical distinction directs ethical obligations and clinical responsibilities, including the possible use of deep brain stimulation (DBS) for (MCS) individuals.

11 In his 2004 Allocution on the care of patients in a persistent vegetative state, Pope John Paul II stressed the intrinsic value and personal dignity of every human being. The Pope claimed,

> no matter what the concrete circumstances of his or her life . . . the administration of water and food, even when provided by artificial means, always

> represents a natural means of preserving life, not a medical act. Its use, furthermore, should be considered, in principle, ordinary and proportionate, and as such morally obligatory, insofar as and until it is seen to have attained its proper finality, which in the present case consists in providing nourishment to the patient and alleviation of his suffering.
>
> (*Origins* 33, April 8, 2004: 737, 739–40)

In 2007, the CDF affirmed the position in the following: "A patient in a 'permanent vegetative state' is a person with fundamental human dignity and must, therefore, receive ordinary and proportionate care which includes, in principle, the administration of water and food even by artificial means" (Congregation for the Doctrine of the Faith, *Responses to Certain Questions of the United States Conference of Catholic Bishops Concerning Artificial Nutrition and Hydration* (August 1, 2007). Of course, the debate continues. See Hamel, R.'s (2007). The CDF statement on artificial nutrition and hydration: What should we make of it. *Health Care Ethics USA*, *15*(4), 5–7. See also Boyle, J.'s (2017). A catholic approach to withholding medically provided food and water. In Eberl, J. (Ed.), *Contemporary controversies in catholic bioethics* (pp. 425–441). Springer.

12 The unilateral withdrawal of life-sustaining treatment is difficult in itself. Its withdrawal under crisis conditions magnifies the difficulty. The conditions of the recent pandemic required intense scrutiny of the permissibility of withdrawal of life-saving treatment. In "Is It Ethical to Unilaterally Withdraw Life-Sustaining Treatment in Triage Circumstances" (*Journal of the Catholic Health Association of the United* States (2021) 29:1), Jason and Eberl and G. Kevin Donovan examine several policies proposed by Catholic health care institutions as they attempted to apply the principle of double effect to address the allocation of limited resources, including ventilators, in the situation of unprecedented need of the COVID-19 pandemic. Eberl and Donovan remind the decision-makers that their focus must remain on the good of the patient at hand. The overriding principle for the unilateral removal of the ventilator is its physiological futility.

10 Issues at the End of Life

The Catholic tradition understands death as a hinge moment; it is the moment of passage from mortal life to eternal life. The *Book of Wisdom* prefigures this understanding. The author of the *Wisdom* text wrote:

> But the souls of the just are in God's hands, and no torment, in death itself, has power to reach them. Dead? Fools think so; think their end loss, their leaving us, an annihilation; but all is well with them. The world see nothing but the pains they endure; they themselves have eyes only for what is immortal; so light their suffering, so great the gain they win! God, all the while, did but test them, and testing them found them worthy of him. His gold, tried in the crucible, his burnt sacrifice, graciously accepted, they do but wait for the time of their deliverance; then they will shine out, these just souls, unconquerable as the sparks that break out, now here, now there, among the stubble.
>
> (*Wisdom* 3: 1–7)

While death entered the world with sin, Christ, through his suffering and death, made eternal life with God possible for humanity. As Christ suffered too, so must humanity, but in this suffering the human spirit is tempered and the human soul is cleansed so as to be worthy of God. With death, the trajectory of the relationship from God – in creation – to God – in redemption – is complete.

The focus of this final chapter is death and care for the dying in the twenty-first century. It will progress in the following order:

(A) Observations on the progression of the human encounter with dying and death;
(B) Examination of the very modern issue of the medical determination of death;
(C) Discussion of the contemporary medical, ethical, and legal issues dealing with the end of life;

DOI: 10.4324/9781003627197-10

(D) Afterword: reflection on the Catholic understanding of death as it responds to the challenge of dying in the face of medical, ethical, and legal pressures in the contemporary culture.

(A) Observations on the Human Encounter With Dying and Death

Dying is a natural process and death is its end. Human beings are made of corruptible matter which inevitably disintegrates. It is possible to hold this disintegration in abeyance, but not forever. For most of the history of humanity, death and dying were everywhere. Men, women, and children died and there was little that anyone could do about it. Pregnancy and childbirth had high rates of mortality and morbidity for mothers and their children. Death in infancy was common. The accounts of the lives of the founding mothers, as well as the founding fathers, provide stark testimony to this sad situation. Malnourishment, disease, famine, and starvation took their toll and life expectancy reached hardly beyond a few decades. The social constructs surrounding death were simple. In the best of circumstances, people died at home surrounded by family and attended by clergy. Physicians, with their limited arsenal of tools, stepped aside.

In modern history, really only in the last 70 or so years, death has been held in abeyance by the marvelous advances of medical science. First came antibiotics, and then increasingly sophisticated technologies including ventilators, feeding tubes, and transplantation expertise made possible by immunosuppressant drugs followed, and now the possibility of tinkering with the building codes and signals of life, the genes. It is often the case that the results have been spectacular in offering renewed life to those who have suffered illness and traumatic injury. On the other hand, it is sometimes the case that there is no possible renewal of human life and treatment risks the prolongation of dying. Death, when it occurs, becomes an affair of technology and of medical specialists. It is viewed sometimes as a failure for medicine and technology. Death has been far removed from the home, family, and clergy into the hospital. In some instances, death is achieved only when the battle is called to a halt in an arena surrounded by medical personnel and machines.

Human satisfaction with this new technology and this new construct has been short-lived. The lingering and litigated deaths of Karen Ann Quinlan, Nancy Cruzan, and others – some perhaps in our own families – have caused a reappraisal of this technological construct. While it is still important to acknowledge that technology is great, it is also appropriate to acknowledge that sometimes technology does not serve the human good. Technology used to prolong dying when the downward spiraling of the dying process has been entered and when dying is imminent seems inimical to the human good. So far human history has recorded three phases in its encounter with death: (1) death is everywhere and humans are powerless in the face of its onslaught; (2) death is an enemy and the powerful tools of science and medicine can defeat it; and (3) death is inevitable and separation is painful but there are ways to understand dying and death and to mitigate its pain and suffering. This human response to dying and the transition to each of the phases have been propelled by human understanding and desires. The first phase was marked by the need and the desire for more medicine. The second phase witnessed the need and the desire for more and better medicine. The third phase is the present and what is needed in addition to the gains of medicine is not more medicine but more *than* medicine. However, there is uncertainty as to what that more is. So, the search has begun for a new construct, but in the meantime there is a vacuum. A few things have been tried; some have been successful and some have not. But whatever the construct may be, it must be set within an understanding of the occurrence of death as a physiological event.

(B) Determining Death

The determination of death used to be a simple matter, that is, the patient stopped breathing and the heart stopped beating or the heart stopped beating and the patient stopped breathing, eventually, the organs of the body including the brain, ceased functioning and cellular disintegration began. These clinical signs that a person died are designated the cardiopulmonary standard. Advances in technology changed that simple determination. In some cases, the use of machines to sustain respiration and administration of vasopressors to maintain circulation gave the illusion of life where human life was no longer possible. The continuation of the use of these machines in these circumstances seemed inappropriate. In other cases, the pressure for organs suitable for transplantation, initiated a press for a speedy declaration of death before the deterioration of the organs had begun. The success of immunosuppressant drugs to forestall rejection in organ transplantation increased the pressure of the therapeutic imperative to retrieve organs in the best possible condition. The complexity and number of patients and families confronted with both these problems, both the determination of donor death and the need for salvageable organs, reached a level that drew the attention of the medical profession.

1. *Report of the* Ad Hoc *Committee of the Harvard Medical School to Examine the Criteria of Brain Death*

To deal with both these issues of the appropriate declaration of death and transplantation, but more precisely their potential intersection with patients whose brain had suffered irreversible injury so as to be incapable of integration of the bodily functioning of the organism but whose lung and heart functions were machine dependent, Dr. Henry K. Beecher convened a committee at Harvard Medical School. In his letter of September 29, 1967 to the Standing Committee on Human Studies, Beecher identified the issue as the ethical problems created by the hopelessly unconscious individual (Beecher, 1968, p. 6). At the request of Dr. Beecher, Dr. Robert Ebert, Dean of Harvard Medical School, invited those who would constitute an *ad hoc* subcommittee to study the issue. The Committee of approximately thirty people, some from the Medical School, others from the University and from affiliated institutions, met as scheduled on October 19, 1967. In his letter of invitation, Dr. Ebert wrote:

> Dr. Beecher's presentation re-emphasized to me the necessity of giving further consideration to the definition of brain death. As you are well aware, many of the ethical problems associated with transplantation and other developing areas of medicine hinge on appropriate definition.
>
> With its pioneering interest in organ transplantation, I believe the faculty of Harvard Medical School is better equipped to elucidate this area than any other single group.
>
> (Kopp, p. 7)

Initial correspondence among the attendees continued to identify two major issues. The first is the determination and declaration of death as brain death; the second is the retrieval of organs for donation. The subsequent correspondence continued to express some concern with the perception of the relationship between the declaration of brain death and the retrieval of organs. In July 1968, Dr. Ebert wrote the following to Dr. Beecher:

> I have only one issue to raise, but I think it of some importance. I would urge the re-writing of the item 2 on page 1. At present it reads as follows: 'An issue of secondary but by no means minor importance is that with increased experience and knowledge and development in transplantation, there is a greater need for tissues and organs of, among others, the patient whose cerebrum has been hopelessly destroyed in order to restore those who are salvageable.' The connotation of this statement is unfortunate, for it suggests that you wish to redefine death in order to make viable organs more readily available to persons requiring transplants. Immediately the reader thinks how this principle might be abused. Later . . . this suspicion is allayed by the suggestion that the physicians pronouncing death should not be involved in the transplantation procedure. Nonetheless, the total impact of the whole statement has been weakened.
>
> (Kopp, p. 8)[1]

The paper that was issued from the work of the committee was titled *A Definition of Irreversible Coma: Report of the Ad Hoc Committee of the Harvard Medical School to Examine the Criteria of Brain Death* (*Report*). It was published as a special communication in the Journal of the American Medical Association (*JAMA*, Vol. 205, No. 6.) The *Report*, following the suggestion of Dr. Ebert, attended first to the suffering of the patient, "who suffered permanent loss of intellect" (*Report*, 337) and the burden on families. Only then did the *Report* turn to the recovery of organs for transplantation by noting that obsolete criteria for determination of death can cause controversy. The *Report*, in offering irreversible coma as the new criterion for death, claims that the condition is found in patients "*who have no discernible central nervous system activity*" (italics in original) (*Report*, 337) and who have no possibility regaining brain function. The *Report* delineates the clinical characteristics that must be present to confirm the condition of irreversible coma. The first three clinical measures are diagnostic and the fourth is confirmatory. The diagnostic criteria are (1) complete unreceptivity and unresponsitivity; (2) no movements or spontaneous breathing; and (3) no reflexes. The fourth measure, electroencephalogram, properly administered and monitored, is to serve as confirmatory. All the tests are to be repeated again in 24 hours before a final determination may be made by the physician. Once that final determination is made, death is declared and only then is the respirator to be turned off. At the core of this understanding of whole brain death are two notions: (1) the brain is the operator of integration for the organism as a whole and (2) consequent to the failure of the functioning of the brain both the circulatory system and respiratory system will cease to function within a limited time span. While the *Report* acknowledges the complexity of values – religious, moral, and legal – surrounding the death of any person, it clearly affirms that the assessment that the central nervous system is so damaged that it can no longer function and that there is no possibility of recovery is a medical judgment to be determined only by a physician. The *Report* says, "It is recommended as a part of these procedures that judgment of the existence of these criteria is solely a medical issue" (*Report*, 1968, p. 339).

In support of the unique role of medicine, the *Report* indicates that the law and the Catholic moral traditions both turn to medical expertise to be the determiners of the fact that death has occurred. The *Report* quotes *Black's Law Dictionary* (fourth edition, 1951) to reinforce this claim in the following:

> The cessation of life; the ceasing to exist; *defined by physicians* as a total stoppage of the circulation of the blood and the cessation of animal and vital functions consequent thereupon, such as respiration, pulsation, etc. [italics added in original].
>
> (*Report*, 1968, p. 338)

In a gesture to ethics embedded in a religious Catholic tradition as operative in supporting the unique role of medicine, the *Report* turns to the 1957 allocution, *The Prolongation of Life*, of Pope Pius XII. This allocution addressed to a gathering of physicians in response to questions addressed to the Holy Office by Dr. Bruno Haid, chief of anesthesiology at the University of Innsbruck's surgery center. Haid's questions arose in the situation in which the patient, in the hopes of eventual recovery, has been maintained on artificial respiration equipment and is now judged to be beyond recovery. In his response the Holy Father clearly indicated that "[i]t remains for the doctor, and especially the anesthesiologist, to give a clear and precise definition of 'death' and the 'moment of death' of a patient who passes away in a state of unconsciousness" (Pope Pius XII, 1957). In addition, the Holy Father maintains that the determination of the fact of death in a particular case belongs neither to the competence of the Church nor to the deduction from religious or moral principles. It is a natural law question and its answer is to be resolved by human reason as it confronts human nature. Its resolution belongs to the domain of medical practice.

In addition to the question of the proper expertise and authority, the Holy Father offered several critical observations in the described situation. These observations include the obligation to accede to and be provided with ordinary care, the informed consent of the patient, the obligation of the family or surrogate of the patient to exercise substituted judgment on behalf of the incompetent patient, the distinction between the function of the organism as a whole as distinct from continuing activity of individual organs, and appropriate response in the situation of uncertainty. The Holy Father maintained that human reason, as well as Christian morals, requires that ordinary means be taken to preserve life and health. He described ordinary means as a function of "persons, places, times, and culture . . . means that do not involve grave burden for oneself or another" (Pope Pius XII, 1957). The discussion of consent of the patient in relation to the duties of the physician implies that the informed decision of the patient directs the action of the physician in regard to any means beyond those considered ordinary. Moreover, if the patient has been rendered incompetent, the family assumes the duty of directing action according to the expressed choices of the patient. A distinction is made between the vital functions of the organism as a whole and the spontaneous function of individual organs within the organism. The functioning of the individual organs may continue for a time even in the absence of support of the organism as a single totality when the external support ceases operation. The allocution recognizes that in some cases insoluble doubt may occur. In these instances, the presumptions operative in the facts at hand are controlling. These presumptions are to be found in the medical assessment and the law as incorporating the medical judgment.

In summary, the *Report* of the *ad hoc* Committee (1) lists a set of clinical criteria for the declaration of death as a neurological event; (2) sets up a complex clinical procedure to guide that determination; (3) defends the unique role of medicine to define those procedures; and (4) creates a new and powerful concept that came to be known as brain death.

2. *Uniform Determination of Death Act*

In the 1970s, following the publication of the *Report*, many state legislatures and some courts recognized this new and additional set of clinical signs for the determination of death. The cardiopulmonary standard was joined by, and for the most part at least in the public mind, replaced by the whole brain death standard. In 1981, in order to provide a uniform standard for the determination of death the National Conference of Commissioners on Uniform State Laws approved and proposed a model state law for the determination of death. The Commissioners were joined in this effort with the cooperation of the American Medical Association, the American Bar Association, and the President's Commission for the Study of Ethical Problems in Medicine and Biomedical and Behavioral Research. The result of their work was the Uniform Determination of Death Act (UDDA). The UDDA set forth the following: an individual who has sustained either (1) "irreversible cessation of circulatory and respiratory functions," or (2) "irreversible cessation of all functions of the entire brain, including the brainstem," is dead (President's Commission, 1981). With the publication of the UDDA, the public, if not all of the medical profession, seemed to understand and accept these standards for the determination of death. The visual imagery utilized by the Commission facilitated this understanding. The imagery offered the notion that there are two possible windows for viewing the interior biological life of a person. When one window is obstructed, as is the case with the artificial maintenance of circulation and respiration, then the other window, the measure of brain activity, is used to provide the requisite view. Questions remained as to whether these were two related measures when taken together permitted the declaration of death or whether each standard stood on its own as a single determiner of the occurrence of death.

While there continues to be general consensus on the understanding of death as being in accordance with accepted medical standards, the advance of technology and the needs of sick patients sometimes press for a broadening of the criteria for the determination of death. The pressure is most acute in two distinct instances. One continues to be the need for a declaration of death for organ removal for transplantation and the other is the cessation of life-sustaining treatment, including nutrition and hydration, in patients who do not meet the criteria of whole brain death. In the presence of these practices and the experiences of physicians, new concerns arose about the adequacy and appropriateness of the brain death standard. Some argued for a less stringent standard such as higher brain death or loss of personal life as evidenced by an awareness of an historical self. Others argued for a more stringent standard including total brain death and the permanent loss of vital function. The less stringent standard might provide more organs appropriate for transplantation at the cost of less protection and less respect for the life of the patient whose organs are to be removed. The more stringent standard permits the loss of organs that might serve the good of patients needing them for the continuation of life, but more protection for the dying patient. Among the practices that raised concern was the appearance of rushing the declaration of death to ensure the viability of the organs for transplantation. Recall that the Harvard *Report* required extensive clinical diagnostic and confirmatory tests over a period of 24 hours. Among the experiences was that of the survival of patients, some for weeks or months or years, who had been diagnosed as brain dead. These challenges served as catalysts for further examination of the issue of whole brain death.

3. *President's Council on Bioethics*

The President's Council on Bioethics (PCBE), in the presence of advances in critical care medicine, the successes in organ transplantation, and the reported challenges presented by the use of the neurological criteria in determination of death at the interface of these, took up, once again, the appropriate standard for the declaration of death. In its 2008 report, *Controversies in the Determination of Death* (CDD), the PCBE clearly acknowledged that the passage from life to death is most often a process that reaches an irreversible end and the central issue is when is it appropriate to refer to this person who was alive as now someone who is dead. The long-recognized standard of irreversible cessation of circulation and respiration provides clear evidence of the occurrence of death. Hence, the PCBE considered its central question to be the adequacy of the physiological and philosophical reasons put forth to assess that a patient who has suffered total brain failure is dead. Note that the PCBE uses the term "total brain failure" rather than "brain death." Furthermore, the PCBE cautioned that philosophical concepts proposed, as important as they are, as referencing the occurrence of death must be rooted in clinical reality. This assertion of the necessity of observation of specific and measurable clinical facts in the occurrence and declaration of death led the PCBE to reject the notion that death might be considered a social or legal construct untethered to the physiology of the situation. Furthermore, the PCBE maintained that in the case of uncertainty about whether a patient is known to be dead, that patient should be considered alive. This eminently practical rule allows the question of whether a person is living or dead to be revisited, while a too quick declaration of death for the purpose of removal of salvageable life-sustaining organs, may, in itself, make the harvesting of organs the cause of death.

The PCBE recognized and explored the two opposing positions regarding the soundness of the biological justification of the whole brain death standard, that is, the irreversible loss of all brain function. Central to the objections presented by the many critics, including A.D. Shewmon, of the neurological standard is the fact that somatic integrity appears to persist even in the presence of what appears to be the loss of total brain function. Shewmon and others offered as evidence for the integration of the organism by its own internal somatic mechanism the following clinical observations:

- Homeostasis of a countless variety of mutually interacting chemicals, macromolecules, and physiological parameters, through the functions especially of liver, kidneys, cardiovascular and endocrine systems, but also of other organs and tissues (e.g., intestines, bone, and skin in calcium metabolism; and cardiac atrial natriuretic factor affecting the renal secretion of renin, which regulates blood pressure by acting on vascular smooth muscle);
- Elimination, detoxification, and recycling of cellular wastes throughout the body;
- Energy balance, involving interactions among liver, endocrine systems, muscle, and fat;
- Maintenance of body temperature (albeit at a lower-than-normal level and with the help of blankets);
- Wound healing, capacity for which is diffuse throughout the body and which involves organism-level, teleological interaction among blood cells, capillary endothelium, soft tissues, bone marrow, vasoactive peptides, clotting and clot lysing factors (maintained by the liver, vascular endothelium, and circulating leucocytes in a delicate balance of synthesis and degradation), etc.;
- Fighting of infections and foreign bodies through interactions among the immune system, lymphatics, bone marrow, and microvasculature;
- Development of a febrile response to infection;
- Cardiovascular and hormonal stress responses to unanesthetized incision for organ retrieval;
- Successful gestation of a fetus in a [brain dead] pregnant woman;
- Sexual maturation of a [brain dead] child;
- Proportional growth of a [brain dead] child over time.

(Shewmon, p. 56)

In addition to these, three other observations are presented: (1) the continuation of the inherent rhythmicity of the heart muscle, (2) the fact that in the early development of the organism, its embryonic stage, the heartbeat precedes the development and functioning of the central nervous system, and (3) uncertainty of and inability to test for the validity of predictions of survival time. Some who object to the neurological determinants claim that the presence of these observations, inasmuch as they suggest uncertainty about the status of a particular patient, requires caution about, perhaps even a staying of, the declaration of death. Nonetheless, this uncertainty does not require interventions that are either extraordinary or futile, that is, either burdensome or ineffective. These questions repeat concerns that were voiced by Hans Jonas in the earliest days following the publication of the Harvard criteria. Jonas carefully took measure of the proper question in the face of what he called "marginal ignorance" in the following:

> And here the question is not: has the patient died? But: how should he – still a patient – be dealt with? Now *this* question must be settled, surely not by a definition of death, but by a definition of man and of what life is human. That is to say, the question cannot be answered by decreeing that death has already occurred and the body is therefore in the domain of things; rather it is by holding, e.g., that it is humanly not justified – let alone demanded – to artificially prolong the life of a brainless body . . . On that philosophical ground . . . the physician can, indeed should, turn off the respirator and let the "definition of death" take care of itself by what then inevitably happens.
>
> (Jonas, 1980a, p. 138)

Those who support continuation of the neurological standard, as proposed in the Harvard criterion as confirmed by repeated clinical testing, argue that the consequence of whole brain death is the inevitable cessation of functioning of the organism as a whole. The brain is the integrator of all the vital activities of the organism. They, including Bernat, Culver, and Gert, claim that continuation, by technological support, of circulation and respiration are not signs of life but artifacts of that technical support. Removal of that support will result in loss of those functions as vital functions, including the loss of somatic integration, of this particular organism. In this view, the brain is viewed as the integrator of all bodily functions. The brain is understood as the engine which drives and maintains the persistence of the organism as a whole. That claim is clearly expressed in the following:

> This criterion [whole brain death] is perfectly correlated with the permanent cessation of functioning of the organism as a whole because

> the brain is necessary for the functioning of the organism as a whole. It integrates, generates, interrelates, and controls complex body activities. A patient on a ventilator with a totally destroyed brain is merely a group of artificially maintained subsystems since the organism as a whole has ceased to function.
>
> (Bernat, 1981, p. 391)

The PCBE found acceptable the biological justification for this neurological standard even as it found imprecision in the expression of this standard. In its report, the PCBE affirmed the 1981 Uniform Determination of Death Act. Recall that the UDDA affirmed the traditional cardiopulmonary standard of loss of heart and lung function as a sign that death has occurred and, as well, the standard of irreversible loss of all brain function including brain stem. This last, which the PCBE designated as total brain failure (CDD, p. 19) as a sign of the death of a person, is followed by the usual markers of loss of heart and lung function.

Nonetheless there were several concerns that presented to the PCBE for their scrutiny. The first was the adequacy of the reasoning to defend the whole brain death determination. The second was the matter of fact that in some cases irreversible loss of total brain function occurs while technical assistance maintains circulation and breathing. The third was the concern about the organ procurement practice of controlled donation after cardiac death (controlled DCD). The fourth was the concern about the end of life care of the patient who is now considered eligible for the donation of major organs.

The progression of their study through the examination, including the explication of the physiology of respiration and circulation, provided the PCBE the opportunity to address the multifaceted opposing sides of the neurological standard as well as other difficult issues such as the persistent vegetative state, the total temporary loss of the respiration ability, and the condition often referred to as locked-in syndrome (LIS). In regard to the first issue the adequacy of the reasoning, both physiological and philosophical, to defend the total brain failure determination of death, the PCBE attempted to develop a more precise understanding of the situation of the patient that permits referring to a human being as having died. Here they examined the integrated systems including the heart and circulatory system, the lungs and respiratory system, and the central nervous system, especially as it functions in breathing. These are the systems that support the vital functions of the organism. However, the total failure of the brain and the irreversibility of that failure will result in the subsequent failure, unless supported mechanically, of the circulatory and respiratory systems. The focus of the PCBE shifted from the concept of the brain, a single albeit complex organ, as integrator to the concept of the vital work, that is, the interrelated systems of heart and lungs and brain, of the organism in the preservation of life of the organism as a whole as it responds in and to its environment. The PCBE concluded that the cessation of these integrated functions distinguishes the dead from the living. The PCBE proposed the following:

> The work of the organism, expressed in its commerce with the surrounding world, depends on three fundamental capacities:
>
> 1. Openness to the world, that is, receptivity to stimuli and signals from the surrounding environment.
> 2. The ability to act upon the world and to obtain selectively what it needs.
> 3. The basic felt need that drives the organism to act as it must, to obtain what it needs and what its openness reveals to be available.
>
> (CDD, p. 61)

In regard to the second, that is, ventilation and circulation maintained mechanically and chemically, the PCBE affirmed the matter of fact that in some cases of irreversible loss of total brain function in which technical assistance is maintaining circulation and breathing, that assistance is medically ineffective and burdensome and, therefore, ought to be discontinued to allow the occurrence of death. These cases, however, must be distinguished from those instances in which there is brain injury, whether to the brain stem or to the higher brain, which require temporary or permanent technological assistance.

In regard to the third, the concern about the organ procurement practice of controlled donation after cardiac death (controlled DCD), the PCBE urged caution. Donation after cardiac death (DCD) is a new protocol applied when there is severe neurologic injury but the patient does not yet meet the criteria for brain death. In this procedure the technology used to support breathing and circulation is removed in a surgical environment and the transplant team awaits asystole, usually three to five minutes to remove salvageable organs. Asystole in this circumstance is considered the irreversible stoppage of the heart as capable of contributing to the life of this particular patient. The impossibility of this particular heart to contribute to this particular life does not preclude the possibility that this heart can serve life in another, healthier, organism. In its concern about the end of life care of the patient who is now considered eligible for the donation of major organs, the PCBE reiterated the essential dignity of the human person both in this patient soon to be dead and in the family members whose mourning and respect for their loved one will be interrupted by the required surgical process. To these concerns, the PCBE added its cautious support for the continuation of the organ transplant program as currently operative as a contribution to the social good.

In concluding its work, the PCBE recommended the reaffirmation of both the neurological standard and the cardiopulmonary standard for the determination of death as appropriate to the particular patient. The PCBE understood the neurological standard to encompass total brain function failure including the brain stem and they understood the pragmatic issue of accepting the neurological standard to protect the current established practices directing organ transplantation. The PCBE understood the cardiopulmonary standard to encompass the cessation of the respiratory and cardiac capacities and the irreversibility of the cessation of those functions. In addition the PCBE reaffirmed the necessity and ethical propriety of the application of the traditional legal requirement of the dead donor rule (DDR) prior to the harvesting of transplantable organs and, as well, the impermissibility of the use of patients in a permanent vegetative state as a source of transplantable organs.

As was their custom throughout their tenure (2000–2008), the PCBE appended the personal statements of members of the Council to their reports. Dr. Pellegrino, chair of the Council, added a lengthy and significant statement to the report on controversies surrounding death. While Pellegrino agreed with the Council's recommendations, he expressed some concern with the adequacy of the arguments advanced by members of the Council. His concerns focused on the following: "(1) the matter of definition, (2) the significance of the DDR, (3) the relative merits of the neurological and cardiopulmonary standard, and (4) the places of prudential reasoning and futility in remedying some of the problems with both standards" (CDD, p. 107).

In regard to the matter of "definition" of death Pellegrino distinguished between philosophical and empirical understandings of death. The philosophical, Pellegrino maintained, is conceptual as it attempts to list the negative descriptors or predicates that distinguish death from life. The empirical is substantive or realistic as it lists a set of observable properties as clinical criteria. Pellegrino maintained that any proposed philosophical conceptual definition must be rooted in these clinical criteria as referencing indisputable objective signs of death. He listed four philosophical accounts: (a) loss of somatic integration; (b) loss of capacity for engagement with the environment; (c) loss of higher brain function; and (d) loss of animation of the body by the soul, and he finds each wanting. The loss of the somatic integrative function consequent on brain death as determinant of death has been cast into doubt by concerns with this account of death that have been put forward since the emergence of the neurological criteria. The role of the brain as sole integrator has been challenged by clinical observation more likely to be considered significant than to be passed off as merely anecdotal. The notion of engagement with the environment was expanded and refined by the work of the PCBE to permit the declaration of death for those patients who suffered "loss of capacity by the apneic patient for active spontaneous engagement with the environment through the function of breathing . . . even if respiratory and cell metabolism are sustained by mechanical ventilation" (CDC, pp. 109–110). Excluded from this category of patients are those who, while maintaining cognitive function, suffer respiratory paralysis and who require significant life support. This last category includes patients who are suffering from conditions, whether permanent or temporary, such as locked in syndrome (LIS), spinal cord injuries, and poliomyelitis.

Also excluded are those patients whose higher brain functions appear to be lost and who are considered unable to relate to the human community or unable to relate to a continuous personal self. This loss of mental capacity, higher brain function, as the criterion for the determination of death proposes that a patient be declared dead when the parts of the brain which serve as the material basis for cognitive capacity such as the cerebral cortex cease functioning. This distinction would permit a declaration of death for patients whose brain stem is still operative and supporting spontaneous respiration. Declaration of death for these patients is impossible under both the neurological and the cardiopulmonary standards, and hence unethical and a violation of the prescriptive code of the medical profession. The press for the use of higher brain function criterion is fueled in part by the need for salvageable organs for transplantation and in part by a concern for the quality of life of the patient who has suffered traumatic brain injury such as to render the patient incapable of inter or intra personal life.

The final philosophical criterion, that is, the departure of the soul as the principle of animation from the body, has its source in rich and ancient philosophical and religious traditions, but provides no empirical or observable clinical facts. Pellegrino concluded that in the presence of doubt about the declaration of death, whether from the neurological standard or the cardiopulmonary standard, resort is to be made to the judgment of practical reason that follows from a sufficient degree of moral certainty. He maintained that the exercise of prudence activated by both the precautionary principle ("when in doubt, act to avoid the gravest danger" (CDD, p. 115)) and the proportionality principle ("properly balance the benefits and burdens of treatment" (CDD, p. 115)). The proportionality principle avoids the error of inaction and the loss of salvageable organs. The precautionary principle avoids the error of premature action and the consequence of death by organ removal. Together these principles can serve the good of the dying and the good of the patient in need of a life-sustaining organ.

In service of the application of these principles, Dr. Pellegrino appends his developed notion of clinical futility in the decision process in the care of the patient who is beyond medical rescue in the following:

> Clinical futility is present when any medical intervention is: (1) *ineffective*, i.e., unable to change the natural history of a disease or its trajectory towards death; (2) *non-beneficial*, i.e., unable to satisfy any good or value perceived by the patient or his or her surrogate; and (3) *disproportionately burdensome* to the patient, physically, psychologically, or financially. Balancing the relationship among those three criteria is at the heart of the prudent, precautionary, and proportionate action. This formulation accommodates the physician's expertise with respect to effectiveness, the patient's values with respect to benefits, and it results in shared decision making regarding the proportionality of benefits and burdens.
>
> (CDD, p. 116)

The assessment of futility renders further treatment inappropriate and requires its withdrawal. To continue treatment would be to harm the patient.

The complexity of issues surrounding dying and death requires the judgment of practical wisdom. Practical wisdom requires maturity and competence to judge in the particular circumstances what is the best choice. In the specific situation involving the care of the dying, both the dying patient who is beyond the curative capacity of medicine and the dying patient who needs the donation of an organ, practical wisdom strains to protect both patients. Practical wisdom is guided by an absolute rule and a set of prudential concerns. The absolute rule is the dead donor rule and it must be applied without compromise. The prudential rules require care for the dying and protection of salvageable organs. At a minimum, the prudential rules require respect of a sufficiently appropriate time of observation and deliberation in the declaration of death in the process of controlled donation after death. The allotted time should be sufficient to lean toward the life of the dying patient in the presence of doubt. Throughout this process, there must be sufficient attention to the concern for the family whose attendance of their dying relative and later dead relative has been interrupted.

(C) New Constructs for Dying and Death

In the presence of the remarkable advances of science and medicine, which have extended the temporal span of human life, dying and death remain as the process of reaching the end of natural life and the gateway to eternal life. Both are inevitable and they call forth the application of human reason to construct ways of dealing with them in a manner that respects human dignity and respects the gift of life. Among the new constructs that have been attempted to navigate the complexity of issues at the end of life are shared decision-making, physician-assisted suicide, hospice care, and palliative care.

(1) Shared Decision-Making at the End of Life

In an effort to share decision-making at the end of life, patients and physicians began conversations about appropriate care at the end of life. In order to provide some guarantee that these decisions be effective, recourse was made to the tools of the law. Conversation turned to living wills, power of attorney for health care decisions, and advance directives. The United States Congress responded to this perceived need by passage of the Patient Self-Determination Act.

In 1990, the Patient Self-Determination Act became law and the law became operative in 1991. The law allows a patient to write advance directives to guide medical care in future situations when the patient is both terminally ill and incompetent. It also allows the patient to designate a surrogate decision-maker to speak on behalf of the patient in accord with the previously articulated lived values and choices as substituted judgment when the patient is no longer competent or capable. A substituted judgment is the expression by the surrogate of the known wishes and values that the patient would have applied in the particular situation had the patient been able to express them. If the preferences and values of the patient are unknown, the surrogate is expected to make a best interest judgment, that is, an assessment of what would be the choice of a reasonable person in this situation. Further, the law requires hospitals and all health care institutions receiving Medicare and Medicaid funds to put into place procedures for recording, storing, and making available the advance directives.

This effort was lauded on many fronts. The Ethical and Religious Directives for Catholic Health Care Services that guide health care in Catholic Institutions address the issues of advance directives and surrogate decision-makers in the following:

> 24. In compliance with federal law, a Catholic health care institution will make available to patients information about their rights, under the laws of their state, to make an advance directive for their medical treatment. The institution, however, will not honor an advance directive that is contrary to Catholic teaching. If the advance directive conflicts with Catholic teaching, an explanation should be provided as to why the directive cannot be honored.

25. Each person may identify in advance a representative to make health care decisions as his or her surrogate in the event that the person loses the capacity to make health care decisions. Decisions by the designated surrogate should be faithful to Catholic moral principles and to the person's intentions and values, or if the person's intentions are unknown, to the person's best interests. In the event that an advance directive is not executed, those who are in a position to know best the patient's wishes – usually family members and loved ones – should participate in the treatment decisions for the person who has lost the capacity to make health care decisions.

Nonetheless, the Patient Self-Determination Act and its offspring, advance directives and living wills, have created as many problems as they have solved. Both have caused a great deal of confusion. In accordance with the provisions of the Patient Self-Determination Act, the expressed choices in the advance directive become operative only in the situation when the patient is both incompetent and terminally ill. Outside that limited situation, advance directives do not apply inasmuch as it is presumed that the patient is capable, even if not competent, of expressing choices in regard to level of care and inasmuch as there is a presumption that some choices are appropriate for the terminally ill patient that are not appropriate outside that situation. Furthermore, there is no guarantee that the expressed choices will be carried out or that the choices are appropriate to the contemporaneous medical condition of the patient.

The law requires that the choices be (1) consistent with the principles of the standard practice of medicine, (2) in conformity with statutory law, and (3) in conformity with the policies of the particular health care institution. The first protects the medical profession and the physician from the reduction of the practice to a set of technical skills which serves the will of the patient who, almost without exception, is untrained in the art of medicine. The second implements the *parens patriae* obligations of the state to protect the lives of its citizens. The third protects the ethical and legal commitments of the institution, especially religious institutions, providing health care. In addition, the application of the stated desires of the incompetent and terminally ill patient often requires the persistent intervention of the family of the patient. There is no guarantee that the choices of the patient will be consistent with the choices of the family. Moreover, the Patient Self-Determination Act seems to canonize the "right to choose" without asking what is chosen and what is the justification for what is chosen. It focuses on choice as controlling rather than on the obligation to choose rightly and wisely.

The limitations of advance directives, including the resistance of patients to confront their own dying and death, generated considerable dissatisfaction for families and in medical practice. The proposed remedies subsequent to this state of affairs were at polar opposites. At one pole, the writing of advance directives was considered a useless exercise marked by hubris. It was considered useless because it is impossible to know the circumstances of one's dying and death. The hubris was the result of thinking that one's life is one's own and to be disposed of as one chooses. At the other pole, the limitations of the advance directive spawned a new initiative in the form of a new instrument of choice the Physician Orders for Life Sustaining Treatment (POLST). This initiative and its paradigmatic form were the work of a task force at the Center for Ethics in Health Care at Oregon Health Sciences University. In 1991, the task force produced a pilot instrument, the Medical Treatment Coversheet. The purpose of the coversheet was to reduce and consolidate the information contained in multiple documents such as advance directives and living wills to a single page which would be prominently displayed in the chart of the patient. In 1995, the task force's POLST form was released for use in the state of Oregon. Since that time, the POLST initiative has spread to many states and has been adopted as law in a number of states. Sometimes it is designated POLST; other times it is called MOLST, Medical Orders for Life Sustaining Treatment; and in some states it utilizes the name of the state, for example, in Pennsylvania it is Pennsylvania Orders for Life Sustaining Treatment. It is claimed that the unique advantage of the POLST is that the form is distinctive; that it is simple because of its check box response form; that it is in the chart; that it is portable; and that, as physician orders, it is actionable. Additional support for the POLST paradigm can be found in federal efforts, including the *Personalize Your Care Act*, by members of the U.S. House of Representatives. This Act includes funding, under Medicare and Medicaid coverage, for consultation provided by physicians with patients for the purpose of voluntarily drafting of advance care plans and directives. In addition the Act provides grants to educational groups to facilitate the composition of POLST documents.

Generally, the POLST form has several distinct sections and there are some variations within the sections. The POLST form from the state of Pennsylvania can serve as an example. It has two major sections (A) and (B). Section (A), deals with cardiopulmonary resuscitation in the situation where a person has no pulse and is not breathing. There are two options: (A-1) CPR/attempt resuscitation and (A-2) DNAR/do not attempt resuscitation. The directive to allow natural death is generally appended to the DNAR order in Section A-2. If Section (A) does not apply, then attention is directed to Section (B). Section (B) directs allowable medical interventions for the patient who has a pulse and is breathing. The check box options here are: (B-1) comfort measures only; (B-2) limited additional interventions;

and (B-3) full treatment. In some forms Section (B-1) is accompanied by the directive that the patient prefers no hospital transfer and in other forms Section (B-1) is accompanied by the option to transfer if necessary for appropriate comfort care. The limited additional interventions Section (B-2) provides the opportunity to opt into or out of a variety of interventions including cardiac monitors, IV fluids, intubations, mechanical ventilators. Comfort care remains an integral part of Section (B-2) along with a notation to transfer to a hospital if that is appropriate but to avoid admission to intensive care if that is a possible. Section (B-3) directs full treatment which includes hospital transfer and intensive care. Additional sections, such as directives in regard to antibiotic administration and artificially administered nutrition and hydration, are found in many POLST forms. The section on the use of antibiotics includes the following options: (1) no antibiotics; use other means to relieve symptoms; (2) determine the limited use of antibiotics as medically appropriate for comfort care; and (3) use antibiotics as medically indicated if life can be prolonged. If the POLST form has a section on the administration of artificially delivered nutrition and hydration, in addition to the check-off boxes, it usually contains the caveat to always offer food and liquids by mouth if that is possible. The options offered are (1) no artificial nutrition and hydration by tube; (2) nutrition and hydration by tube for a trial period; and (3) long-term artificial administration of nutrition and hydration. Some POLST forms have small sections for summary of patient goals of care. In addition, there is generally open-ended space provided in each section for additional orders.

All forms have check-off-boxes to indicate discussion occurred with patient or with appropriate decision-maker for an incompetent or incapable patient such as parent of a minor, guardian, spouse, health care agent. The implementation of this discussion is generally the work of designated facilitators, such as social workers, admission coordinators, chaplains, administrators, who are expected to have had the requisite training. All POLST forms require the signature and dating by a physician or other clinician such as a registered nurse practitioner (ARNP) or an appropriately credentialed physician assistant (PA-C). Some POLST forms require the signature of the patient or the signature of the surrogate of the patient; others only recommend the signature of the patient or surrogate. Some POLST forms have statutory authority as having legislative approval; some do not.

The POLST initiative, as well as the Patient Self-Determination Act, represents efforts to plan rationally for the inevitability of dying and death. Neither were intended to prolong dying or to hasten death.[2] Nonetheless, there are some concerns with the implementation and use of POLST. The advance directive and living will provided for in the Patient Self-Determination Act intended that these documents be the work of thoughtful discussion between the physician and the patient and between the patient and family. The POLST document appears to be the result of an admission related conversation between the patient or the patient's surrogate and a designated facilitator. The advance directives are designed to become applicable only when the patient is both terminally ill, defined as six months or less to live, and unconscious. The POLST contains no such limitation, either as to time or condition, in its application and appears to extend the time frame for application in the form of the question of possible death of the patient within a year or even within two years. Advance directives as law and as hospital and health care institutions policies contain specific language that requires the advance directive to be in conformity with the standards of care of the medical profession, the requirements of law, and the policies of the hospital. These requirements and these protections are not part of the stand-alone POLST paradigm. The relationship between an existing advance directive and the signed POLST form has not been clarified; hence the possibility of conflict is present with no determination of how that conflict might be resolved. It may be the case that an advance directive, if there is one, needs to be attached to the POLST form and filed electronically with that form. Most POLST orders contain an initial directive which says: "**First** follow these orders. **Then** contact physician" (bold in the original). The appropriateness of following this order requires a reasonable and informed judgment that the imminent situation requires application of the particular directives contained in the POLST document.

Notwithstanding the existence and practical reasonableness of forms and opportunities to voice choices for care at the end of life, there remains a persistent set of fears as people grow older. Among them are (1) the fear of dying too soon; (2) the fear of a prolonged period of dementia before death; and (3) the fear of enduring unbearable pain in the last days of the dying process. The POLST paradigm seems to put the patient at some risk for the first when there is no certainty of the enduring choices of the patient as might have been expressed in an advance directive. It will be important for those charged with overseeing medicine and its practices to be mindful of the frequency of the withdrawal of treatment that results in death as the choice of the surrogate on the basis of the POLST directives. The central concern of the second fear is the inability of the patient to make choices, including the choice of nutrition and hydration, at the advanced stage of dementia. At an advanced stage of decline, a prudential judgment would have to be made by the clinician and surrogate as to what constitutes ordinary care for this particular patient. Among the options for care are: the delivery of nutrition and hydration through medical devices (PEG tube, nasogastric tube, IV delivery), the feeding of the patient by another, and the offering of food and drink to the patient. If the POLST form and/or the advance directive are to be effective here, these nutrition and hydration options have to be made explicit. One suggestion to overcome this ambiguity for the person prior to the onset of this severely impaired cognitive state is an additional check-off box with three options: (1) continue nutrition and hydration as long as it is beneficial to the person; (2) continue nutrition and hydration for a limited time, as specified, until a reevaluation determines whether or not it benefits the person; and (3) do not offer any assisted nutrition and hydration, but continue to offer food and water.

For Catholics and Catholic health care institutions, the Ethical and Religious Directives at 56, 57, and 58 provide moral guidance in these situations with the Catholic tradition's distinction between ordinary and extraordinary care. These directives are the following:

> 56. A person has a moral obligation to use ordinary or proportionate means of preserving his or her life. Proportionate means are those that in the judgment of the patient offer a reasonable hope of benefit and do not entail an excessive burden or impose excessive expense on the family or the community.
>
> 57. A person may forgo extraordinary or disproportionate means of preserving life. Disproportionate means are those that in the patient's judgment do not offer a reasonable hope of benefit or entail an excessive burden, or impose excessive expense on the family or the community.
>
> 58. In principle, there is an obligation to provide patients with food and water, including medically assisted nutrition and hydration for those who cannot take food orally. This obligation extends to patients in chronic and presumably irreversible conditions (e.g., the "persistent vegetative state") who can reasonably be expected to live indefinitely if given such care. Medically assisted nutrition and hydration become morally optional when they cannot reasonably be expected to prolong life or when they would be "excessively burdensome for the patient or [would] cause significant physical discomfort, for example resulting from complications in the use of the means employed." For instance, as a patient draws close to inevitable death from an underlying progressive and fatal condition, certain measures to provide nutrition and hydration may become excessively burdensome and therefore not obligatory in light of their very limited ability to prolong life or provide comfort.

Note that the application of these directives requires a prudential judgment of what serves this patient as a person at this moment; that the directives focus first on reasonable benefit to the person; and, finally, there is the consideration of burden and expense on the family and the community.

The final concern for an aging population lies in the real, even if rare, possibility of unbearable and unremitting pain in the last days of life, that is, should it be the situation that none of the analgesics normally offered at this stage provides relief for the patient. If this is the case, then the choice of sedation to unconsciousness until death, not sedation to cause death, must be an option. Here the principle of double effect is operative. This purely methodical principle rests on the common sense perception that the human agent is responsible for acts and omissions and also, to some degree, for the consequences of action. It recognizes also that in this imperfect and complicated world, an action may have more than one effect. The foreseen effects of an action may be both good and bad. The principle states the conditions under which it is permissible to engage in an act which has these two foreseen effects. The conditions are (1) the act itself must be good or indifferent; (2) the good effect is not produced by means of the bad effect; (3) only the good effect and not the bad effect is directly intended; and (4) there is a proportionate reason for placing the action and permitting the bad effect. Here the principle is applied in order to relieve pain in the dying patient.

The *Ethical and Religious Directives for Catholic Health Care Services* permit the prescription of those medications which have as the intended effect the mitigation of the pain of the patient and the bad, although not intended, effect of depressing the respiratory system or interfering with a vital function resulting in the death of the patient. If no currently available medications are capable of relieving the pain, the option of sedation to unconsciousness until death is to be made available. The good of the mitigation of the pain is permissible, even though death may be the foreseen result. The *Ethical and Religious Directives for Catholic Health Care Services* address the issue of pain relief in the following:

> 61. Patients should be kept as free of pain as possible so that they may die comfortably and with dignity, and in the place where they wish to die. Since a person has the right to prepare for his or her death while fully conscious, he or she should not be deprived of consciousness without a compelling reason. Medicines capable of alleviating or suppressing pain may be given to a dying person, even if this therapy may indirectly shorten the person's life so long as the intent is not to hasten death. Patients experiencing suffering that cannot be alleviated should be helped to appreciate the Christian understanding of redemptive suffering.

This directive recognizes that the dignity of the person requires that the patient (1) be kept free of pain; extreme pain can interfere with the person's cognitive capacity; (2) be able to prepare appropriately for death; (3) be prescribed medication to relieve pain even if the appropriate medication shortens life; (4) be rendered unconscious for the compelling reason of mitigating pain unable to be assuaged by any other medical means; and (5) be offered the opportunity to choose suffering, as did Christ, for the sake of salvation.

(2) *From Euthanasia to Physician-Assisted Suicide*

The human concern and struggle for a good and dignified death, euthanasia, is perennial. In the contemporary era, the solutions range from acceptance of the natural status of dying to suicide by one's own hand or with assistance of a third party, most often a physician. The range of euthanasia options between simply dying on one hand and various forms of killing are understood in such descriptors as active or passive and voluntary, involuntary, or nonvoluntary. The active/passive descriptors rest, respectively, on the distinction between killing and allowing death to occur. The killing of active euthanasia is direct and the agent can be self (suicide) or by another (homicide). Passive euthanasia is understood as taking no means to prevent the occurrence of death from an existing terminal pathology. The morality of passive euthanasia depends on the ordinary/extraordinary care distinction. The descriptors voluntary, involuntary, and nonvoluntary are a function of informed consent. Voluntary refers to the choice of the person as the agent of a free and informed choice. This would require that the person be situated so as to be capable of making a free and informed choice. Involuntary refers to an action that opposes the expressed free and informed decisions of the person. Nonvoluntary refers to actions for which the subject of the action is unable, either because incompetent or not capable, to form or act upon a free and informed decision. From this list of descriptors, physician-assisted suicide is to be understood as the voluntary active killing of the patient by the patient – suicide – with the assistance of the technical skills of a medical professional. The physician becomes an immediate formal and material cooperator in the act. The assistance of the physician is claimed as necessary because these skills guarantee accomplishment of the chosen end.

Recourse to suicide, even though proscribed by most religious traditions, including the Catholic tradition, and restricted by civil authorities, has been present throughout human history. And while no longer considered a criminal act, attempted suicide or serious suicidal ideation are considered an indication of mental distress and a cause for psychiatric evaluation and protective confinement in most jurisdictions in the United States. In 1997, the United States Supreme Court rulings, *Glucksberg v. Washington* and *Vacco v. Quill*, found no federal right in the U.S. Constitution to medical assistance in suicide. Nonetheless, interest in some states pushed the movement forward and in 1994 Oregon passed its *Death with Dignity Act* and implemented that act in 1997.

The philosophical arguments that have been put forth in favor of physician-assisted suicide are powerful and they are interwoven with the call for compassion. Compassion is a rich human emotion which allows us to share in the sorrow of each other and binds us in solidarity with each other as we struggle through life. But, compassion as a motive for action is only one element in the determination of the integral goodness of an act. The heart must be informed by reason and reason must examine carefully the adequacy of the motive, the object of the act, the circumstances, and the consequences. Here the object of the act is killing – the killing of the self – with the cooperation of the physician. Robert Jay Lifton's account in *The Nazi Doctors* (Lifton, p. 51ff) of compassion as the moving force for the medically encouraged and state authorized killing of handicapped children with the consent of the parents signals the danger of such killing. These were children whose lives were described as having existence but not life. Their compassionate killing marked a change in attitude for the medical profession. It was, in the words of Leo Alexander, "the small beginning" (Alexander, p. 43). The killing quickly progressed to the compassionate killing of impaired adults and eventually to the ruthless killing of 12 million – 6 million Jews and 6 million others – Poles, Priests, Jehovah Witnesses, homosexuals, political dissidents.

The debate on physician-assisted suicide is situated within a matrix framed by a set of legal, philosophical, medical, practical, and economic arguments. The legal arguments in the United States center on (a) the protection found in the liberty claim and the equality claim in the 14th Amendment to the Constitution, specifically in the due process clause and the equal protection clause, (b) on rulings found in several Supreme Court decisions, notably *Cruzan* and *Planned Parenthood v. Casey,* and (c) on common law notions of freedom from unconsented touching. The central philosophical notion is that of the exercise and limits of autonomy of all interested parties. In medicine, the major issue is the role of physicians in providing care to vulnerable patients. Within the profession itself, perturbations are caused by the nutrition/hydration debate, by the distinction between withholding and withdrawal of treatment, by the issue of pain management, by the confusion of the role of the profession, and by the fear of litigation which taints all of these medical concerns. The prohibitive cost of health care at the end of life is a legitimate pressing concern for families as well as for society.

In the debate in the United States, the legal issues, specifically liberty and equality, are similar to the issues that are central to the debate in other developed nations. However, the liberty and equality claims must be set within the limitations of the obligations of the civil authority and the commitments of the professions. Closer scrutiny of those arguments, as they are claimed to be embedded in the provisions of the 14th Amendment of the Constitution, is an appropriate starting point to examine the philosophical and legal notions which are easily expanded to the general argument. The Fourteenth Amendment was added to the Constitution in 1868, in the wake of the American Civil War, to guarantee to former slaves the rights accorded to all citizens. The two critical clauses of the 14th amendment, for purposes here are these: "nor shall any state deprive any person of life, liberty, or property, without due process of law; nor deny to any person within its jurisdiction the equal protections of the laws." The first clause under consideration has been designated the "substantive due process clause" inasmuch as there has been an attempt to render substantively the notion of liberty. What is it that citizens are at liberty to do? What, if any, are the limits on liberty? Specifically, in regard to the question of medical assistance in suicide, the question is: is the notion of liberty broad enough to encompass the assistance by physicians or other medical personnel in accomplishing suicide for a sick person. A decision of the United States Supreme Court, *Planned Parenthood v. Casey* (1992) described a particular understanding of that liberty as it applies in reproductive decisions in these terms, "the right to define one's own concept of existence, of meaning, of the universe, and of the mystery of human life" (*Casey*, 505 U.S. 833, 1992). Proponents of the right to assistance in suicide have attempted to make this the broad understanding of liberty apply in the pursuit of their goal. Is that the correct understanding of liberty and can it be extended to include the liberty to end human life? Scrutiny of the passage shows it to be so capacious as to be without limit and open to any choice. Subsequent Supreme Court decisions, *Glucksberg v. Washington* (liberty claim) and *Vacco v. Quill* (equality claim) made short work of what has now been named with considerable derision "the mystery passage." In these decisions (9–0) the Supreme Court held that the liberty that is meant in the constitution is the notion of ordered liberty, liberty that is balanced by rights and duties of others and by the rights and duties of citizens. And if there be any room for commonsense in the debate, then the observation that liberty cannot be exercised without life has meaning.

The second clause of the 14th amendment, the equal protection clause, is understood by those who argue for physician-assisted suicide in this way: since the desired end or object of the act is death, it matters not how death is accomplished. In some, death will be accomplished by the withdrawal of treatment and, in others, death will be accomplished by a lethal dose of medication. If the withdrawal of treatment is allowed so that death may follow, so too should the dispensation of lethal medication. This, they argue, is to treat the dying equally. This argument fails in an important distinction, namely, that distinction between allowing death to occur and killing. In the former, death as a natural occurrence follows from the underlying pathology or the failure of organ systems. Technology and medical interventions, which no longer serve the good of the person, are withdrawn in order to avoid the prolongation of the dying process. These technological medical interventions, which once served life, now are deemed medically inappropriate and burdensome by the profession and the family. They are ineffective; offer no benefit to the person; and may impose a burden on the person, the family, and the health care resources.

The decision to withdraw treatment, but continue care, is consistent with the ordinary/extraordinary care distinction in the Catholic tradition. Furthermore, the integral goodness of the act is preserved inasmuch as, the object as care of the patient, the intention as allowing natural death to occur, and the circumstances that is the person is dying are all good. In the latter instance of physician-assisted suicide, the patient is intentionally assisted in suicide – self-killing – by a medical professional. Moreover, the act lacks integral goodness inasmuch as the intention is to directly kill. Finally, it is a violation of the commitment of the medical profession as its role has been traditionally understood. This commitment to refrain from physicians' being agents of killing guided the medical profession in the West for centuries in the Hippocratic Oath. While the Oath has been jettisoned, the American Medical Association, at this point, rejects the participation of physicians in patient suicide. Here the medical profession, even when its powers are limited, maintains a tradition which is committed to care, to cure when possible, to cope when cure is not possible, and to care, when that is all that is possible.

Against the right to assistance in suicide by medical personnel as a liberty right and an equality claim are asserted the rights and obligations of the state. The state, in the exercise of its *parens patriae* role, articulates at least six obligations that fall within its province. These obligations are made explicit in Supreme Court decisions including, most recently, *Vacco v. Quill* and *Glucksberg v. Washington*. The obligations are (1) the preservation of life of the person, (2) the discouragement of suicide, (3) the protection of third-party interests, (4) the integrity of the medical profession, (5) protection of the vulnerable ill, including the elderly and members of minority communities, from untoward pressure of others, and (6) protection of the citizens of the nation from abuses observed in other nations. The obligation of the state to preserve the lives of its citizens is one of its fundamental duties. In fulfillment of that obligation to defend life, the state has in place a range of protections from prohibitions against killing to welfare laws to sustain life for those who cannot care for themselves. The reciprocal obligation of the citizen and of the polity, respectively, to live and to protect life is as ancient as the *Politics* of Aristotle and as new as the constitution of any emerging nation. Life is the fundamental right. Without the protection and exercise of the right to life, the exercise of any other right, liberty or property, is impossible.

The state takes seriously its role in the protection of citizens against suicide. The reason for this concern on the part of the state is that careful study of suicide, in such reports as the New State Task Force Report of 1994, revealed suicide attempts to be an act of desperation most often committed by people (95%) who are suffering from treatable clinical depression. The Task Force, having come to the realization that suicide is most often not a rational act, reached the unanimous conclusion that suicide should not be made legal and that medical professionals ought not be permitted to facilitate the act. Now it is true that suicide was decriminalized in most jurisdictions in the United States in 1970. Nonetheless, the decriminalization of suicide was not meant to and does not legalize the act of suicide. Recognition of the illness of the person committing suicide, the extravagance of decreeing criminal penalties for a sick person who committed suicide, and concern for the consolation of grieving family members moved the law to decriminalize suicide. The expectation that attended the decriminalization was that the medical community, along with the cooperation of families and appropriate social and religious agencies, would find medical, familial, social, and religious interventions to care for depressed or mentally ill patients to protect them from the harm of suicide.

Third-party interests to be protected by the state include the interests of children or spouses who might be financially or emotionally dependent on the person contemplating suicide. Third-party pressures on a sick person contemplating suicide may be the pressure of family members to balance needs and interests such as care of the sick family member versus the education of a child, the pressure of poverty, the pressure of dependence including the stigma of loss of function, the pressure of being a member of a minority, the pressure of being a woman, the pressure of an insurance carrier who denies treatment coverage, and the pressure experienced by the authority of a medical professional whose suggestion that life be ended is perceived by the patient as a prescription. Inasmuch as these pressures interfere with the exercise of informed consent by inhibiting freedom, the state prudentially expresses a concern about these potential constraints.

The concern of the state for the integrity of the medical profession is an important state interest. The medical profession has had in its origin and continues to have in its commitment service to the life and health of patients. Affirmation of this dedication is clearly articulated in the AMA Code of Medical Ethics (A-02 Edition) which says, "[p]hysician-assisted suicide is fundamentally incompatible with the physician's role as healer, would be difficult or impossible to control, and would pose serious societal risk."

In these 1997 U.S. Supreme Court decisions, *Glucksberg v. Washington* and *Vacco v. Quill*, the Court also expressed concern about its observations of the experiences in Europe, especially the Netherlands, with euthanasia and physician-assisted suicide. An account follows of the Dutch experience, along with the experience of the state of Oregon, which legalized physician-assisted suicide in 1994 and implemented the practice in 1997.

(a) The Netherlands Experience

The observation of practices surrounding death and dying in other nations and polities can be instructive for nations considering the adoption of the new practices. The Netherlands may serve as a case study of the practice of active euthanasia and assisted suicide by physicians. The practice of euthanasia and physician-assisted suicide has had general acceptance in the Netherlands, despite the fact that both practices were forbidden by law until very recently. This was the progression. In 1981, the Royal Dutch Medical Association, despite the fact that both euthanasia (Article 293) and physician-assisted suicide (Article 294) were illegal, issued a set of guidelines for these practices. Physicians who followed the guidelines are required to report participation in these practices and have been promised immunity from prosecution. The guidelines require four conditions be met before euthanasia be performed. They are (1) the patient must be a mentally competent adult; (2) the patient must request euthanasia voluntarily, consistently, and repeatedly over a reasonable time and the request must be documented; (3) the patient must be suffering intolerably, with no prospect of relief, although the disease need not be terminal; and (4) the doctor must consult with another physician not involved in the case. (The combination of the possibility of making a voluntary informed decision and of being in the condition of suffering intolerable pain presents a problem.)

The bioethical world watched the experiment in the Netherlands. Many bioethicists thought that because of the unique nature of the homogeneous society and culture of the Netherlands, the country might serve as a model for the successful implementation of the medically assisted delivery of death. That assessment changed with the publication of the Remmelink Report. Professor Jan Remmelink, former Attorney-General of the High Council of the Netherlands, was appointed to head a commission to investigate the medical practice of euthanasia. The Remmelink Report presented these data: in 1990, there were 2300 deaths (1.9%) caused by voluntary euthanasia and in 1995, there were 3100 deaths (2.3%) deaths caused by voluntary euthanasia; in 1990, there were 400 deaths (0.3%) by way of physician-assisted suicide and in 1995, there were 540 deaths (0.4%) by way of physician-assisted suicide; in 1990, there were 1000 deaths (0.8%) from nonvoluntary euthanasia and in 1995, there were 945 deaths (0.7%) resulting from nonvoluntary euthanasia. The deaths from nonvoluntary euthanasia are startling as is the incremental growth in deaths resulting from voluntary euthanasia and from physician-assisted suicide. Furthermore, with the passage of time, the categories for permissible euthanasia have been expanded. In 1994, suffering was expanded to include unbearable mental suffering. In 2000, the *New England Journal of Medicine* reported significant clinical problems with the completion experience of euthanasia and assisted suicide in the Netherlands (Groenewoud, pp. 551–56). These problems occurred in 7% of the cases of assisted suicide and 16% of the cases of euthanasia. Some of the attempts at assisted suicide became cases of euthanasia because of complications with completion and some of the euthanasia attempts experienced problems of longer than expected time of death, failure to induce coma, or the awakening of the patient after coma induction.

In 2001, the practices of euthanasia and physician-assisted suicide were made legal in the Netherlands. The legalization of both occasioned a widening of eligibility, both in the age requirement and the condition requirement, for these practices. To the condition of terminal illness "tiredness of living" has been added as a sufficient reason. Another significant addition in the new law is its expansion of euthanasia and physician-assisted suicide to minors between the ages of 12 and 16 with the consent of parents. Since 2007, the Netherlands has reported significant increases in both numbers and categories. The increments in numbers and the categories suggest the occurrence of the downward slide on a slippery slope. In 2012, the group *Right to Die Netherlands* developed a mobile clinic with twenty-three doctor/nurse teams to deliver its services.

A further expansion of the euthanasia movement in the Netherlands can be seen in the Groningen Protocol of 2005. The Groningen Protocol applies the practice of euthanasia to newborns, and by logic if not by law, to children under the age of 12. The protocol was ratified by the Dutch Pediatric Society. The requirements are similar to those, although absent informed consent, applied to adults. They include: the hopelessness of the condition, the presence of unbearable suffering, poor expected quality of life, the consent of the parents, appropriate medical consultation, careful execution of the termination, and the reporting to the office of the medical examiner who sends the report to a regional review committee. If the regional review committee, composed of a doctor, a lawyer, and an ethicist, should judge that the termination was improperly done, the review committee would be required to alert the district attorney. Physicians who support the Groningen Protocol in the Netherlands report that the numbers of children euthanized are declining because of wider acceptance of prenatal screening and abortion.

(b) The Oregon Experience

The state is exercising due diligence in the performance of its *parens patriae* role when it factors into its deliberations its obligations to protect its citizens in the light of these worrisome observations of practices in the Netherlands. Despite the concerns expressed by the U.S. Supreme Court in *Glucksberg v. Washington* and *Vacco v. Quill*; despite the findings of the

New York Task Force in *When Death Is Sought*: and despite the widespread publication of the results of the experiment in the Netherlands there was considerable pressure exerted in some states to legalize physician-assisted suicide. In 1994 Oregon, by way of public referendum, passed its *Death with Dignity Act* (DWDA). Following Court challenges and a second referendum in 1997 Oregon implemented the Act. Since 1997 medical assistance in suicide has become law in Washington (2008), Vermont (2013), California (2015), Colorado (2016), Hawai'i (2018), New Jersey (2019), and Maine (2019). In 2009, physician-assisted suicide was recognized in Montana by Court decision as not being illegal inasmuch as there are no laws in the state which forbid the practice.

Oregon's DWDA Act allows terminally ill adult Oregonians to obtain and use prescriptions from their physicians for self-administered, lethal doses of medications. The State of Oregon has declared that ending one's life in accordance with the DWDA law does not constitute suicide. The requirements for eligibility for the procedure, which begins with requesting a prescription for a lethal medication, in Oregon are: a patient must be an adult (18 years of age or older); a resident of Oregon; competent or capable – defined as able to make and communicate health care decisions; and have been diagnosed with a terminal illness that will lead to death within six months. The procedure as set out in the law is the following: (1) the patient must make two oral requests to his or her physician, separated by at least 15 days; (2) the patient must provide a written request to his or her physician, signed in the presence of two witnesses; (3) the prescribing physician and a consulting physician must confirm the diagnosis and prognosis; (4) the prescribing physician and a consulting physician must determine whether the patient is capable; (5) if either physician believes the patient's judgment is impaired by a psychiatric or psychological disorder, the patient must be referred for a psychological examination[3]; (6) the prescribing physician must inform the patient of feasible alternatives to DWDA, including comfort care, hospice care, and pain control; and (7) the prescribing physician must request, but may not require, the patient to notify his or her next-of-kin of the prescription request. No physician is required to take part in the process. In 2023, the Oregon Legislative Assembly passes House Bill 2279, which removed the residential requirement for patients seeking the assistance of physicians to accomplish their suicide.

The data presented here are from the January 2024 report on the Oregon Public Health Division site. The charts show the progression of participation in the DWDA from its inception in 1998 until the end of 2023 (https://www.oregon.gov/oha). Oregon reports that since the law passed, 4274 people have had prescriptions written under the Death with Dignity Act. To date, 2847 patients died from ingesting the prescribed medications. The chart here lists recipients of DWDA prescriptions; DWDA deaths; and attending physicians (2018–2023).

Year	*Prescription Recipients*	*DWDA Deaths*	*Attending Physicians*
1998	24	16	n/a
1999	33	27	n/a
2000	39	27	22
2001	44	21	33
2002	58	38	33
2003	68	42	42
2004	60	37	40
2005	65	38	40
2006	65	46	41
2007	85	49	46
2008	88	60	60
2009	95	59	64
2010	97	65	59
2011	114	71	62
2012	116	85	62
2013	121	73	62
2014	155	105	83
2015	218	135	106
2016	204	139	101
2017	218	158	92
2018	261	178	108
2019	296	193	113
2020	373	259	142
2021	384	255	132
2022	433	304	145
2023	560	367	167
TOTAL	4,274	2,847	

Figure 10.1 Oregon Death With Dignity Act: Prescription Recipients, Deaths, Attending Physicians

From the inception of Oregon's DWDA in 1998 to 2023, there has been a marked increase in the number of prescriptions written (from 24 to 560) in and the number of deaths by assisted suicide (from 16 to 367). In 2019, just one patient requesting lethal prescriptions was referred for psychiatric evaluation. In 2023, three patients requesting lethal prescriptions were referred for psychiatric evaluation. The end of life concerns as expressed by the patient in order of frequency were: loss of autonomy (91.6%); less able to engage in activities making life enjoyable (88.3%); loss of dignity (63.8%); losing control of bodily functions (46.6%); burden on family and friends (43.3%); concern about or inadequate pain control (34.3%);

financial implications (8.2%). Most of the underlying illnesses (65.9%) were forms of cancer. Other illnesses reported included heart disease (10.1%); chronic respiratory disease (6.8%); and amyotrophic lateral sclerosis (5.7%). In the 2023, Report 56.4% of patients were male and 43.6% were female. This is a slight shift from 2019, which reported that 50% were male and 50% were female. There was an increase in the number of patients enrolled in Medicare, Medicaid and other governmental programs from 56.7% on average from 1998–2021 to 80.1% in 2022 to 78% in 2023 with a corresponding decrease in the numbers of those enrolled in private insurance from 42.3% on average from 1998–2021 to 19.9% in 2022 to 22% in 2023. The Oregon Health Authority reported that during 2023, the rate of deaths under the auspices of the Death with Dignity Act was 0.8% of total deaths in the State. A total of 167 physicians participated in the writing of prescriptions in 2023. The approximate number of physicians practicing in Oregon in 2023 was 6,700. The physicians participating in DWDA represent approximately 2.5% of practicing physicians. At least one physician wrote 76 prescriptions. The attending physician, that is the prescribing physician, was present at time of death in 44 cases (12%) in that same year. Approximately half (51%) of the physicians involved in physician-assisted suicide in Oregon practice in the Portland Metro area.

Since its inception in 1997, there have been concerns with the implementation, regulation, and oversight of the DWDA. The law, described by the Oregon Health Authority as a permissive law, does not include any oversight or regulation that is distinct from any other kind of medical care. The implementation of DWDA is determined on an individual basis by qualified patients and licensed physicians. The attending physician determines if the patient meets the criteria, including the residency criterion, set forth in the act. There is no minimum residency requirement; the attending physician determines if residency has been established. In January 2020, a revision to the waiting period in the application of DWDA became effective. This change exempted patients from the waiting periods – 15 days between the first and second oral requests for the DWDA medication and 48 hours from the time of the patient's written request for the DWDA medication and the writing of the prescription – if their life expectancy was determined as less than the waiting period.

The Oregon Health Authority has the responsibility of recording the data on participation and issuing an annual report. On its site, the OHA claims that it "does not investigate whether patients met the DWDA criteria, nor how their diagnosis, prognosis, and treatment options were determined." While participating patients are reported to the Oregon Health Authority by name, the law guarantees the confidentiality of all participating patients. The identity of individual patients is not recorded in any manner. The collection of names by the State permits verification by cross-checking the death certificates. The OHA recommends that physicians record as the cause of death the underlying medical pathology and that they designate the manner of death as natural.[4] The confidentiality of participating physicians is protected by encoding their names. All source documentation is destroyed, approximately one year, after the release of Annual Report.

Physician-assisted suicide represents a stage in the Promethean myth of modern curative medicine that offers the promise of human salvation – the deliverance from suffering – in more and better medicine. In 1979, Dr. André Hellegers, just before his own death, warned about the inevitable consequences of the displacement of the Catholic traditional caring task of medicine by the curing goal. Hellegers said,

> As the caring branches of medicine were gradually pushed aside by the curing ones, there seemed to be less use for the Christian virtues. I think that shortly the need of those old Christian virtues will return and once again be at a premium.
>
> Our patients will need a helping hand and not a helping knife. . . . We must either recapture the Christian virtues of care or we shall be screaming to be induced into death to reach the discomfort free society. (Hellegers, p. 101)

If suicide, physician-assisted suicide, and euthanasia understood as killing the vulnerable are judged irrational, unethical and dangerous and if the prolongation of the dying process by technological interventions is judged unethical, how then ought the dying be cared for until death be accomplished? To respond to this real need, two significant movements have emerged in the field of care of the dying. The first is the hospice movement and the second is the palliative care movement as an out-growth of the hospice movement.

(3) *The Hospice Movement and Palliative Care*

Hospice as a modern movement in medical care originated with the work of Cicely Saunders, nurse, social worker, physician, researcher, entrepreneur, Dame of the Order of Saint Gregory the Great, Dame of the British Empire, and winner of the prestigious Templeton Prize in Religion. Her work, beginning in 1963, at Saint Joseph Hospice in London, sparked her interest in pain relief for those with terminal illnesses. Her complex background and training provided her with insights about the pain that terminally ill patients experienced. She developed the notion of total pain which encompasses physical suffering, mental distress, emotional difficulties, and as well, social and familial problems. She saw the necessity of putting multidisciplinary teams in place to address this total pain. In 1967, she had sufficient resources to establish Saint Christopher's Hospice. In 1987, the Royal College of Physicians acknowledged palliative care as a medical specialty. In 2010, the Cicely Saunders Institute was established at King's College London. It provides a complete multi-professional environment for researchers, practitioners, teachers, and patient care.

The catalyst for the hospice movement in the United States was supplied by Florence Wald, former Dean of the Nursing School at Yale, who started the first American hospice unit. She was inspired by the work described by Dame Saunders's lecture in 1963 at Yale. Wald invited Saunders to come to Yale as visiting faculty in 1965. In 1968 Wald resigned her position as Dean and went to London to observe the practices at Saint Christopher's Hospice. She returned to the United States to form an interdisciplinary team of doctors, clergy, and nurses to study the needs of and to care for dying patients. She and her team founded the first hospice in Branford, Connecticut which provided in-home care for the dying. By 1980, the hospice at Branford provided inpatient as well as home care for the dying. In 1982, the United States Congress required Medicare to pay for hospice care. In 2006, the American Board of Medical Specialties recognized hospice and palliative care as a medical specialty.

As did Saunders, Wald's concern was the amelioration of the pain of terminally ill patients so that their final days might be spent preparing for death in a dignified way. The apothegm of the hospice movement, do nothing which hastens death and do nothing which prolongs dying, has its origin in the oft repeated quote of Dame Saunders, *You matter because you are you, and you matter to the end of your life. We will do all we can not only to help you die peacefully, but also to live until you die.* At its best, the hospice movement offers care, comfort care, and company to the dying. The problem with the hospice movement is that it takes time and enduring care, which require patience and commitment, and we are not a patient people.

The growth of the Hospice Movement prompted the development and expansion of palliative care medicine. The central focus of the palliative care approach is directed at improving the quality of life for patients and their families facing the problems associated, not only with dying, but with persistent pain that often accompanies life-threatening, serious or chronic illness. The palliative care movement recognizes that physical pain is one part of the suffering endured by those suffering life-threatening illness and by those facing terminal illness. A multidisciplinary palliative care team, comprised of physicians, nurses, pharmacists, social workers, chaplains, physical therapists, occupational therapists, and the family, focuses on symptoms such as nausea, depression, and pain, as well as, emotional, psychological, and spiritual distress. Palliative care itself is not directed at cure. At its farthest extreme palliative care may include palliative sedation, deep continuous sedation, in its treatment arsenal. Palliative sedation is to be distinguished from euthanasia which directly intends the death of the patient. Palliative sedation intends the amelioration of the pain of the patient even as it acknowledges the possibility of the shortening of the life of the patient as an indirect and unintentional effect of the sedation. This is an appropriate application of the principle of double effect. Since its inception as a hospital based palliative care consult service in 1985 at Wayne State University, the palliative medicine movement has expanded throughout the United States both as a comprehensive integrated medical program within hospitals and as independent specialty teams. In 2006, palliative care became a board certified subspecialty of internal medicine. In 2011 JACO, the Joint Commission that accredits and certifies health care programs, initiated an Advanced Certification Program for Palliative Care that recognizes hospital inpatient palliative care programs. To obtain this certification, a hospital must show superior patient and family centered care and enhancement of the quality of life for patients with serious illness.

(D) Afterword – Reflection on the Catholic Understanding of Death

In the face of these contemporary challenges, Catholics are called upon to witness their beliefs in their living and dying and to express their beliefs, as a contribution to the common good, in the public square. Dying is natural and death is its end. But, death is not the ultimate end of for human life; it is a passage. Hence, death is not the ultimate evil. Human life is a gift, albeit a finite gift, to each individual. It is to be lived as a particular gift with hope sustained by faith that surely holds that our end lies in eternal and joyful union with God. So life is to be held and lived as a gift with all its particularities and commitments. The death of any person is the death and the loss of a unique person whose life touched countless others. So death is to be experienced as pain both by the dying and by those who remain. In the pain there is something that can unite us with Christ, and something to be offered to God as a sharing in the pain of Christ. Pain is not only something to be avoided; it is also something that can be offered. It is right for human beings to mourn death and the losses that are brought on by death. Professor Gil Meilaender suggests that dying and death are to be approached as neither the greatest evil nor the ultimate good. Meilaender reminds us that, "even in the most dignified of deaths, we need to recognize the presence of a hostile power, the 'last enemy' from which Jesus himself shrank, a power that cannot be overcome simply by dying" (Meilaender, p. 6). Death is not the ultimate good. C.S. Lewis in *Miracles* suggests the appropriate manner for the Christian to countenance death. Lewis wrote this about differing attitudes toward death:

> One is the lofty view, which reached its greater intensity among the Stoics, that Death "doesn't matter," that is "kind nature's signal for retreat," and that we ought to regard it with indifference. The other is the " natural point of view . . . that Death is the greatest of evils . . . . The first idea simply negates, the second simply affirms, our instinct for self-preservation; neither throws any new light on Nature, and Christianity countenances neither. Its doctrine is subtler. On the one hand Death is the triumph of Satan, the punishment of the Fall, and the last enemy. . . On the other hand, only he who loses his life will save it. We are baptized into the *death* of Christ, and it is the remedy for the Fall. Death is . . . the thing Christ came to conquer and the means by which he conquered.
>
> (C.S. Lewis, pp. 129–130)

To walk that fine line requires that there may be no direct killing either by others or by oneself, no assistance in suicide and, at the same time, no prolongation of dying. To do either rejects the gift of human life as created life. The exact and powerful conceptual tools of the Catholic tradition, such as the distinction of ordinary care and extraordinary care and the principle of double effect, assist clear understanding and appropriate care. Catholics ought to know these principles because they should have been taught these principles. They must be applied with resolute firmness. The goodness of life and the goodness and sorrow attending its earthly end must be affirmed. It is, perhaps, in dying that the experience, finally, of human nature as created and radically dependent is affirmed. We need to acknowledge our finitude and affirm that death is not our end. We shall die and we need to prepare for death. This preparation for death is a lifelong project. It is both appropriate and prudential to use the God given gift of reason to prepare for death. Part of this preparation includes discussion with family members and with care givers of what might constitute appropriate treatment at the end of life. It is an act of love to have this discussion and concretize this discussion in a document to be action-guiding at the difficult time when death is at hand. Catholics ought to live and die in such as way as to model the belief that Jesus took on our human nature to show the path to God. Jesus healed but he also suffered and died. In His suffering and dying, Jesus, from the depths of His humanity, called out for consolation. In Gethsemane, He asked to be rescued, "My Father . . . take this cup of suffering from me." He revealed to His friends His grief and anguish. He said, "The sorrow in my heart is so great that it almost crushes me."

He asked them to stay with Him and He is sorely disappointed by their failure to remain with Him. He experienced abandonment and, close to the end, He cried out to His heavenly Father, "*Eli, Eli, lema sabachthani.*" And, at last, He placed Himself into His Father's care. Jesus experienced sadness in his dying and we shall experience sadness in our own dying. Those who love us will experience sadness and loss in the knowledge of our dying, just as the disciples experienced sadness in the dying of the Christ. We should not abandon each other in this. The dying have much to teach the living as they patiently endure dependence and care. And the living may learn to become truly compassionate when they attend as caring people – to touch, to wash, to anoint, and to be present to the dying.

Fr. Richard McCormick, eminent Catholic moral theologian who died in 2000, sketched out a careful path for us. In his words and in his living to the very end, he reminded us frequently that dependency, whether from age or illness, is a call to cling to the power of God. He, when speaking of physician-assisted suicide as an act of isolation and abandonment said, "[r]ejection of our dependence means ultimately rejection of our interdependence and eventually of our very mortality" (McCormick, 1991, p. 1133). And when he addressed the issue of cessation of no longer beneficial nutrition and hydration, he reminded us that we, as a people who say we believe in life after death, ought to act as if we actually believe that (McCormick, 1992, p. 214). He warned us too that failure to attend these distinctions and failure to use the intellectual tools and concepts of the Catholic tradition might force the holders of the Catholic tradition to flee it.

Finally, we ought to recall the words of Jesus:

> Do not let your hearts be troubled. You have faith in God; have faith also in me. In my Father's house there are many dwelling places. If there were not, would I have told you that I am going to prepare a place for you? And if I go and prepare a place for you, I will come back again and take you to myself, so that where I am you also may be. Where I am going you know the way. . . I am the way and the truth and the life. No one comes to the Father except through me.
>
> (*John* 14: 1–6)

Questions for Reflection

1. Review the transitions in the approaches to dying and death in the modern era and the shifting human assessment of the gains and losses found in the transitions. What light do those traditions shed on your approach to your own dying and death and the dying and death of those you love. Where do you find yourself saying: "I wish we could go back to that." Where do you find yourself saying: "I wish we could

move on from that." Where do you find yourself saying: "Isn't there something else?"

2. Why is it important to be precise about (a) the definition of death and (b) the criteria that mark the transition from life to death? What problems have you encountered in areas of medicine, law, theology, or philosophy from imprecise definitions or inadequate criteria?
3. In the search for a new construct to enable human beings to deal with dying and death, the Patient Self-Determination Act became law.

   a. What are its advantages and disadvantages?
   b. Does it overemphasize, underemphasize, or fail to consider any key factors?
   c. What are the key principles in your own construct for dealing with dying and death?

4. Physician-Assisted Suicide has been suggested as an appropriate remedy to the restraining of death. Develop and evaluate the set of arguments that have been brought forth in its defense. Be certain to include the following:

   a. Legal arguments
   b. Philosophical arguments
   c. Medical arguments
   d. Practical arguments
   e. Economic arguments

5. Against the right to assistance in suicide by medical personnel as a liberty right, there are asserted rights and obligations of the state – the *parens patriae* obligations of the state. What do the experiences in the Netherlands and Oregon tell about the relationship between good intentions and public policy in a fallen wowrld? How might those experiences shape the discussions about *parens patriae* obligations in the U.S.A.?
6. Read the Introduction and Directives 55–66 in Part Five, "Issues in Care for the Dying," of the *Ethical and Religious Directives for Catholic Health Care Services*. Are the guidelines helpful in assisting health care practitioners in the care of the dying?
7. What role has the hospice movement played in the search for a new approach to dying and death? What issues still need to be addressed?
8. How should a Christian prepare for death? What is a good death?
9. What obligations do Christians owe the dying?
10. Write your obituary; plan your funeral.

Notes

1 In *Death before dying*. OUP, 2014, Gary Belkin addresses two persistent charges against the work of Dr. Beecher and the Committee. The first charge was that the Committee operated from a strong disposition to declare death for the sake of transplantation. The second was that the Committee did not have empirical evidence for its recommendations. To the first, Belkin maintains that the concern of the Committee was how to move from care to experimentation. To the second, Belkin presents the data of the ten years of clinical experience of the physicians caring for 421 patients at Massachusetts General Hospital.

2 Despite the original intentions of the Patient Self-determination Act and POLST, both seem to lead to the pressure for the physician-assisted suicide, now named medical assistance in dying. The Catholic tradition attempts to distinguish acts that prolong dying and acts that alleviate pain and have the unintended effect of hastening death, and acts that intend and effect death.

3 This would seem to require that one of the physicians be a psychiatrist.

4 Is this a matter of the falsification of medical records?

Bibliography

Alexander, L. (1949). Medical science under dictatorship. *The New England Journal of Medicine*, *241*(2).

American College of Pediatricians. (2017). Gender dysphoria in children. *Statement*. acpeds.org

American Medical Association. (2021a). *AMA principles of medical ethics*. https://www.ama-assn.org/about/publications-newsletters/ama-principles-medical-ethics

American Medical Association. (2021b). *Code of medical ethics opinion 1.1.3*. https://www.ama-assn.org/delivering-care/ethics/patient-rights

American Medical Association. *Medical-futility in end-of life care* (Issued June 1997, based on the report adopted Chicago: December 1996).

American Psychiatric Association. (2013). *Diagnostic and statistical manual of mental disorders* (5th ed.; DSM-5). American Psychiatric Publishing.

American Society of Human Genetics and American College of Medical Genetics. (1995). Points to consider: Ethical, legal, and psychosocial implications of genetic testing in children and adolescents. *American Journal of Human Genetics*, *57*, 1233–1241.

Anderson, J. A., & Kimmelman, J. (2014). Are phase 1 trials therapeutic? Risk, ethics, and division of labor. *Bioethics*, *28*(3), 138–146.

Anscombe, G. E. M. (1981). Mr. Truman's degree. In *The collected philosophical papers of G. E. M. Anscombe* (Vol. III, Ethics, Religion and Politics, pp. 62–71). Blackwell.

Aquinas, T. (1944). Summa theologiae. In A. C. Pegis (Ed.), *Basic writings of St. Thomas Aquinas*. Random House.

Aristotle. (1941a). *Nicomachean ethics. The basic works of Aristotle* (R. McKeon, Ed.). Random House, Inc.

Aristotle. (1941b). *Politics. The basic works of Aristotle* (R. McKeon, Ed.). Random House, Inc.

Aronoff, J. B. (2014). The constitutionality of asexualization legislation in the United States. *St. John's Law Review*, *1*(2), Article 3.

Ashley, O.P., B. M. (1996). *Living the truth in love: A biblical introduction to moral theology*. Fathers and Brothers of the Society of Saint Paul.

Augustine. (1955). The good of marriage. In R. J. Deferrari (Ed.) & Wilcox, M.M., C. T. (Trans.), *Writings of Saint Augustine*. Fathers of the Church.

Baltimore, D., Berg, P., Botchan, M., Carroll, D., Alta Charo, R., Church, G., Corn, J. E., Daley, G. Q., Doudna, J. A., Fenner, M., Greely, H. T., Jinek, M., Steven Martin, G., Penhoet, E., Puck, J., Sternberg, S. H., Weissman, J. S., & Yamamoto,

K. R. (2015). A prudent path forward for genomic engineering and germline gene modification. *Science*, *348*(6230), 36–38.
Barré, J-L. (2005). *Jacques and Raïssa Maritain: Beggars for heaven*. University of Notre Dame Press.
Beecher, H. K. (1968). A definition of irreversible coma: Report of the Ad Hoc committee of Harvard Medical School to examine the definition of brain death. *Journal of the American Medical Association*, *205*(6).
Benedict XVI. (2007, November 30). *Spe salvi* [Saved in hope]. Libreria Editrice Vaticana.
Benedict XVI. (2009, June 29). *Caritas in veritate* [Charity in truth]. http://www.vatican.va/holy_father/benedict_xvi/encyclicals/documents/hf_ben-xvi_enc_20090629_caritas-in-veritate_en.html
Bernat, J. L., Culver, C. M., & Gert, B. (1981). On the definition and criterion of death. *Annals of Internal Medicine*, *94*(3).
Blackless, M., Charuvastra, A., Derryck, A., Fausto-Sterling, A., Lauzanne, K., & Lee, E. (2000). How sexually dimorphic are we? Review and synthesis. *American Journal of Human Biology*, *12*(2), 151–166.
Boyle, J. (2017). A catholic approach to withholding medically provided food and water. In J. Eberl (Ed.), *Contemporary controversies in catholic bioethics* (pp. 425–441). Springer.
Brandt, A. M. (1978, December). Racism and research: The case of the Tuskegee Syphilis study. *Hastings Center Report*, *8*(6), 21–29.
Brugger, E. C. (2016). Are brain dead individuals dead: Grounds for reasonable doubt. *Journal of Medicine and Philosophy*, *41*(3), 329–350.
Buck v. Bell, 274 U.S. 200, (1927).
Burwell v. Hobby Lobby, 573 U.S. 682 (2014).
Byrn v. New York City Health and Hospitals Corp., 31 N.Y. 2d 194, 286 N.E. 2d (1973).
Callahan, D. (1970). *Abortion: Law, choice, and morality*. Macmillan Publishing Co.
Carlson, B. M. (1988). *Patten's foundations of embryology*. McGraw-Hill Publishing Company.
Carlson, J. W. (1989). *Donum vitae* on homologous interventions. *Journal of Medicine and Philosophy*, *14*(5), 523–540.
Carmichael, L. (1970). Onset and early development of behavior. In P. H. Mussen (Ed.), *Carmichael's manual of child psychology* (Vol. I, 3rd ed.). John Wiley and Sons, Inc.
Catholic Church. (2012). *Catechism of the Catholic Church* (2nd ed.). Libreria Editrice Vaticana.
Cavanaugh, T. A. (2006). *Double effect reasoning: Doing good and avoiding evil*. Oxford University Press.
Cavanaugh, T. A. (2018). *Hippocrates' oath and Asclepius' snake*. Oxford University Press.
Center for Disease Control. (n.d.). https://mchb.hrsa.gov/chusa14/health-status-behaviors/infants/preterm-birth-low-birth.html
Center for Disease Control. cdc.gov/nchs/fastats/infertility.htm
Cherry, M. J. (2005). *Kidney for sale by owner: Human organs, transplantation, and the market*. Georgetown University Press.
Cohen, A. (2016). *Imbeciles: The Supreme Court, American eugenics, and the sterilization of Carrie Buck*. Penguin Press.
Committee on Assessing Genetic Risks, Institute of Medicine. (1994). *Assessing genetic risks: Implications for health and social policy* (Eds., L. B. Andrews, J. E. Fullarton, N. A. Holtzman, & A. G. Motulsky). National Academies Press.

Committee on Science, Engineering, and Public Policy, National Academy of Sciences. National Academy of Engineering, Institute of Medicine, National Research Council. (2002). *Scientific and medical aspects of human reproductive cloning*. National Academy Press.

Condic, M. L. (2008). *When does human life begin: A scientific perspective* (White Paper Series, Vol. 1, No. 1). The Westchester Institute.

Condic, M. L. (2020). *Untangling twinning*. University of Notre Dame Press.

Congregation for the Doctrine of the Faith. (1981). *Donum vitae. Instruction on respect for human life in its origin and on the dignity of procreation*. Daughters of Saint Paul.

Congregation for the Doctrine of the Faith. (2007, August 1). *Responses to certain questions of the United States conference of Catholic Bishops concerning artificial nutrition and hydration*. Liberia Editrice Vaticana.

Congregation for the Doctrine of the Faith. (2008, September 8). *Dignitas personae. Instruction of certain bioethical questions*. Liberia Editrice Vaticana.

Craig, D. (2014). *Health care as a social good*. Georgetown University Press.

Cruzan v. Director, Missouri Department of Health, 497 U.S. 261 (1990).

Curlin, F., & Tollefsen, C. (2021). *The way of medicine: Ethics and the healing professions*. University of Notre Dame Press.

Dobbs v. Jackson Women's Health Organization, No. 19–1392, (597 U.S. 215, 2022).

Doe v. Bolton (410 U.S. 179, 1973).

Donadio, R., & Goodstein, L. (2010, November 21). *In rare cases pope justifies the use of condoms* (p. A1). New York Times.

Donceel, J. (1970). Immediate animation and delayed hominization. *Theological Studies*, *31*(1).

Dossabhoy, S. S., Feng, J., & Desai, M. S. (2018). The use and relevance of the Hippocratic oath in 2015-a survey of US medical schools. *Journal of Anesthesia History*, *4*(2), 139–146. https://doi.org/10.1016/j.janh.2017.09.005

Dougherty, C. (2009). Ethical dimensions of health care rationing. In M. M. Hogan & D. Solomon (Eds.), *Medical ethics at Notre Dame: The J. Philip Clarke family lectures*. The Notre Dame Center for Ethics and Culture.

Eberl, J. T. (Ed.). (2017). *Contemporary controversies in Catholic bioethics*. Springer.

Eberl, J. T., & Kevin Donovan, G. (2021). Is it ethical to unilaterally withdraw life-sustaining treatment in triage circumstances. *Journal of the Catholic Health Association of the United States*. https://www.chausa.org/publications/health-progress/article/pandemic-coverage/is-it-ethical-to-unilaterally-withdraw-life-sustaining-treatment-in-triage-circumstances; https://pubmed.ncbi.nlm.nih.gov/33539842/

Eisenstadt v. Baird (405 U.S. 438 1972).

Emon, A. M. (2004–2005). Natural law and natural rights in Islamic law. *Journal of Law and Religion*, *20*(2), 351–395.

Engelhardt, T. H. (1974). The ontology of abortion. *Ethics*, *84*(3), 217–234.

Fajgenbaum, D. (2019). *Chasing my cure*. Ballantine Books.

Fehring, R., & Schlidt, A. (2001). *Trends in contraceptive use among Catholics in the U.S.A*. Marquette University Nursing School Publications.

Finnis, J. M., & Grisez, G. (1981). The basic principles of natural: A reply to Ralph McInerny. *American Journal of Jurisprudence*, *26*(1).

Fins, J. (2015). *Rights come to mind: Brain injury, ethics, and the struggle for consciousness*. Cambridge University Press.

Flannery, K. L. (2019). *Cooperation with evil: Thomistic tools of analysis*. The Catholic University of America Press.

Francis. (2016, March 19). *Amoris laetitia. W2.vatican.va. Apostolic exhortation on love in the family*. http://w2.vatican.va/content/francesco/es/apost_exhortations/documents/papa-francesco_esortazione-ap_20160319_amoris-laetitia.html

Francis. (2019, April 13). *Address to the Italian association for the donation of organs, tissues and cells*. Liberia Editrice Vaticana.

Galton, F. (1869). *Hereditary genius: An inquiry into its laws and consequences*. Macmillan.

Ginsburg, R. B. (1985). Some thoughts on autonomy and equality in relation to *Roe v. Wade*. *North Carolina Law Review*, *63*(2), 375–386.

Graaf, G., Buckley, F.F., & Skotko, B.G. (2015). Estimates of the live births, natural losses, and elective terminations with down syndrome in the United Sates. *American Journal of Medical Genetics Part A, 167A*, 756–767.

Granfield, D. (1971). *The abortion decision*. Doubleday & Company, Inc.

Griswold v. Connecticut (381 U.S. 479 1965).

Groenewoud, J. H., van der Heide, A., Onwuteaka-Philipsen, B. D., Willems, D. L., van der Maas, P. J., & van der Wal, G. (2000). Clinical problems with the performance of Euthanasia and physician-assisted suicide in the Netherlands. *The New England Journal of Medicine*, *342*(8).

Hamel, R. (2007). The CDF statement on artificial nutrition and hydration: What should we make of it. *Health Care Ethics USA*, *15*(4), 5–7.

Hamel, R., & Walter, J. (Eds.). (2007). *Artificial nutrition and hydration and the permanently unconscious patient: The Catholic debate*. Georgetown University Press.

Hauerwas, S. (2008). *Living gently in a violent world: The prophetic witness of weakness*. InterVarsity Press.

Hauerwas, S. (2009). Practicing patience: How Christians should be sick. In M. M. Hogan & D. Solomon (Eds.), *Medical ethics at Notre Dame: The J. Philip Clarke family lectures*. The Notre Dame Center for Ethics and Culture.

Hippocrates. (1923). *Volume 1: Ancient medicine. The Loeb classical library*, No. 147 (W. H. S. Jones, Trans.). Harvard University Press.

Hogan, M. M. (1997). Tris Engelhardt and the queen of hearts. In B. P. Minogue, G. Palmer-Fernandez, & J. E. Reagan (Eds.), *Reading Engelhardt*. Kluwer Academic Publishers.

Hogan, M. M. (2002). *Marriage as a relationship: Real and rational*. Marquette University Press.

Hogan, M. M., & Solomon, D. (2008). *Medical ethics at Notre Dame: The J. Philip Clarke Family Lectures 1988–1999*. The Notre Dame Center for Ethics and Culture.

The Holy Bible. (1950). (R. Knox, Trans.). Sheed & Ward, Inc.

Institute of Medicine (US). (2000). *Committee on non-heart-beating transplantation II: The scientific and ethical basis for practice and protocols*. National Academies Press (US).

John Paul II. (1981, November 22). *Familiaris consortio* [The role of the Christian family in the modern world]. Vatican.

John Paul II. (1993, August 6). *Veritatis splendor* [The splendor of truth]. Vatican.

John Paul II. (1995, March 25). *Evangelium vitae* [The gospel of life]. Vatican.

John Paul II. (1998, September 14). *Fides et Ratio* [Faith and reason]. Vatican.

John Paul II. (2000, August 29). Address the Italian association for the donation of organs, tissues and cells. Vatican.

John Paul II. (2004). Address to the participants in the international congress on "life-sustaining treatments and vegetative state: Scientific advances and ethical dilemmas." *Origins*, *33*, 737, 739–740.

Jonas, H. (1980a). Against the stream: Comments on the definition and redefinition of death. In *Philosophical essays: From current creed to technological man* (pp. 134–142). University of Chicago Press.

Jonas, H. (1980b). Philosophical reflections on experimenting with human subjects. In *Philosophical essays: From current creed to technological man* (pp. 105–133). University of Chicago Press.

Jones, R. K., Finer, L. B., & Singh, S. (2010). *Characteristics of U.S. abortion patients, 2008*. Alan Guttmacher Institute.

Kant, I. (1999). *Foundations of the metaphysics of morals* (L. W. Beck, Trans.). Harcourt Brace.

Klitzman, R. (2008). *When doctors become patients*. The Oxford University Press.

Kopp, V. J. (1997). Henry Knowles Beecher and the redefinition of death. *Bulletin of Anesthesia History*, *15*, 6–8.

Lawrence v. Texas, (539 U.S. 558, 2003).

Le Fort, Gertrud von. (2010). *The eternal woman*. Ignatius Press.

Leo XIII. (1879, August 4). *Aeterni patris* [On the restoration of Christian philosophy]. Vatican.

Lewis, C. S. (1947). *Miracles*. Macmillan.

Lewis, R. (1992). *Beginnings of life*. Wm. C. Brown Publishers.

Lifton, R. J. (1986). *The nazi doctors: Medical killing and the psychology of genocide*. Basic Books.

Lombardo, P. (2011). The constitutionality of asexualization legislation in the United States. In *A Century of Eugenics in America*. Indiana University Press.

Lonergan, S. J., Bernard, J. F. (1964). *Insight: A study of human understanding*. Philosophical Library Inc.

Lonergan, S. J., Bernard, J. F. (1967a). Cognitional structure. In F. E. Crowe (Ed.), *Collection* (pp. 221–239). Herder and Herder.

Lonergan, S. J., Bernard, J. F. (1967b). Finality, love, marriage. In F. E. Crowe (Ed.), *Collection*. Herder and Herder.

Lonergan, S. J., Bernard, J. F. (1972). *Method in theology*. Herder and Herder.

Lysaught, M. T. (2011). Moral analysis of a procedure at phoenix hospital. *Theology Faculty Research and Publications*, *373*. https://epublications.marquette.edu/theo_fac/373

Maimonides, M. (1917). Oath of Maimonides. (H. Friedenwald, Trans.). *Bulletin of the Johns Hopkins Hospital*, *28*, 260–261.

Majority Report. (1967, April 19). Pontifical commission for the study of the problems of population, family and births. *National Catholic Reporter*.

Mangan, J. T. (1970). The wonder of myself: Ethical-theological aspects of direct abortion. *Theological Studies*, *31*(1).

Maritain, R. (2016). *We have been friends together*. Saint Augustine Press.

Masek, L. (2018). *Intention, character, and double effect*. University of Notre Dame Press.

Maslow, A. H. (1959). *New knowledge in human values*. Harper and Row.

Mayer, L. S., & McHugh, P. R. (2016, Fall). Sexuality and gender: Findings from the biological, psychological, and social sciences. *The New Atlantis*, Number 50.

McCormick, S. J., Richard A. (1991a). Physician-assisted suicide: Flight from compassion. *Christian Century*.

McCormick, S. J., Richard A. (1991b). Who or what is the pre-embryo. *Kennedy Institute of Ethics Journal*, *1*(1), 1–15.

McCormick, S. J., Richard A. (1992). Moral considerations Ill considered. *America*.

McCormick, S. J., Richard A. (1995). Does Christianity make a difference? *Christian Bioethics*, *1*(1), 97–101.

McCormick, S. J., Richard A. (1996, July 20). Authority and leadership: The moral challenge. *America*.

McInerny, R. (1980). The principles of natural law. *American Journal of Jurisprudence*, *25*(1), Article 1.

McInerny, R. (2003). *The very rich hours of Jacques Maritain*. University of Notre Dame.

Meilaender, G. (2008). Death and dignity: Apart and not a part. In M. M. Hogan & D. Solomon (Eds.), *Medical ethics at Notre Dame: The J. Philip Clarke Family Lectures*. The Notre Dame Center for Ethics and Culture.

Minority Report. (1967, April 19). Pontifical commission for the study of the problems of population, family and births. *National Catholic Reporter*.

Model Penal Code of the American Law Institute. (Proposed Draft, 1962). *Offenses against the Family*. American Law Institute. § 230.

Murphy, W. F., Jr. (2017). The disease-prevention use of condoms: Why it is not forbidden according to catholic doctrine. In J. T. Eberl (Ed.), *Contemporary controversies in catholic bioethics* (pp. 269–285). Springer.

National Center for Health Statistics. (n.d.). cdc.gov/nchs/fastats/infertility.htm

National Research Council. (2002a). *Report of the National Academy of Science: Scientific and medical aspects of human reproductive cloning*. The National Academies Press.

National Research Council. (2002b). *Scientific and medical aspects of human reproductive cloning*. The National Academies Press. https://doi.org/10.17226/10285

National Research Council Committee for the Study of Inborn Errors of Metabolism. (1975). *Genetic screening programs, principles and research*. National Academy of Sciences.

New York State task force on life and law report: Guide to ventilator allocation, 2015. http://www.health.ny.gov/regulations/task_force/reports_publications/docs/ventilator_guidelines.pdf

Newman, J. H. (1891). *An essay on development of Christian Doctrine*. Longmans, Green and Co.

Noonan, J. T. (1970). *The morality of abortion: Legal and historical perspectives*. The Belknap Press of Harvard University Press.

Noonan, J. T. (1986). *Contraception: A history of its treatment by the Catholic theologians and canonists*. Harvard University Press.

Noonan, J. T. (1993). Development in moral doctrine. *Theological Studies*, *54*(4), 666–677.

Noonan, J. T. (2005). *A church that can and cannot change: The development of catholic moral teaching*. University of Notre Dame Press.

Obergefell v. Hodges (576 U.S. 644, 2015).

O'Connor v. Donaldson (*422 U.S.* 563, 1975).

Oregon Health Care Plan. (n.d.). https://www.oregon.gov/oha/hpa/dsi-herc

O'Rourke, K. D., de Blois, J., & Norris, P. (1994). *A primer for health care ethics*. Georgetown University Press.

Paul VI. (1968). *Humanae vitae*. In *Acta Apostolicae Sedis* (Vol. 60, p. 481). Vatican.

Paul VI. Vatican II. (1965a, December 7). *Gaudium et Spes*: Pastoral constitution on the Church in the modern world. Vatican.

Paul VI. Vatican II. (1965b, November 18). *Dei verbum*: Dogmatic constitution on divine revelation. Vatican.

Pellegrino, E. D. (2008). Does being a Christian physician really matter? In M. M. Hogan & D. Solomon (Eds.), *Medical ethics at Notre Dame: The J. Philip Clarke Family Lectures*. The Notre Dame Center for Ethics and Culture.

Pellegrino, E. D., & Pellegrino, A. A. (1988). Humanism and ethics in roman medicine: Translation and commentary on a text of Scribonius Largus. *Literature and Medicine: Literature and Bioethics*, 7, 22–38.

Pennsylvania Statute: 20 PA CSA 5431(a)(6).

Pinckaers, O.P., S. (2003). *Morality: A catholic view* (O. P. Michael Sherwin, Trans.). St. Augustine Press.

Pius XI. (1930, December 30). *Casti connubii: Christian marriage to the venerable brethren, patriarchs, primates, archbishops, bishops, and other local ordinaries enjoying peace and communion with the apostolic see*. Vatican.

Pius XI. (1931, May 15). *Quadragesimo anno: In the fortieth year*. Vatican.

Pius XII. (1944). *Sentence of the holy roman Rota* (Acta Apostolicae Sedis, Vol. 36, pp. 179–200). Vatican.

Pius XII. (1951a). *Address to the Midwives* (Acta Apostolicae Sedis, Vol. 43, pp. 835–854). Vatican.

Pius XII. (1951b). *Address to the association of large families and the family front* (Acta Apostolicae Sedis, Vol. 43, pp. 855–860). Vatican.

Pius XII. (1952). *Address to the first international congress on the histopathology of the nervous system* (Acta Apostolicae Sedis, Vol. 44, pp. 779–789). Vatican.

Pius XII. (1954). *Address to the twenty-sixth congress of the Italian society of urologists* (Acta Apostolicae Sedis, Vol. 45, pp. 673–679). Vatican.

Pius XII. (1956). *Address to the second world congress on fertility and sterility* (Acta Apostolicae Sedis, Vol. 48, pp. 467–474). Vatican.

Pius XII. (2 mars 1957–1ermars 1958). *Discours et messages-radio de S.S. Pie XII, Dix-neuvième année de Pontificat* (pp. 615–621). Vatican.

Pius XII. (2 mars 1957–1ermars 1958). *The prolongation of life. Discours et messages-radio de S.S. Pie XII, Dix-neuvième année de Pontificat*. Vatican.

Pius XII. (1958a). *Address to the seventh international congress of hematology* (Acta Apostolicae Sedis, Vol. 50, pp. 732–740). Vatican.

Pius XII. (1958b). Address to the tenth national congress of the Italian society of plastic surgery (Acta Apostolicae Sedis, Vol. 50, pp. 952–961). Vatican.

Planned Parenthood of Central Missouri v. Danforth (428 U.S. 52, 1976).

Planned Parenthood of Southeastern Pennsylvania v. Casey (505 U.S. 833, 1992).

Plato. (1978). The republic. In P. Shorey (Trans.), E. Hamilton & H. Cairns (Eds.), *The collected dialogues of Plato*. Princeton University Press.

Pontifical Council on Justice and Peace. (2004, April 2). Compendium of the social doctrine of the catholic church. Vatican.

President's Commission for the Study of Ethical Problems in Medicine and Biomedical and Behavioral Research. (1981). *Defining death: Medical, legal and ethical issues in the determination of death*. U.S. Government Printing Office.

Ramsey, P. (1970). *The patient as person: Explorations in medical ethics*. Yale University Press.

Religious Freedom Restoration Act. Pub. L. No. 103–141, 107 Stat. 1488 (November 16, 1993), codified at 42 U.S.C. § 2000bb through 42 U.S.C. § 2000bb-4.

Religious Land Use and Institutionalized Persons Act (RLUIPA), Pub.L. 106–274 (text), (September 22, 2000) codified as 42 U.S.C. § 2000cc et seq.

Report of the Ad Hoc committee of the Harvard Medical School to examine the criteria of brain death, a definition of irreversible coma. (1968). *JAMA*, *205*(6), 337–340.

Report of the National Academy of Science: Scientific and medical aspects of human reproductive cloning. (2002). National Academies Press.

Report of the President's Council on bioethics. Human cloning and human dignity. (2002). The President's Council on Bioethics.

Report of the President's Council on bioethics: Controversies in the determination of death. (2008b). The President's Council on Bioethics.

Report of the President's Council on bioethics: The changing moral focus of newborn screening. (2008a). The President's Council on Bioethics.

Roe v. Wade, (410 U.S. 113, 1973).

Rosen, R. (2015, April 15). The best doctor is also a Philosopher (57K; translation P. N. Singer). In *Galen on science and the humanities* (Kemp Lecture). University of Missouri.

Shewmon, A. D. (2008, December). The brain and somatic integration: Insights into the standard biological rationale for equating 'brain death' with death. *The Journal of Medicine and Philosophy*, *26*(5) (2001), 457–478) in *Controversies in the determination of death: A White paper by the President's council on bioethics* (p. 56). The President's Council on Bioethics.

Smith, J. (2011, June). Fig leaves and falsehoods. *First Things*.

Swinton, J. (2004). *Critical reflection on Stanley Hauerwas' theology of disability*. Routledge.

Tollefsen, C. (Ed.). (2007). *Artificial nutrition and hydration: The new catholic debate*. Springer.

Tollefsen, C. (Ed.). (2017). The use of a condom to prevent HIV among married couples. In J. T. Eberl (Ed.), *Contemporary controversies in catholic bioethics* (pp. 255–268). Springer.

Tooley, M. (1983). *Abortion and infanticide*. Clarendon Press.

Tribe, L. (1998). On not banning cloning for the wrong reasons. In M. Nussbaum & C. R. Sunstein (Eds.), *Clones and clones: Facts and fantasies about human cloning*. W.W. Norton.

UAW v. Johnson Controls, Inc. (111 U.S. 1196 EPD 40, 605,1991).

Union Pacific Railway Company v. Botsford 141 U.S. 250 (1891).

United States Conference of Catholic Bishops. (2018). *Ethical and religious directives for catholic health care services* (6th ed.), United States Conference of Catholic Bishops.

United States v. Karl Brandt, et al., (1946, October–1949, April). Trials of war criminals before Nuremberg military tribunals under control council law no. 10.

Vacco v. Quill (521 U.S. 793, 1997).

Veatch, R. (2012). *Hippocratic, religious, and secular medical ethics*. Georgetown University Press.

Warren, M. A. (1973). On the moral and legal status of abortion. *The Monist*, *57*(1), 43–61.

Washington v. Glucksberg (521 U.S. 702, 1997).

Whitemore, T. D. (2009). Response to Charles Dougherty. Ethical dimensions of health care rationing. In M. M. Hogan & D. Solomon (Eds.), *Medical ethics at Notre Dame: The J. Philip Clarke family lectures*. The Notre Dame Center for Ethics and Culture.

Wojtyla, K. (1981). *Love and responsibility*. Farr Farrar, Straus and Giroux, Inc.

Index

Page numbers in *italic* indicate a figure and page numbers in **bold** indicate a table on the corresponding page. Page numbers followed by n refer to a note.

Made in the USA
Las Vegas, NV
19 September 2026

ea2ec4ea-76e9-4a00-92d4-cce2e24f863eR01